Inducing Targeted Protein Degradation

Inducing Targeted Protein Degradation

From Chemical Biology to Drug Discovery and Clinical Applications

Edited by Philipp Cromm

WILEY-VCH

Editor

Dr. Philipp Cromm
Bayer AG
Research & Development, Pharmaceuticals
Muellerstrasse 178
13342 Berlin, Germany

Library of Congress Card No.: applied for

British Library Cataloguing-in-Publication Data
A catalogue record for this book is available from the British Library.

Bibliographic information published by the Deutsche Nationalbibliothek
The Deutsche Nationalbibliothek lists this publication in the Deutsche Nationalbibliografie; detailed bibliographic data are available on the Internet at <http://dnb.d-nb.de>.

Print ISBN: 978-3-527-35013-1
ePDF ISBN: 978-3-527-35017-9
ePub ISBN: 978-3-527-83621-5
oBook ISBN: 978-3-527-83620-8

Cover Design: FORMGEBER, Mannheim, Germany

Typesetting Straive, Chennai, India
Printing and Binding CPI Group (UK) Ltd, Croydon, CR0 4YY

C117918_041122

Contents

Preface

Dear Targeted Protein Degradation Enthusiasts,

Thank you for deciding to read this book! I am very delighted to see that we share the passion for targeted protein degradation (TPD). We – all contributing authors and I – hope you will enjoy reading our take on this exciting and rapidly evolving field! By making the conscious decision for this book I trust you have a general interest in TPD, have come across the concept beforehand, and are now looking to deepen and/or broaden your knowledge. I feel very honored you chose this book over all the other great options out there. So, what can you expect from the following chapters?

My goal for this book was to provide a broad and diverse overview of this still very young but skyrocketing field. I wanted to provide you with a bird's-eye view of the topic by collecting perspectives from various angles including both academia and industry. Furthermore, as TPD is still in its early years, I wanted the younger generation of scientists to share their thoughts on the matter, with most of them having been involved hands-on in the groundbreaking work that got the ball rolling and all of us very excited. I hope you will recognize a few of the contributors by name from some of the early works in the field when you yourself were eagerly reading up and devouring the latest news on TPD. A lot of these early pioneers have since moved on to pursue their own careers in academia or industry and continue to shape the TPD field with their contributions and ideas. So stay tuned for what the next wave of science will bring!

I want to thank all contributors of this book for their hard work and effort to assemble each individual chapter. I hope all contributions will merge into a good overall fit to provide a comprehensive overview of the TPD field. The chapters will take you on a journey from the fundamentals of protein homeostasis and E3 ligase biology to various aspects of TPD like mono- and heterobifunctional degraders, ternary complexes, computational modeling, covalent-, CNS-, and RNA targeting; before at last reaching the world of clinical candidates: how to profile, understand, and identify your candidate on the way to human clinical trials. Along the way, we are always aiming to share our best guesses about future developments in the field and are as excited as you are to see if they become reality one day.

I wish you a great time reading the book and hope you will enjoy it as much as I did! Once again, a great THANK YOU to everyone involved in realizing and publishing this book and to you for the trust you put in me by deciding to read it!

Sincerely,
Philipp Cromm

1

Targeted Protein Degradation – The Story So Far

Daniel H. O Donovan, Laura M. Luh and Philipp M. Cromm

Bayer AG, Research and Development, Pharmaceuticals, Drug Discovery Sciences, Müllerstraße 178, 13353, Berlin, Germany

1.1 Introduction to Targeted Protein Degradation (TPD)

Protein homeostasis is a pivotal process in cells comprising protein production and removal. The cell has two major pathways to achieve the latter; primarily, the ubiquitin proteasome system (UPS) that degrades the vast majority of all proteins, or alternatively lysosomal degradation and autophagy, capable of degrading whole organelles such as mitochondria [1, 2]. The UPS is centered around the 76 amino acid small protein ubiquitin that is attached or removed from other proteins as a post-translational modification (PTM) and encodes via a complex pattern of ubiquitination the fate of the target protein [3, 4]. Ubiquitination is achieved by the concerted actions of a series of ubiquitin ligases (E1, E2, and E3) that add ubiquitin chains to substrates, thereby marking them for proteasomal degradation. Autophagy is the second major protein degradation pathway and is a self-degrading mechanism in which a cytoplasmic material is sequestered in double-membrane vesicles and delivered to the lysosome for degradation. Using chemical biological tools to control these endogenous degradation machineries is the hallmark of targeted protein degradation (TPD). While conventional small molecules generally block the activity of a protein, small-molecule degraders aim to eliminate or deplete the protein of interest (POI) following the paradigm of event-driven pharmacology [5–7]. This exciting concept not only expands the drug discovery toolbox but also enables broadening of druggable space and has therefore drawn tremendous attention within both the pharmaceutical industry and academia in recent years. The TPD concept is emerging as a new therapeutic modality with many such compounds entering the clinic and a multitude of start-up companies arising with a focus on TPD.

There are essentially two classes of small-molecule protein degraders: monovalent and bivalent degraders. Destabilizers such as small-molecule hydrophobic tags

Inducing Targeted Protein Degradation: From Chemical Biology to Drug Discovery and Clinical Applications, First Edition. Edited by Philipp Cromm.

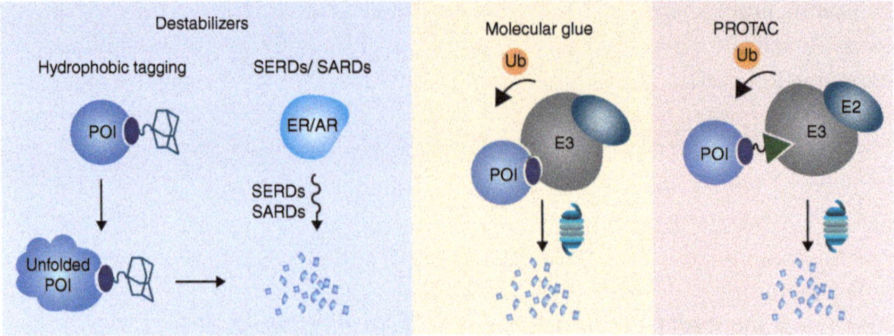

Figure 1.1 Schematic representation of different TPD approaches. While the complete molecular machinery by which HyTags and SERDs induce protein degradation remains unclear, molecular glues and PROTACs act via a E3-ligase-mediated mechanism resulting in proteasomal degradation.

(HyTags) or selective estrogen receptor degraders (SERDs) as well as molecular glue degraders represent monovalent molecules, while proteolysis targeting chimeras (PROTACs®) and related technologies comprise the class of bifunctional degraders (Figure 1.1) [8]. This chapter aims to provide a brief overview of the milestones in TPD achieved to date, including recent clinical advances and the enticing opportunities beyond proteasomal degradation.

1.1.1 What Can Be Expected from this Book?

This book aims to provide a comprehensive overview of the field of TPD. The journey toward controlling protein abundance and function began long before the current excitement around TPD, which has seen a surge in activity during the past 5–10 years. Thus, several techniques modulating protein levels were already established in the early 2000s, consisting mostly of chemical biology tools [9].

To appreciate the rationale behind TPD, one must first familiarize oneself with the cellular machinery controlling protein degradation. The complex cellular processes driving protein degradation, i.e. the UPS and E3 ubiquitin ligases, are highlighted in the contributions of Doris Hellerschmied and Vincenzo D'Angiolella in Chapters 2 and 3, respectively. For a detailed understanding of the molecular mechanisms and structural complexity of the degrader machinery, Morgan Gadd presents Chapter 4 on ternary complexes of small-molecule degraders. Although today we still rely on structural biology to unravel the machinery of ternary complexes, computational approaches are being refined to predict the ternary interaction of a degrader and its protein targets. John Karanicolas in Chapter 5 provides an overview of the current efforts on ternary complex prediction and what we might expect in the future. Switching gears to molecular glue degraders, Cristina Mayor-Ruiz in Chapter 6 explains how the field is progressing from serendipitous discovery to the directed and rational hunt for novel molecular glue degraders. After discussing the general principles of TPD, a specialized discourse on TPD in neurodegenerative diseases and covalent protein degraders is provided by Fleur Ferguson and Xiaoyu Zhang in Chapters 7 and 8, respectively.

Controlling protein levels before the protein is translated from RNA provides another means to achieve TPD. The current approaches to modulate protein abundance by addressing RNA are highlighted in Chapter 9 by Andrei Ursu. The concept of inducing novel protein–protein interactions (PPIs) to facilitate the transfer of a ubiquitin onto a POI has sparked the creative mind of several groups to harness the concept either for additional PTMs or other forms of protein degradation. Thus, George Burslem provides an overview of heterobifunctional molecules beyond PROTACs in Chapter 10.

As the main goal of this book is to provide a summary of the TPD field from all angles (including both academia and the industry), the transition of small-molecule protein degraders from chemical biology tools to drug discovery and clinical applications is an essential part of the story. Proof-of-concept (PoC) studies that often originated within academic groups provide the foundation to generate excitement and ultimately produce convincing preclinical data. However, to develop viable clinical candidate degraders, many additional parameters need to be optimized and other challenges must be addressed. To shed light on the path towards clinical candidate development, a team from Boehringer Ingelheim provides an overview of TPD in drug discovery in Chapter 11, while a team from Roche digs deep into the drug metabolism and pharmacokinetic (DMPK) properties and hurdles associated with small-molecule protein degraders in Chapter 12. Finally, in Chapter 13, a team from Arvinas shares their views on their exciting journey of TPD from a chemical biology tool to a clinical candidate.

1.2 Development of Targeted Protein Degradation: Chronology and Milestones

Despite the recent explosion in interest in TPD, the first protein degrader drugs appeared more than 30 years ago with the development of selective estrogen receptor degraders (SERDs) for the treatment of breast cancer (Figure 1.2). Shortly before the launch of fulvestrant as the first SERD drug, the first paper describing PROTACs was published in 2001. However, it was not until 2004 with the advent of cell-permeable PROTACs that the current "gold rush" slowly began to take shape. Since the late 2000s, advances have been reported with increasing frequency, beginning with the recruitment of new E3 ligases (cereblon [CRBN], von Hippel–Lindau [VHL], and cellular inhibitor of apoptosis protein [cIAP] binding warheads) and the burgeoning development of new modalities for TPD such as HyTags and IMiD molecular glues. In 2015, PROTACs took a leap forward toward drug-like therapeutics with the first *in vivo* efficacy experiments. Just four years later in 2019, ARV-110 became the first PROTAC to enter human clinical trials for degradation of the androgen receptor (AR) to treat prostate cancer. The following year, the first non-oncology PROTAC entered the clinic (KT-474), an IRAK4 degrader for immune-mediated inflammatory diseases, and today, there are more than 20 PROTACs and molecular glues in ongoing clinical trials. It is clear from the ever-increasing pace of development that we are still in the expansion phase for this promising class of therapeutic agents, and we expect many more advances in the coming years.

1.2.1 Milestone 1: Early Monovalent Protein Degraders – The Surprising Biology of Fulvestrant

In the early 1990s, researchers discovered a strange phenomenon while studying the anti-estrogen breast cancer drug today called fulvestrant (known then as ICI 164,384, Figures 1.2 and 1.3). In a radioligand displacement experiment, fulvestrant showed twofold weaker binding when compared to the endogenous agonist ligand estradiol (K_d values of 1.9 and 0.9 nM, respectively). Despite this fact, cells treated with fulvestrant showed a profound reduction in their response to stimulation with estradiol [10]. From the standpoint of classical pharmacology, this posed a conundrum; as an antagonist, fulvestrant would be expected to exert its effect through an occupancy-driven mechanism. A competitive antagonist would occupy the binding site and therefore block the binding and stimulatory effect of estradiol, while an allosteric modulator could bind to an orthosteric site to modify protein dynamics and modulate the pharmacological response. However, fulvestrant did something else; somehow, the compound elicited a significant reduction in estrogen receptor (ER)

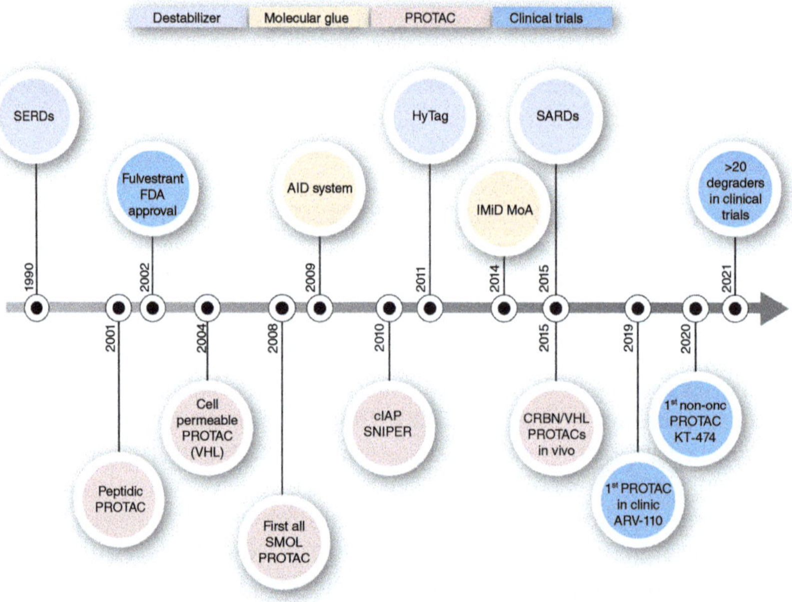

Figure 1.2 Timeline highlighting key achievements of the TPD field. SMOL, small molecule.

Figure 1.3 Structure of the SERD fulvestrant, a marketed breast cancer drug.

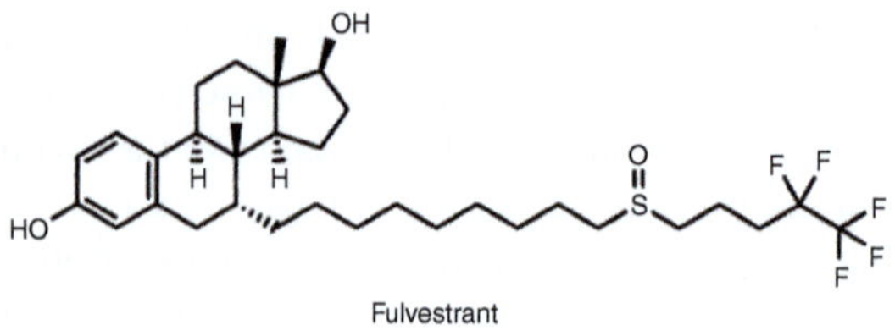

levels as confirmed by Western blot analysis, immunoprecipitation, and radiography [11]. Here was a drug that abrogated protein function not by merely occupying the active site and blocking its function but by directly reducing the quantity of protein within the cell. The disappearance of the receptor led to an insufficient quantity of protein to elicit an agonist response, thereby halting ER signaling by a new mechanism of action. Researchers dubbed these new compounds SERDs, and SERD molecules are still among the foremost treatments for ER-positive breast cancer today.

Since these early discoveries, there has been significant progress in our understanding of SERDs and related molecules. Researchers have demonstrated that proteasomal degradation of ER is linked to receptor dimerization and nuclear localization [12], and new ER receptor degraders have been designed through improved understanding of protein–ligand interactions at the molecular level (see 1.2.6) [13]. However, despite over two decades of research, the molecular biological cascade by which fulvestrant exerts its mechanism of action has not yet been fully elucidated.

Nonetheless, research teams took inspiration from the growing understanding of proteasomal degradation to create new methods of targeted degradation. In 2009, Nishimura et al. described the auxin-inducible degron (AID) system by which small-molecule plant hormones ("Auxins") could be harnessed to induce degradation (Figure 1.2) [14]. In these studies, researchers transplanted the plant-specific auxin-dependent degradation to other eukaryotic cell lines, including yeast cells and engineered cell lines derived from higher organisms including mouse, monkey, and human. The method was later adapted using the clustered regularly interspaced short palindromic repeats (CRISPR)/Cas9 gene editing system to enable endogenous tagging of human and mouse cells, thereby expanding the utility of the AID system for the functional analysis of POIs [15].

In 2011, Crews and coworker described another new approach to targeted protein degradation (TPD) using hydrophobic tagging (HyTag). In its original incarnation, the target protein for the HyTag approach was a bacterial dehalogenase (HaloTag), which could be fused to a protein of interest, initially using green fluorescent protein (GFP), which enabled the facile quantification of protein levels (Figure 1.1). The tagged fusion protein could then be engaged using a chloro-alkyl bearing small molecule (the HyTag), which reacted specifically with the HaloTag protein. The HyTag also includes a linker moiety (derived from polyethylene glycol, PEG) and terminates in a lipophilic chemical group, such as an adamantyl residue. Treatment of these engineered cells with HyTag molecules enabled specific degradation of the protein of interest via the proteosome, presumably through recognition of the HyTag-bearing target as a misfolded protein (Figure 1.1). To illustrate the therapeutic potential of this modality, the authors also extended the method to the degradation of tagged $HRAS^{G12V}$ (GTPase HRas protein), a mutant protein that is a key driver in several tumor types [16, 17].

Inspired by the earlier discovery of fulvestrant as an ER degrader, in 2015, the Crews laboratory combined their HyTag approach with a ligand that engaged the AR, a key pharmacological target in the treatment of prostate cancer. The high-affinity AR ligand RU5906324 was combined with a PEG-based linker and the hydrophobic tag to create a new series of selective AR degraders termed SARDs, by analogy with the earlier SERD acronym. The administration of SARDs to LNCaP prostate cancer cells showed dose-dependent degradation of the AR and a concomitant arrest of cell proliferation. SARD molecules remain a potential source of new therapies for the treatment of prostate cancer.

1.2.2 Milestone 2: The First PROTACs – From Peptidic Degraders to Chemical Biology Tools

Looking back into the development of TPD, the birth of PROTACs can be identified with the 2001 PNAS publication by Crews and Deshaies describing chimeric molecules targeting the POI protein methionine amino peptidase 2 (MetAP2) in tandem with the E3 ligase Skp1–cullin–F box (SCF) complex to elicit ubiquitination and degradation [18]. Why did this initial publication not create the wave of excitement around TPD, which we see today, and instead flew under the radar for almost 15 years? The answer may lie in the structure of the first PROTAC molecule (Figure 1.4). Despite its seminal role in the development of TPD, the compound was not in the least drug-like and incorporated many chemical features that severely limited its range of applications. To engage the F box protein β-TRCP, a doubly phosphorylated 10 amino acid peptide was used, while the MetAP2 protein was engaged using the covalent natural product ovalicin, with both entities tethered together using a polyglycine suberate linker. Consequently, the first PROTAC was covalent on the target site (and therefore not substoichiometric) and not cell permeable, restricting the PoC experiments to be carried out *in vitro* in *Xenopus* egg extracts. Nevertheless, this publication provided the first example of small-molecule-induced protein degradation without the need for genetic modification of any of the involved proteins. Although its longevity was not obvious in 2001 the PROTAC concept had arrived and was here to stay.

At this point, we must also give credit to the work that paved the way to this initial publication. In 1995, Gosink and Vierstra were able to redirect the specificity of ubiquitination of an E2 enzyme and subsequent adenosine triphosphate (ATP)-dependent degradation *in vitro* by creating a chimera of the E2 ligase and a POI targeting peptide via genetic modification [19]. Similarly, in 2000, Zhou et al.

Figure 1.4 Structure of the first PROTAC reported in 2011. The amino acids of the β-TRCP targeting peptide as well as the poly glycine linker are depicted in a single-letter code.

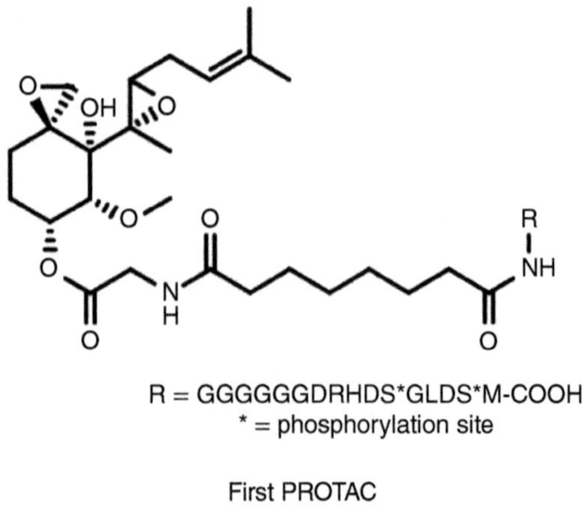

reported the degradation of a target protein after genetically fusing its peptide ligand to a subunit of an E3 ligase complex [20].

After the initial PoC study with MetAP2 in 2001, the next milestone achieved by Crews and coworkers was the degradation of the ER and the AR using two non-covalent PROTACs based on their previously used bisphosphorylated β-TRCP (F-box/WD repeat-containing protein 1A) engaging decapeptide [21]. While already espousing catalytic potential, these PROTACs were still not cell permeable and therefore needed to be microinjected into cells. The first cell-permeable PROTACs were reported in 2004 [22]. Thus, Crews and Deshaies abandoned the bisphosphorylated β-TRCP decapeptide for a heptameric hydroxyproline containing a HIF1α-derived peptide sequence engaging the E3 ligase VHL, which was fused to an octa D-Arg sequence to obtain cell permeability. These tool PROTACs achieved proteasome-dependent degradation of FK506 binding protein (FKBP)-fused constructs as well as AR degradation at high μM concentration and were the first PROTACs engaging VHL instead of β-TRCP, thereby demonstrating that additional E3 ligases are amenable to induced TPD.

Another key step was the transition from cell-based experiments to *in vivo* efficacy, which was partly achieved in 2013 by a less celebrated, albeit fascinating story from the Crews lab reporting conditional PROTACs [23]. A "bait" sequence comprising the tyrosine phosphorylation sequence of either TrkA or ErbB3 was coupled with the peptide ligand for VHL and octa D-Arg. Inside the cell, the "bait" tyrosine phosphorylation sequence is activated by phosphorylation, and the phosphorylated tyrosine sequence is subsequently bound by the actual target protein FRS2α or PI3K. After binding to the "bait" sequence, the target is finally ubiquitinated by VHL and then degraded by the proteasome. Despite limited statistical significance, the conditional PI3K PROTAC showed hints of *in vivo* efficacy after repeated intraperitoneal dosing in a xenograft model. However, all of these early peptide-based PROTACs suffered from poor bioavailability and limited potency, which restricted them from achieving their full potential and generating excitement within the budding TPD community.

The first "all-small-molecule" PROTAC was reported by the Crews lab as early as 2008 (Figure 1.2) [24]. Comprising the MDM2 inhibitor nutlin and a non-steroidal AR ligand connected via a PEG linker, this PROTAC was able to induce the degradation AR at 10 μM in HeLa cells. The choice of MDM2 as the E3 ligase was somewhat surprising; however, in 2008, the nutlins were among the only well-characterized small-molecule E3 ligase binders available. However, MDM2 is a relatively poor E3 ligase and indeed nutlins themselves can induce AR degradation [25, 26], and so the explosion of interest in PROTACs was again unduly postponed.

1.2.3 Milestone 3: Improving Drug-Like Properties – SNIPERs and Peptidomimetic VHL Binders

The endeavor toward more drug-like PROTACs continued in 2010 with a publication from Itoh et al. recruiting the ubiquitin ligase cellular inhibitor of apoptosis protein 1 (cIAP1) to degrade the cellular retinoic acid binding proteins (CRABP-I and -II) via their respective binders methyl bestatin (MeBS) (cIAP1) and *all-trans*

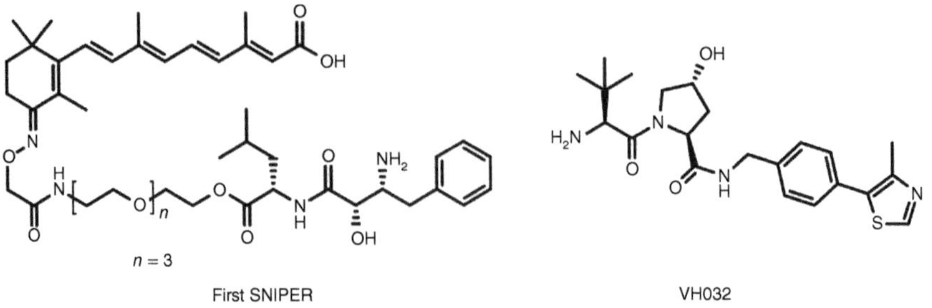

Figure 1.5 Structure of the first SNIPER targeting the E3 ligases cIAP1 and CRABP-I and II and the VHL peptidomimetic VH032.

retinoic acid (ATRA) (cellular retinoic acid-binding protein [CRAPB]-I,II, Figure 1.5) [26]. The target scope of these MeBS degraders was expanded to retinoic acid receptor (RAR) as well as ER and AR, and the acronym SNIPER (specific and non-genetic IAPs-dependent protein erasers) was coined in 2011 [27]. However, while these MeBS SNIPERs or PROTACs showed cellular activity without recourse to microinjection or cell penetrating peptides, unfortunately these compounds induce autoubiquitination and degradation of the IAP E3 ligase itself, thereby hampering the potency of the resultant degraders (DC_{50} values in the μM range).

While SNIPERs were making their debut, Ciulli and Crews were focused on VHL and committing significant effort to convert the heptameric hydroxyproline containing HIF1α peptide into a smaller, more drug-like peptidomimetic using fragment-based drug discovery (FBDD) [28, 29]. They solved numerous crystal structures and tested many substituents around the hydroxyproline core pharmacophore to develop the predecessors of today's well-known VHL ligand VH032 (Figure 1.5). Despite having no direct connection to TPD, this groundbreaking work paved the way for future success in the field.

1.2.4 Milestone 4: PROTACs on the Rise – Small-Molecule Degraders Achieve *in vivo* PoC

Despite the PROTAC concept having been established as early as 2001, the TPD field as we know it today was spurred primarily by two key publications from the Bradner and Crews labs in the spring of 2015 [30, 31]. Winter et al. used the IMiD thalidomide to engage the E3 ligase CRBN and induced the selective degradation of BRD4 *in vitro* and *in vivo*, showing efficacy in a leukemia xenograft model (Figure 1.6) [30].

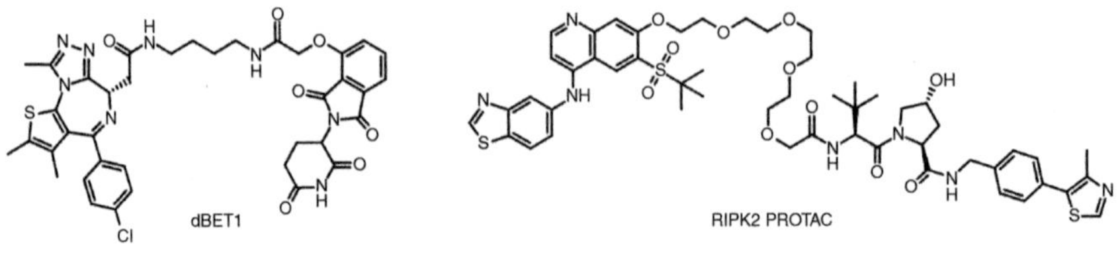

Figure 1.6 Chemical structures of the *in vivo* PROTACs dBET1, engaging CRBN, and the RIPK2 degrader PROTAC engaging VHL.

In another study, Bondeson et al. made use of the previously identified VHL peptidomimetics to degrade the estrogen-related receptor alpha (ERRα) as well as the serine-threonine kinase RIPK2 in various mice tissues and showed that substoichiometric amounts of PROTACs can be sufficient to reach full ubiquitination (Figure 1.6) [31]. Together, these two publications were able to fulfill three important criteria that had previously held the excitement around PROTACs in check: (i) PROTACs are able to induce the ubiquitination of superstoichiometric quantities of their target protein, (ii) PROTACs display very high degradation selectivity across the whole proteome, and (iii) PROTACs can be drug-like and efficacious *in vivo*, showing broad tissue distribution as well as delayed leukemia progression in mice.

That same year, a third publication from Arvinas sparked further excitement around PROTACs and the prospect of achieving clinical use [32]. Lu et al. reported data on how a BRD4-based CRBN PROTAC outperforms its parent small-molecule BRD4 inhibitor in various Burkitt's lymphoma cell lines *in vitro*. These three reports revived the field of small-molecule-induced protein degradation and provided momentum as the pharma industry began to recognize the therapeutic potential of TPD versus traditional small-molecule drugs. The interest continued to grow as Arvinas provided the first data for an orally available AR degrader outperforming the marketed anti-androgen enzalutamide in a prostate cancer xenograft model.

Shortly after VHL- and CRBN-based degraders had proven their ability to induce *in vivo* target degradation, IAP engaging degraders (SNIPERs) followed suit [33]. In 2018, Ohoka et al. identified an IAP-based ER degrader and demonstrated *in vivo* degradation and efficacy in an ER-positive breast cancer xenograft model. In these studies, the authors moved away from MeBS (used for the first IAP PoC degrader) and focused instead on the peptidomimetic IAP antagonist LCL161. Further variation of the IAP ligand identified ER SNIPERs with superior degradation activity and reduced autoubiquitination and degradation of the IAP E3 ligases [34]. Nevertheless, for some time, IAP PROTACs remained inferior to the VHL- and CRBN-based PROTACs reported since 2015. Like VHL, the IAP ligands represent peptidomimetics comprising an essential N-terminal *N*-methyl alanine, a feature that hampers their potential to achieve oral bioavailability. However, in a recent groundbreaking effort, researchers at GSK identified an extremely long-lasting IAP-based RIPK2 degrader that maintained RIPK2 protein ablation for more than 96 hours after a single subcutaneous dose [35]. The effect could be prolonged to more than 60 days using a slow release formulation [36].

In addition to the two "workhorse" E3 ligases VHL and CRBN (and to some extent IAP), many groups have continued to work on making additional E3 ligases accessible for TPD. A lot of exciting work has come from the labs of Benjamin Cravatt and Daniel Nomura utilizing the power of chemoproteomics and covalent ligand screening to identify novel ligands for E3 ligases [37, 38]. Various members of the CUL4-associated factor (DDB1- and CUL4-associated factor homolog protein [DCAF]) and RING finger protein (RNF) families have been successfully recruited for TPD using covalent binders and fragments. Further details on covalent degraders and the identification of E3 binders using chemoproteomics are reported in Chapter 8 of this book authored by Xiaoyu Zhang.

1.2.5 Milestone 5: Sticking It to the Man! Molecular Glues

In addition to SERDs and PROTACs, molecular glues represent another family of degraders currently generating excitement in both academia and the pharmaceutical industry. At a time when the PROTAC concept was still gathering momentum, research into the MoA of the small-molecule drug thalidomide opened the door to the fascinating world of small-molecule PPI inducers today termed molecular glues (Figure 1.2) [39–42]. The concept of inducing neoprotein–protein interactions has been known since the elucidation of the MoA of cyclosporin A and FK506 in 2021 [43, 44]. However, the realization that the small and simple molecules of the immunomodulatory imide drug (IMiD) family (e.g. thalidomide, pomalidomide, and lenalidomide, Figure 1.7) exert their effect via degradation of the transcription factors Ikaros (IKZF1) and Aiolos (IKZF3) came as a great surprise [45, 46]. All the more significant is that such protein targets were previously thought to be "undruggable." The IMiD drugs reshaped the protein surface of the E3 ligase CRBN to selectively recruit neosubstrates for ubiquitination and subsequent proteasomal degradation. Lenalidomide (Revlimid®) has since emerged as a best-selling drug, earning more than US$ 12 billion in revenue in 2020 alone. A detailed understanding of the IMiD MoA informed by multiple ternary complex X-ray structures has enabled the field to further flourish, with multiple IMiDs now in clinical trials (Table 1.3) [47, 48]. By tuning their structures and molecular properties, these compounds display distinct degradation selectivity to various members of the Ikaros family of zinc finger proteins and beyond.

Molecular glues are particularly attractive for drug discovery because of their lower molecular weight and improved drug-like properties versus bifunctional modulators such as PROTACs. However, until recently, the discovery of molecular glue degraders was driven primarily by serendipity. In addition to the IMiD drugs, this was also true of the discovery of the MoA of indisulam, which was revealed to be a degrader of RBM39 via recruiting the E3 ligase DCAF15 [49]. Perhaps, the first "rational" discovery of a molecular glue was the identification of compounds restoring the degradation of mutated β-catenin via its cognate E3 ligase β-TRCP [50]. Recently, work from three independent groups allowed the identification of molecules degrading cyclin K in an E3 agnostic manner [51–53]. The recent progress in the field of molecular glues has driven the foundation of multiple small Biotech companies focused on identifying the next IMiD/CRBN system, as well as expanding the target space and selectivity profiles based on the distinct degron motif identified for all IMiD targets. For further details on molecular glues, we refer the reader to Chapters 4 and 6 authored by Morgan Gadd and Cristina Mayor-Ruiz, respectively.

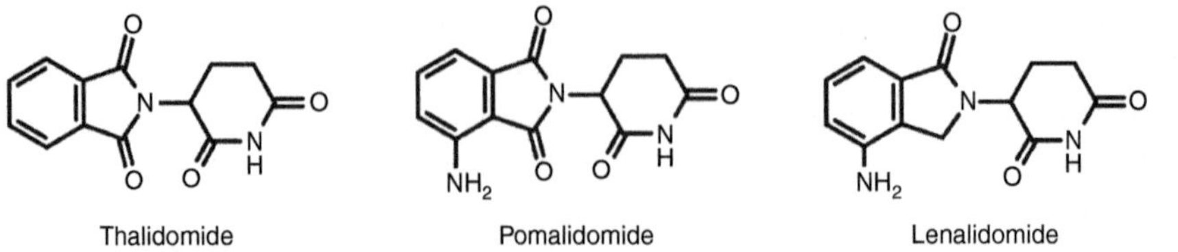

Figure 1.7 Chemical structures of the IMiDs thalidomide, pomalidomide, and lenalidomide.

1.2.6 Milestone 6: Human After All – TPD in Clinical Trials

Possibly, the first example of intentional TPD in human clinical trials was fulvestrant, an ER ligand later found to induce degradation of the target protein (a class of compounds later termed SERDs). Similarly, thalidomide and related molecular glues were identified through serendipitous discovery. In contrast, the current generation of clinical degraders has been purposefully designed to induce degradation, often with an underlying rationale for why TPD might be advantageous compared to traditional occupancy-based inhibition. In the case of bifunctional degraders such as PROTACs, their structural features typically engender "beyond rule-of-5" chemical properties, which brings significant challenges for drug delivery and oral bioavailability [54, 55]. Overcoming this challenge for such molecules and achieving bioavailability is a success story that has allowed these compounds to recently enter human clinical trials (Figure 1.2).

Fulvestrant was the first SERD drug to be approved in the United States in 2002 (Figures 1.2 and 1.3). Although fulvestrant has proven clinically effective, its oral bioavailability is severely limited because of its high lipophilicity, and therefore, the drug must be administered by intramuscular injection. To overcome this limitation, a new generation of SERD drugs is now under development to improve upon the DMPK profile of fulvestrant (Table 1.1) [56]. Several next-generation SERDs are now under clinical evaluation for the treatment of breast cancer, including four

Table 1.1 SERD and SARD degraders in clinical trials.

Drug name	Company	Target protein(s)	Indication(s)	Clinical phase
Camizestrant (AZD9833)	AstraZeneca	ER	Breast cancer	Phase III
Elacestrant (RAD1901)	Radius Health	ER	Breast cancer	Phase III
Rintodestrant (G1T48)	G1 Therapeutics	ER	Breast cancer	Phase I
Giredestrant (GDC-9545)	Roche Genentech	ER	Breast cancer	Phase III
Amcenestrant (SAR439859)	Sanofi	ER	Breast cancer	Phase III
LY3484356	Loxo oncology	ER	Breast cancer	Phase I
Zn-c5	Zentalis	ER	Breast cancer	Phase I
D-0502	InventisBio	ER	Breast cancer	Phase I
Galeterone (TOK-001)	University of Maryland	AR	Prostate Cancer	Phase II
ASC-J9	AndroScience	AR	Acne vulgaris	Phase IIb (discontinued)
AZD3514	AstraZeneca	AR	Prostate cancer	Phase I (discontinued)

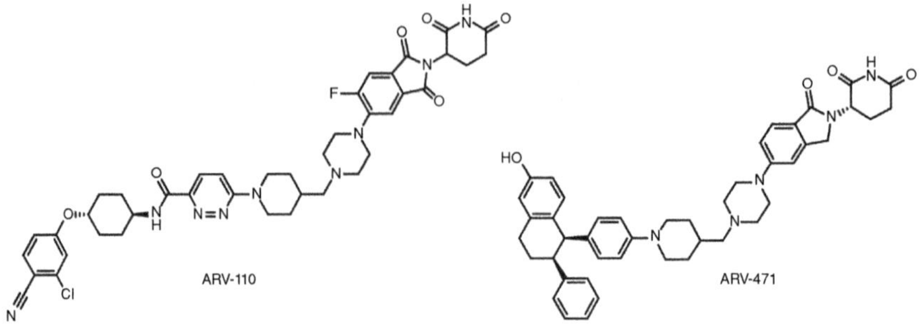

Figure 1.8 Chemical structures of the first two PROTACs to enter clinical trials; the AR degrader ARV-110 and the ER degrader ARV-471.

compounds currently in phase III trials. In contrast with SERDs, there has been less progress in the clinical development of SARD drugs targeting the AR. AZD3514 was under development as a first-in-class, orally bioavailable SARD for the treatment of prostate cancer and entered phase I trials in 2010, where it showed moderate antitumor activity but caused significant nausea and vomiting precluding further investigation [57]. ASC-J9 is another SARD that was under clinical evaluation for the topical treatment of acne vulgaris. Although the compound showed improved efficacy compared with placebo, its clinical development has not progressed beyond phase IIb (Table 1.1) [58].

In 2019, the first bifunctional degraders entered human clinical trials. Like SARD drugs, ARV-110 targets the AR for the treatment of prostate cancer, while ARV-471 is an ER degrader for the treatment of breast cancer (Figure 1.8). Both drugs have since demonstrated the proof of mechanism, providing useful levels of pharmacokinetic exposure and the modulation of hormone-related biomarkers in clinical volunteers, allowing these drugs to progress to phase II trials [59, 60]. These pioneering studies aimed to tackle their respective cancer indications via clinically validated protein targets, a strategy that helped to minimize the risk of failure by ensuring that their novel mode of action was counterbalanced by proven disease biology. Since 2019, more than 10 additional bifunctional degraders have entered the clinic, including several compounds that target novel biological pathways (Table 1.2) [61]. Although many of these degraders focus on oncology indications, both KT-474 from Kymera® and NX-5948 (Nurix®) target autoimmune diseases, thus demonstrating the potential for TPD in therapeutic areas other than cancer.

Molecular glues have also played a significant role in the transition of TPD to the clinic. Inspired by the earlier IMID drugs such as thalidomide, researchers have designed new compounds that specifically degrade protein targets linked to lymphoma, leukemia, and solid tumors (Table 1.3) [61]. In contrast to bifunctional degraders, the physicochemical properties of molecular glue degraders comply more closely with Lipinski's "rule of 5," [55], providing an advantage for achieving a pharmacokinetic profile with efficacious clinical exposure. Although the rational design of molecular glue degraders remains a challenge, recent advances may facilitate their discovery and development in the future [51, 62].

Table 1.2 Bifunctional degraders in clinical trials.

Drug name	Company	Target protein(s)	Indication(s)	Clinical phase
ARV-110	Arvinas	AR	Prostate cancer	Phase II
ARV-766	Arvinas	AR	Prostate cancer	Phase I
ARV-471	Arvinas	ER	Breast cancer	Phase II
AC682	Accutar	ER	Breast cancer	Phase I
CC-94676	Bristol Myers Squibb	AR	Prostate cancer	Phase I
AC0176	Accutar	AR	Prostate cancer	Phase I
HP-518	Hinova Pharmaceuticals	AR	Prostate cancer	Phase I
GT20029	Suzhou Kintor Pharmaceutical	AR	Androgenic alopecia, Acne	Phase I
DT2216	Dialectic	BCL-XL (B-cell lymphoma-extra large protein)	Liquid and solid tumors	Phase I
KT-474	Kymera	IRAK4	Autoimmune diseases	Phase I
KT-413	Kymera	IRAK4	DLBCL (diffuse large B-cell lymphoma)	Phase I
KT-333	Kymera	STAT3	Solid and liquid tumors	Phase I
NX-2127	Nurix	BTK	B-cell cancers	Phase I
NX-5948	Nurix	BTK	B-cell cancers, autoimmune diseases	Phase I
FHD-609	Foghorn	BRD9	Synovial sarcoma	Phase I

1.2.7 Milestone 7: Beyond the Proteasome – Inducing Proximity to Modulate Protein Levels

In the wake of the excitement generated by TPD and the realization that functional neo-PPIs can be induced via bifunctional molecules, additional strategies to rationally modulate protein levels have been discovered [63, 64]. In 2018, the Disney lab reported the recruitment of an RNA nuclease to degrade the microRNA-96 (miR-96) resulting in increased levels of the pro-apoptotic transcription factor FOXO1 and coined the term ribonuclease targeting chimeras (RIBOTAC) for ribonuclease targeting chimeras [65]. Additional PoC work followed; however, at this point of time, RIBOTACs might still be considered as chemical biology tools rather than upcoming therapeutics [66, 67].

Moving beyond the power of the UPS to degrade and remove disease-causing proteins, other groups have focused on the second major mammalian degradation machine; the lysosomal pathway [68, 69]. In 2020, Banik et al. reported that by engaging the cell surface mannose-6-phosphate receptor (M6PR), the internalization of

Table 1.3 Molecular glue degraders in clinical trials.

Drug name	Company	Target protein(s)	Indication(s)	Clinical phase
Avadomide CC-122	Bristol Myers Squibb	IKZF1, IKZF3, DNA-PK	Lymphoma	Phase II
DKY709	Novartis	IKZF2	Solid tumors	Phase I
CC-90009	Bristol Myers Squibb	GSPT1	Acute myeloid leukemia	Phase I
Mezigdomide CC-92480	Bristol Myers Squibb	IKZF1, IKZF3	Multiple myeloma	Phase I
Iberdomide CC-220	Bristol Myers Squibb	IKZF1, IKZF3	CML (chronic myeloid leukemia), NHL (non-Hodgkin's lymphoma)	Phase I
CC-99282	Bristol Myers Squibb	IKZF1, IKZF3	Lymphoma	Phase I
CFT7455	C4 Therapeutics	IKZF1, IKZF3	Multiple myeloma and Lymphoma	Phase I
BTX-1188	BioTheryX	IKZF1, IKZF3, GSPT1	Acute myeloid leukemia, NHL	Phase I

protein cargo and its subsequent degradation via the lysosome can be triggered [70]. They named their system lysosome targeting chimeras (LYTACs, Figure 1.9). LYTACs are capable of degrading extracellular as well as membrane proteins and thereby address a niche that PROTACs and molecular glues are unable to reach, as the latter modalities are restricted to intracellular targets. LYTACs were further expanded to include the asialoglycoprotein receptor (ASGPR), which is exclusively expressed on hepatocytes via *N*-acetylgalactosamine (GalNAc). The Biotech company LYCIA Therapeutics® was later founded based on LYTAC technology [71]. Besides LYTACs, sweeping antibodies or Seldegs have also been reported to degrade extracellular protein constructs [68]. For membrane-bound POIs, antibody-based PROTACs (AbTACs) have been employed by the Wells lab, which comprise bispecific antibodies of which one arm is designed to engage the POI while the other arm recruits a membrane-bound E3 ligase to induce ubiquitination on the cytosolic side [72].

Further applications of lysosomal degradation include the so-called autophagy targeting chimeras (AUTACs) and autophagy tethering compounds (ATTECs, Figure 1.9) [69, 73, 74]. While AUTACs are in principle capable of degrading everything within the cell, including whole-cell organelles (e.g. mitochondria), their full MoA remains unknown. ATTECs on the other hand simultaneously engage the LC3 as well as their protein target and have been successfully applied to induce the degradation of mutant Huntington (mHTT) protein via autophagy.

Modulating POI levels has emerged as an exciting playground for novel chemical biology tools, and their use has consequently helped to better understand the

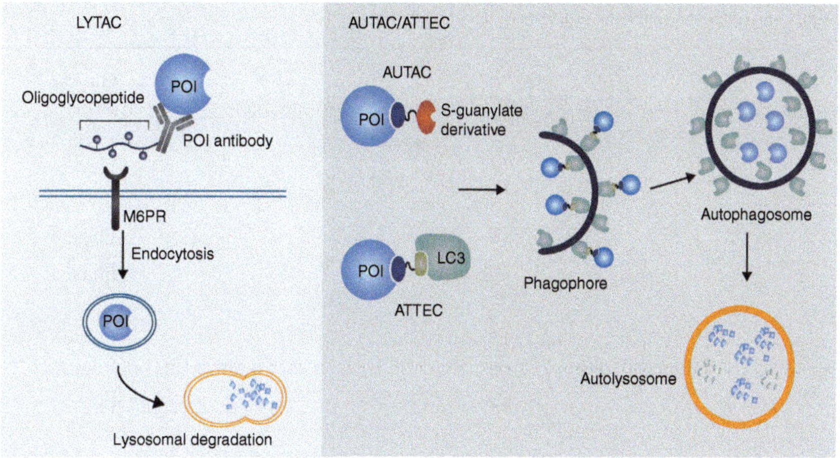

Figure 1.9 Schematic representation of LYTAC and AUTAC/ATTEC mode of action.

biological processes behind protein degradation. However, in their current state, many of these techniques do not yet provide the necessary features to advance to the preclinical stage.

1.2.7.1 Is TPD Just the Beginning? Bifunctional Modulators of Post-transcriptional Modification

Alongside the development of bifunctional degraders that induce ubiquitination (e.g. PROTACs), there have been significant advances in the design of bifunctional compounds that induce other types of protein modification. This includes phosphorylation, dephosphorylation, deubiquitylation, and acetylation, all of which have been achieved via bifunctional modulators analogous to PROTACs. In contrast to polyubiquitination, which results in degradation, these modulators can drive a variety of cellular phenotypes. While PROTACs that have made the transition to clinical development, the therapeutic potential of these agents remains in its infancy – no such bifunctional modulators have yet reached the clinic, despite their potential to modify disease states in cell-based models. As such, the field continues to develop rapidly.

In 2020, a collaboration between Genentech® (USA) and Pharmaron® (China) reported the development of bifunctional compounds that engage the ubiquitously expressed phosphatase PP1 using a peptidic warhead linked to a POI ligand binding to either protein kinase B (AKT) or epidermal growth factor receptor (EGFR), both of which are kinases of therapeutic interest [75]. In this case, the phosphatase warhead plays a similar role to the E3 ligase binding component found in PROTACs. The authors termed these compounds PhoRCs (phosphatase recruiting chimeras, Figure 1.10). In the first instance, they demonstrated a concentration-dependent effect upon the phosphorylation of AKT at threonine 303 and serine 473, both of which are linked to AKT activity. A second PhoRC compound using a targeting

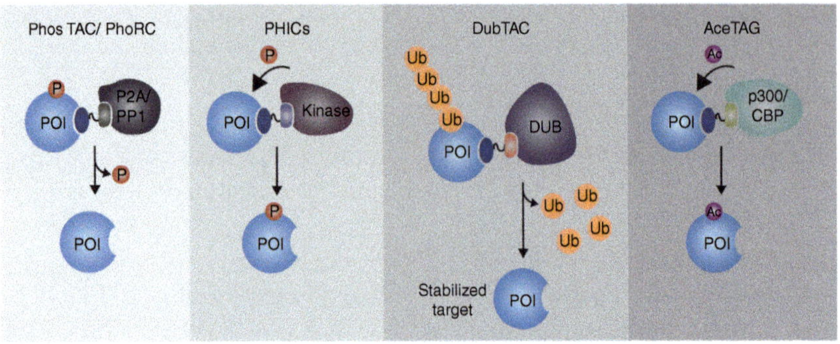

Figure 1.10 Schematic representation of post-translational modification modulators.

ligand derived from the EGFR inhibitor AZD-9291 (Tagrisso) similarly showed decreased levels of EGFR phosphorylation at the tyrosine 1068 residue. Although modest cell activity was demonstrated in this report, the peptidic warhead represents a potential drawback for the PhoRC modality as this feature limits their permeability. Phosphatase ligands with improved physicochemical properties may prove more optimal in the design of future PhoRC compounds.

A related platform recruiting phosphatases for the targeted dephosphorylation of neosubstrates was reported by Crews and coworkers [76]. Termed PhosTACs (phosphorylation targeting chimeras), these compounds rely on the use of tagged proteins – namely, a target phosphatase bearing an FKBP12 tag and a substrate bearing a HaloTag. In this way, a bifunctional compound linking a high-affinity FKBP12 ligand to a chloroalkane binding to the HaloTag can artificially induce ternary complex formation to drive dephosphorylation. The authors exemplified their platform with the fusion proteins for the phosphatase PP2A and either of two substrates: PDCD4 and FOX03a. In both cases, successful dephosphorylation was demonstrated in engineered HeLa cells by Western blot.

Around the same time as the publication of PhoRCs and PhosTACs, a team from the Broad Institute (USA) reported the inverse protein modification, in this case, co-opting kinase proteins for the phosphorylation of a neosubstrate [77]. These compounds were titled phosphorylation-inducing chimeric small molecules (PHICs), phosphorylation-inducing chimeric small molecules (Figure 1.10). In initial studies, the target protein for phosphorylation was the bromodomain-containing protein BRD4 for which a high-affinity ligand (S)-JQ1 and an inactive tool compound (R)-JQ1 were already available. To illustrate the generality of the PHIC modality, phosphorylation was demonstrated in cell-free experiments using two different kinases, AMP-activated protein kinase (AMPK) or protein kinase C (PKC), neither of which are known to interact with BRD4 under normal conditions. By linking a kinase ligand with (S)-JQ1, the resulting PHICs induced phosphorylation as demonstrated via immunoblotting for phospho-Ser484/488 of BRD4. In contrast, PHICs using the inactive isomer (R)-JQ1 showed no phosphorylation. Unfortunately, in cell-based experiments, these initial PHICs proved inactive, possibly owing to differences in the subcellular localization of the BRD4 and the target kinases. The authors then generated PHICs that recruited AMPK kinase for the phosphorylation of the neosubstrate Bruton's tyrosine kinase (BTK) to successfully achieve intracellular phosphorylation. This report expands upon the toolbox of bifunctional modulators but also highlights the potential limitations of such approaches.

As with phosphorylation and dephosphorylation, recent advances have extended upon PROTAC-induced ubiquitination to enable the reverse transformation: deubiquitylation. Termed deubiquitinase-targeting chimeras (DUBTACs, Figure 1.10), these molecules enable targeted protein stabilization (TPS), the inverse of TPD [78]. Using a chemoproteomic approach pioneered in their labs, Nomura and coworkers first discovered a covalent ligand that binds to an allosteric site on OTUB1, a highly expressed deubiquitinating enzyme (DUB) that cleaves K48-linked ubiquitin chains. The OTUB1 recruiting ligand was then linked to a ligand derived from lumacaftor, a cystic fibrosis drug that engages the protein cystic fibrosis transmembrane conductance regulator (CFTR). The resulting DUBTAC compounds therefore induce ternary complex formation between OTUB1 and CFTR, driving deubiquitylation and stabilizing the CFTR protein in a disease-relevant bronchial epithelial cell line.

Acetylation is another post-transcriptional modification that has yielded bifunctional modulators termed AceTAGs (acetylation tagging system, Figure 1.10) [79]. In this case, the authors recruited the highly homologous lysine acetyltransferase (KAT) proteins p300/cyclic adenosine monophosphate response element CREB-binding protein (CBP) for which a high-affinity targeting ligand was already available. Echoing the earlier PhosTAC approach, the acetyltransferase recruiting warhead was linked to an FKBP12 ligand, which bound to an FKBP12-tag modified target protein. Using this platform, several POI targets could be acetylated in a dose-dependent manner in HeLa cells, including histone H3.3, p65/relA, and p53.

These studies illustrate the growing arsenal of methods to harness post-transcriptional modification for chemical biology. In principle, ternary complex formation between any two proteins could be utilized to induce a wide variety of phenotypes. Although such techniques have not yet made the transition from the laboratory to clinical development, there is clear potential for their future development in the pursuit of new therapeutic agents.

1.3 Conclusion and Outlook

The field of TPD and related technologies is undergoing a period of rapid development. Many such compounds are currently under evaluation in clinical trials or are expected to soon reach the clinic (Tables 1.2 and 1.3). Despite the many new molecules, modalities, and technologies already reported to date, we expect that the current wave of discovery represents just the "tip of the iceberg" with significant progress still to come.

However, despite the present explosion of research, unresolved problems and the need for caution remains. As the first PROTAC drugs proceed through clinical trials, we will come to understand the unique safety concerns associated with this modality. It is still unclear whether recruiting E3 ligases might sequester these proteins from their natural roles within the cell (at the time of writing, primarily VHL and cereblon) to any clinically significant extent. If so, there may be a duality to the safety profile of bifunctional molecules, which incur on-target safety risks for both the protein target and the E3 ligase. There is also a double concern regarding the emergence of resistance, where mutations could emerge in either protein (POI or E3 ligase) to overcome engagement. Initial reports on preclinical resistance have primarily identified mutations of the E3 ligase complexes and other proteins involved in the degradation cascade [80–82]. However, at the current stage of investigation, these reports are inconclusive. The final picture of resistance mutations will be painted only after market approval and long-term investigation in real-world patient populations. For oncology, this could be of particular concern as resistance mutations are often a limiting factor for clinical efficacy and durability of response.

On the topic of safety, there is also a persistent concern in the use of these novel modalities for benign diseases. A quick glance at Tables 1.1–1.3 that describe agents in current clinical trials shows an overwhelming bias toward oncology drugs; this is partly driven by the different safety requirements in indications other than cancer. In addition, cereblon-derived PROTACs and molecular glues continue to bear close chemical similarity to thalidomide, which was withdrawn because of the tragic discovery of its teratogenic effects. The drug discovery community has a moral imperative to ensure that future clinical therapies are safe for patients beyond reasonable doubt.

There has been significant progress in overcoming the oral bioavailability concerns of PROTACs, both for cereblon-derived compounds (e.g. clinical candidates ARV-110 and ARV-471, Figure 1.8) and very recently for PROTACs that engage VHL [83, 84]. Despite these few successful examples, it remains difficult to rationally design compounds that achieve bioavailability. In contrast to traditional drug-like small molecules, the chemical features of PROTACs make this task much more challenging, and the "rules" for future drug design are still under active investigation [54].

Despite these concerns, there is still a great deal of optimism surrounding the field. The rapid evolution of new modes of bifunctional modulation (LYTACs, DUBTACs, etc.) has provided unprecedented access to new biological tools that will likely find applications in target validation, fundamental biology, and ultimately as clinical therapeutic agents. These bifunctional modulators might also follow in the footsteps of small-molecule drugs that eventually gave rise to protein and antibody drugs; thus, researchers have been experimenting with bifunctional proteins that engage targets in a similar manner to PROTACs to enable targeted degradation. The so-called "predator" system reported in 2020 is one such example, in which the authors link the E3 ligase Trim21 to a target protein, enabling proteasomal degradation [85]. Although these technologies are in their infancy, we expect significant progress in the development of protein-based bifunctional degraders in the future.

Despite being a relatively young field of research, TPD has already proven tremendously successful. A multitude of small biotech companies have emerged which specialize in all facets of TPD and beyond, including monovalent molecular glues, bivalent protein degraders, lysosome recruiting LYTACs, and autophagy-inducing molecules.

Many of these companies have already advanced toward clinical investigation of their first assets and have secured multibillion USD funding and/or built successful partnerships with major clinical-stage pharmaceutical corporations. Furthermore, most (if not all) large- or medium-sized pharmaceutical companies are conducting their own work in the field of TPD. The realization that the functional interaction of two protein targets can be successfully induced using synthetic small molecules has revolutionized the current paradigm in pharmaceutical research and sparked a "gold rush" in TPD drug discovery [86]. Although it is impossible to predict the clinical outcome and ultimate success of the all degrader molecules currently under investigation, we believe that the research landscape has already changed for the better, leading researchers to explore new technologies that seemed impossible only a few years ago. These are exciting times to work in TPD and we are keen to see which barriers will be broken and which new possibilities will emerge in the coming years.

References

1 Glickman, M.H. and Ciechanover, A. (2002). The ubiquitin-proteasome proteolytic pathway: destruction for the sake of construction. *Physiol. Rev.* 82 (2): 373–428.

2 Todde, V., Veenhuis, M., and van der Klei, I.J. (2009). Autophagy: principles and significance in health and disease. *Biochim. Biophys. Acta* 1792 (1): 3–13.

3 Komander, D. and Rape, M. (2012). The ubiquitin code. *Annu. Rev. Biochem.* 81 (1): 203–229.

4 Kwon, Y.T. and Ciechanover, A. (2017). The ubiquitin code in the ubiquitin–proteasome system and autophagy. *Trends Biochem. Sci.* 42 (11): 873–886.

5 Cromm, P.M. and Crews, C.M. (2017). Targeted protein degradation: from chemical biology to drug discovery. *Cell Chem. Biol.* 24 (9): 1181–1190.

6 Paiva, S.-L. and Crews, C.M. (2019). Targeted protein degradation: elements of PROTAC design. *Curr. Opin. Chem. Biol.* 50: 111–119.

7 Pettersson, M. and Crews, C.M. (2019). PROteolysis TArgeting Chimeras (PROTACs) – past, present and future. *Drug Discov. Today Technol.* 31: 15–27.

8 Luh, L.M., Scheib, U., Juenemann, K. et al. (2020). Prey for the proteasome: targeted protein degradation – a medicinal chemist's perspective. *Angew. Chem. Int. Ed.* 59 (36): 15448–15466.

9 Banaszynski, L.A. and Wandless, T.J. (2006). Conditional control of protein function. *Chem. Biol.* 13 (1): 11–21.

10 Qian, X.-D. and Abul-Hajj, Y.J. (1990). Synthesis and biological activity of 4-methylestradiol. *J. Steroid Biochem.* 35 (6): 745–747.

11 Gibson, M.K., Nemmers, L.A., Beckman, W.C. Jr. et al. (1991). The mechanism of ICI 164,384 antiestrogenieity involves rapid loss of estrogen receptor in uterine tissue. *Endocrinology* 129 (4): 2000–2010.

12 Osborne, C.K., Wakeling, A., and Nicholson, R.I. (2004). Fulvestrant: an oestrogen receptor antagonist with a novel mechanism of action. *Br. J. Cancer* 90 (1): S2–S6.

13 Mottamal, M., Kang, B., Peng, X., and Wang, G. (2021). From pure antagonists to pure degraders of the estrogen receptor: evolving strategies for the same target. *ACS Omega* 6 (14): 9334–9343.

14 Nishimura, K., Fukagawa, T., Takisawa, H. et al. (2009). An auxin-based degron system for the rapid depletion of proteins in nonplant cells. *Nat. Methods* 6 (12): 917–922.

15 Natsume, T., Kiyomitsu, T., Saga, Y., and Kanemaki, M.T. (2016). Rapid protein depletion in human cells by auxin-inducible degron tagging with short homology donors. *Cell Rep.* 15 (1): 210–218.

16 Neklesa, T.K. and Crews, C.M. (2012). Greasy tags for protein removal. *Nature* 487 (7407): 308–309.

17 Neklesa, T.K., Tae, H.S., Schneekloth, A.R. et al. (2011). Small-molecule hydrophobic tagging-induced degradation of HaloTag fusion proteins. *Nat. Chem. Biol.* 7 (8): 538–543.

18 Sakamoto, K.M., Kim, K.B., Kumagai, A. et al. (2001). Protacs: chimeric molecules that target proteins to the Skp1-Cullin-F box complex for ubiquitination and degradation. *Proc. Natl. Acad. Sci. U.S.A.* 98 (15): 8554–8559.

19 Gosink, M.M. and Vierstra, R.D. (1995). Redirecting the specificity of ubiquitination by modifying ubiquitin-conjugating enzymes. *Proc. Natl. Acad. Sci. U.S.A.* 92 (20): 9117–9121.

20 Zhou, P., Bogacki, R., McReynolds, L., and Howley, P.M. (2000). Harnessing the ubiquitination machinery to target the degradation of specific cellular proteins. *Mol. Cell* 6 (3): 751–756.

21 Sakamoto, K.M., Kim, K.B., Verma, R. et al. (2003). Development of protacs to target cancer-promoting proteins for ubiquitination and degradation. *Mol. Cell. Proteomics* 2 (12): 1350–1358.

22 Schneekloth, J.S., Fonseca, F.N., Koldobskiy, M. et al. (2004). Chemical genetic control of protein levels: selective in vivo targeted degradation. *J. Am. Chem. Soc.* 126 (12): 3748–3754.

23 Hines, J., Gough, J.D., Corson, T.W., and Crews, C.M. (2013). Posttranslational protein knockdown coupled to receptor tyrosine kinase activation with phosphoPROTACs. *Proc. Natl. Acad. Sci. U.S.A.* 110 (22): 8942–8947.

24 Schneekloth, A.R., Pucheault, M., Tae, H.S., and Crews, C.M. (2008). Targeted intracellular protein degradation induced by a small molecule: en route to chemical proteomics. *Bioorg. Med. Chem. Lett.* 18 (22): 5904–5908.

25 Logan, I.R., McNeill, H.V., Cook, S. et al. (2007). Analysis of the MDM2 antagonist nutlin-3 in human prostate cancer cells. *Prostate* 67 (8): 900–906.

26 Itoh, Y., Ishikawa, M., Naito, M., and Hashimoto, Y. (2010). Protein knockdown using methyl bestatin–ligand hybrid molecules: design and synthesis of inducers of ubiquitination-mediated degradation of cellular retinoic acid-binding proteins. *J. Am. Chem. Soc.* 132 (16): 5820–5826.

27 Itoh, Y., Kitaguchi, R., Ishikawa, M. et al. (2011). Design, synthesis and biological evaluation of nuclear receptor-degradation inducers. *Biorg. Med. Chem.* 19 (22): 6768–6778.

28 Buckley, D.L., Gustafson, J.L., Van Molle, I. et al. (2012). Small-molecule inhibitors of the interaction between the E3 ligase VHL and HIF1alpha. *Angew. Chem. Int. Ed.* 51 (46): 11463–11467.

29 Buckley, D.L., Van Molle, I., Gareiss, P.C. et al. (2012). Targeting the von Hippel–Lindau E3 ubiquitin ligase using small molecules to disrupt the VHL/HIF-1alpha interaction. *J. Am. Chem. Soc.* 134 (10): 4465–4468.

30 Winter, G.E., Buckley, D.L., Paulk, J. et al. (2015). Phthalimide conjugation as a strategy for *in vivo* target protein degradation. *Science* 348 (6241): 1376–1381.

31 Bondeson, D.P., Mares, A., Smith, I.E.D. et al. (2015). Catalytic *in vivo* protein knockdown by small-molecule PROTACs. *Nat. Chem. Biol.* 11 (8): 611.

32 Lu, J., Qian, Y., Altieri, M. et al. (2015). Hijacking the E3 ubiquitin ligase cereblon to efficiently target BRD4. *Chem. Biol.* 22 (6): 755–763.

33 Ohoka, N., Okuhira, K., Ito, M. et al. (2017). *in vivo* knockdown of pathogenic proteins via specific and nongenetic inhibitor of apoptosis protein (IAP)-dependent protein erasers (SNIPERs). *J. Biol. Chem.* 292 (11): 4556–4570.

34 Ohoka, N., Morita, Y., Nagai, K. et al. (2018). Derivatization of inhibitor of apoptosis protein (IAP) ligands yields improved inducers of estrogen receptor alpha degradation. *J. Biol. Chem.* 293 (18): 6776–6790.

35 Mares, A., Miah, A.H., Smith, I.E.D. et al. (2020). Extended pharmacodynamic responses observed upon PROTAC-mediated degradation of RIPK2. *Commun. Biol.* 3 (1): 140.

36 Miah, A.H., Smith, I.E.D., Rackham, M. et al. (2021). Optimization of a series of RIPK2 PROTACs. *J. Med. Chem.* 64 (17): 12978–13003.

37 Belcher, B.P., Ward, C.C., and Nomura, D.K. (2021). Ligandability of E3 ligases for targeted protein degradation applications. *Biochemistry* https://doi.org/10.1021/acs.biochem.1c00464.

38 Spradlin, J.N., Zhang, E., and Nomura, D.K. (2021). Reimagining druggability using chemoproteomic platforms. *Acc. Chem. Res.* 54 (7): 1801–1813.

39 Ito, T., Ando, H., Suzuki, T. et al. (2010). Identification of a primary target of thalidomide teratogenicity. *Science* 327 (5971): 1345–1350.

40 Gandhi, A.K., Kang, J., Havens, C.G. et al. (2014). Immunomodulatory agents lenalidomide and pomalidomide co-stimulate T cells by inducing degradation of T cell repressors Ikaros and Aiolos via modulation of the E3 ubiquitin ligase complex CRL4CRBN. *Br. J. Haematol.* 164 (6): 811–821.

41 Lopez-Girona, A., Mendy, D., Ito, T. et al. (2012). Cereblon is a direct protein target for immunomodulatory and antiproliferative activities of lenalidomide and pomalidomide. *Leukemia* 26 (11): 2326–2335.

42 Lu, G., Middleton, R.E., Sun, H. et al. (2014). The myeloma drug lenalidomide promotes the cereblon-dependent destruction of ikaros proteins. *Science* 343 (6168): 305–309.

43 Schreiber, S.L. (2021). The rise of molecular glues. *Cell* 184 (1): 3–9.

44 Schreiber, S.L. (1991). Chemistry and biology of the immunophilins and their immunosuppressive ligands. *Science* 251 (4991): 283–287.

45 Chamberlain, P.P. and Cathers, B.E. (2019). Cereblon modulators: low molecular weight inducers of protein degradation. *Drug Discov. Today Technol.* 31: 29–34.

46 Kozicka, Z. and Thomä, N.H. (2021). Haven't got a glue: protein surface variation for the design of molecular glue degraders. *Cell Chem. Biol.* 28 (7): 1032–1047.

47 Leissing, T.M., Luh, L.M., and Cromm, P.M. (2020). Structure driven compound optimization in targeted protein degradation. *Drug Discov. Today Technol.* 37: 73–82.

48 Chamberlain, P.P., D'Agostino, L.A., Ellis, J.M. et al. (2019). Evolution of cereblon-mediated protein degradation as a therapeutic modality. *ACS Med. Chem. Lett.* 10 (12): 1592–1602.

49 Bussiere, D.E., Xie, L., Srinivas, H. et al. (2020). Structural basis of indisulam-mediated RBM39 recruitment to DCAF15 E3 ligase complex. *Nat. Chem. Biol.* 16 (1): 15–23.

50 Simonetta, K.R., Taygerly, J., Boyle, K. et al. (2019). Prospective discovery of small molecule enhancers of an E3 ligase–substrate interaction. *Nat. Commun.* 10 (1): 1402.

51 Mayor-Ruiz, C., Bauer, S., Brand, M. et al. (2020). Rational discovery of molecular glue degraders via scalable chemical profiling. *Nat. Chem. Biol.* 16 (11): 1199–1207.

52 Slabicki, M., Kozicka, Z., Petzold, G. et al. (2020). The CDK inhibitor CR8 acts as a molecular glue degrader that depletes cyclin K. *Nature* 585 (7824): 293–297.

53 Lv, L., Chen, P., Cao, L. et al. (2020). Discovery of a molecular glue promoting CDK12–DDB1 interaction to trigger cyclin K degradation. *eLife* 9: e59994.

54 Edmondson, S.D., Yang, B., and Fallan, C. (2019). Proteolysis targeting chimeras (PROTACs) in 'beyond rule-of-five' chemical space: recent progress and future challenges. *Bioorg. Med. Chem. Lett.* 29 (13): 1555–1564.

55 Lipinski, C.A., Lombardo, F., Dominy, B.W., and Feeney, P.J. (2001). Experimental and computational approaches to estimate solubility and permeability in drug discovery and development settings. *Adv. Drug Delivery Rev.* 46 (1–3): 3–26.

56 Hernando, C., Ortega-Morillo, B., Tapia, M. et al. (2021). Oral selective estrogen receptor degraders (SERDs) as a novel breast cancer therapy: present and future from a clinical perspective. *Int. J. Mol. Sci.* 22 (15): 7812.

57 Omlin, A., Jones, R.J., van der Noll, R. et al. (2015). AZD3514, an oral selective androgen receptor down-regulator in patients with castration-resistant prostate cancer – results of two parallel first-in-human phase I studies. *Invest. New Drugs* 33 (3): 679–690.

58 Results of ASC-J9-202 Phase 2B Clinical Study. http://www.androscience.com/ 2013 (cited20 January 2022). Available from: http://www.androscience.com/artman/publish/news/Results_of_ASC-J9-202_Phase_2B_Clinical_Study.shtml (accessed 2 June 2022).

59 Petrylak, D.P., Gao, X., Vogelzang, N.J. et al. (2020). First-in-human phase I study of ARV-110, an androgen receptor (AR) PROTAC degrader in patients (pts) with metastatic castrate-resistant prostate cancer (mCRPC) following enzalutamide (ENZ) and/or abiraterone (ABI). *J. Clin. Oncol.* 38 (15_Suppl): 3500.

60 Snyder, L.B., Flanagan, J.J., Qian, Y. et al. (2021). Abstract 44: The discovery of ARV-471, an orally bioavailable estrogen receptor degrading PROTAC for the treatment of patients with breast cancer. *Cancer Res.* 81 (13 Suppl): 44.

61 Békés, M., Langley, D.R., and Crews, C.M. (2022). PROTAC targeted protein degraders: the past is prologue. *Nat. Rev. Drug Discov.* 21 (3): 181–200.

62 den Besten, W. and Lipford, J.R. (2020). Prospecting for molecular glues. *Nat. Chem. Biol.* 16 (11): 1157–1158.

63 Alabi, S. and Crews, C. (2021). Major advances in targeted protein degradation: PROTACs, LYTACs, and MADTACs. *J. Biol. Chem.* 296: 100647.

64 Ng, C.S.C. and Banik, S.M. (2022). Recent advances in induced proximity modalities. *Curr. Opin. Chem. Biol.* 67: 102107.

65 Costales, M.G., Matsumoto, Y., Velagapudi, S.P., and Disney, M.D. (2018). Small molecule targeted recruitment of a nuclease to RNA. *J. Am. Chem. Soc.* 140 (22): 6741–6744.

66 Costales, M.G., Suresh, B., Vishnu, K., and Disney, M.D. (2019). Targeted degradation of a hypoxia-associated non-coding RNA enhances the selectivity of a small molecule interacting with RNA. *Cell Chem. Biol.* 26 (8): 1180–6.e5.

67 Zhang, P., Liu, X., Abegg, D. et al. (2021). Reprogramming of protein-targeted small-molecule medicines to RNA by ribonuclease recruitment. *J. Am. Chem. Soc.* 143 (33): 13044–13055.

68 Ahn, G., Banik, S.M., and Bertozzi, C.R. (2021). Degradation from the outside in: targeting extracellular and membrane proteins for degradation through the endolysosomal pathway. *Cell Chem. Biol.* 28 (7): 1072–1080.

69 Pei, J., Wang, G., Feng, L. et al. (2021). Targeting lysosomal degradation pathways: new strategies and techniques for drug discovery. *J. Med. Chem.* 64 (7): 3493–3507.

70 Banik, S.M., Pedram, K., Wisnovsky, S. et al. (2020). Lysosome-targeting chimaeras for degradation of extracellular proteins. *Nature* 584 (7820): 291–297.

71 Ahn, G., Banik, S.M., Miller, C.L. et al. (2021). LYTACs that engage the asialoglycoprotein receptor for targeted protein degradation. *Nat. Chem. Biol.* 17 (9): 937–946.

72 Cotton, A.D., Nguyen, D.P., Gramespacher, J.A. et al. (2021). Development of antibody-based PROTACs for the degradation of the cell-surface immune checkpoint protein PD-L1. *J. Am. Chem. Soc.* 143 (2): 593–598.

73 Takahashi, D., Moriyama, J., Nakamura, T. et al. (2019). AUTACs: cargo-specific degraders using selective autophagy. *Mol. Cell* 76 (5): 797–810.e10.

74 Fu, Y., Chen, N., Wang, Z. et al. (2021). Degradation of lipid droplets by chimeric autophagy-tethering compounds. *Cell Res.* 31 (9): 965–979.

75 Yamazoe, S., Tom, J., Fu, Y. et al. (2020). Heterobifunctional molecules induce dephosphorylation of kinases-a proof of concept study. *J. Med. Chem.* 63 (6): 2807–2813.

76 Chen, P.-H., Hu, Z., An, E. et al. (2021). Modulation of phosphoprotein activity by phosphorylation targeting chimeras (PhosTACs). *ACS Chem. Biol.* 16 (12): 2808–2815.

77 Siriwardena, S.U., Munkanatta Godage, D.N.P., Shoba, V.M. et al. (2020). Phosphorylation-inducing chimeric small molecules. *J. Am. Chem. Soc.* 142 (33): 14052–14057.

78 Henning, N.J., Boike, L., Spradlin, J.N. et al. (2022). Deubiquitinase-targeting chimeras for targeted protein stabilization. *Nat. Chem. Biol.* 18: 412–421.

79 Wang, W.W., Chen, L.-Y., Wozniak, J.M. et al. (2021). Targeted protein acetylation in cells using heterobifunctional molecules. *J. Am. Chem. Soc.* 143 (40): 16700–16708.

80 Ottis, P., Palladino, C., Thienger, P. et al. (2019). Cellular resistance mechanisms to targeted protein degradation converge toward impairment of the engaged ubiquitin transfer pathway. *ACS Chem. Biol.* 14 (10): 2215.

81 Zhang, L., Riley-Gillis, B., Vijay, P., and Shen, Y. (2019). Acquired resistance to BET-PROTACs(proteolysis targeting chimeras) caused by genomic alterations in core components of E3 ligase complexes. *Mol. Cancer Ther.* 18 (7): 1302–1311.

82 Mayor-Ruiz, C., Jaeger, M.G., Bauer, S. et al. (2019). Plasticity of the cullin-RING ligase repertoire shapes sensitivity to ligand-induced protein degradation. *Mol. Cell* 75 (4): 849–58.e8.

83 Kofink, C., Trainor, N., Mair, B. et al. (2022). A selective and orally bioavailable VHL-recruiting PROTAC achieves SMARCA2 degradation in vivo. *ChemRxiv.* https://doi.org/10.26434/chemrxiv-2022-q63s3.

84 Luo, G., Li, Z., Lin, X. et al. (2020). Discovery of an orally active VHL-recruiting PROTAC that achieves robust HMGCR degradation and potent hypolipidemic activity *in vivo*. *Acta Pharm. Sin. B* 11 (5): 1300–1314.

85 Liu, C., Kuang, J., Qiu, X. et al. (2020). Predator: a novel method for targeted protein degradation. *bioRxiv* 231787. https://doi.org/10.1101/2020.07.31.231787.

86 Garber, K. (2021). The PROTAC gold rush. *Nat. Biotechnol.* 40 (1): 12–16.

2

Cellular Principles of Targeted Protein Degradation

João Diamantino and Doris Hellerschmied

University of Duisburg-Essen, Faculty of Biology, Center of Medical Biotechnology, Universitätsstraße 2, D-45141 Essen, Germany

Protein degradation is a critical aspect of a protein's "life cycle" and an essential process for maintaining cellular protein homeostasis. Co-opting cellular degradation pathways for targeted protein degradation (TPD) requires their detailed molecular understanding and most importantly defining biological effectors that confer substrate selectivity and commitment to degradation. Chemical biology or therapeutic strategies that induce proximity between proteins of interest (POIs) and these biological effectors enable TPD. Conversely, using these chemical biology strategies can support work aimed at understanding cellular degradation pathways. This interrelation creates a powerful cycle in which fundamental cell biology research progresses the development of TPD strategies and vice versa (Figure 2.1).

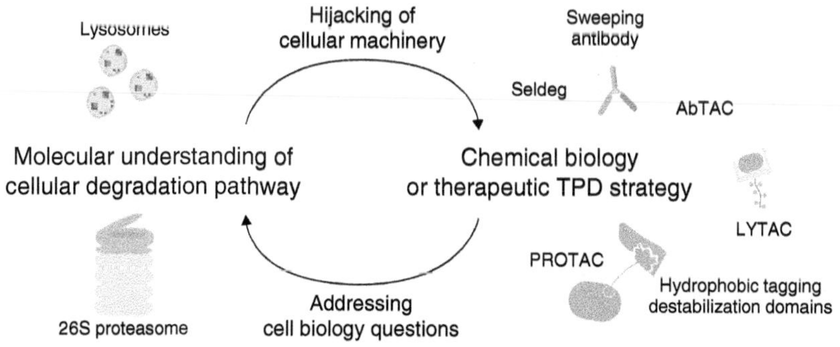

Figure 2.1 Interplay between molecular understanding of cellular degradation pathways and targeted protein degradation (TPD) strategies. TPD approaches rely on the hijacking of cellular degradation pathways to achieve controlled and selective degradation of proteins of interest (POIs), potentially used as a therapeutic strategy or for addressing cell biology questions. Conversely, the use of TPD enhances our understanding of cellular degradation pathways, which can be applied to optimize and develop TPD strategies.

Inducing Targeted Protein Degradation: From Chemical Biology to Drug Discovery and Clinical Applications, First Edition. Edited by Philipp Cromm.

2.1 Basic Principles of Targeting Substrates to the Proteasome and Lysosomes

In eukaryotic cells, two major degradation systems, the proteasome and lysosomes, contribute to regulating the abundance of the proteome [1, 2].

2.1.1 Ubiquitin-Proteasome System (UPS)

The proteasome is a cytosolic and nuclear-localized multi-subunit proteolytic machine [3]. It consists of the 19S regulatory particle, essential for substrate binding and ATP-driven substrate unfolding and the 20S core particle, containing the peptidase activity [3]. Targeting proteins for proteasomal degradation typically requires the activity of the ubiquitination machinery (Figure 2.2). A cascade of ubiquitination enzymes (E1, E2, and E3) mediates the covalent attachment of the small protein modifier, ubiquitin (Ub), to the substrate protein. To this end, the E1 enzyme activates Ub in an ATP-dependent manner and forms a thioester with its C-terminus [4]. Via transthiolation, Ub is transferred to the E2 ubiquitin

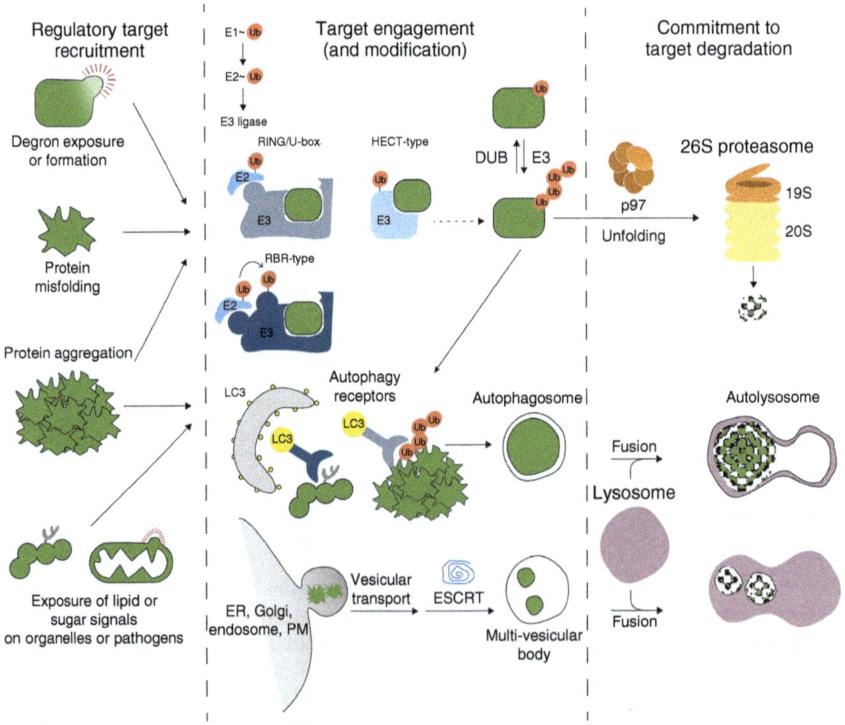

Figure 2.2 Overview of degradation systems in eukaryotic cells. Cellular degradation systems can be divided into three modules conferring substrate selectivity and regulatory checkpoints: regulatory target recruitment, where substrates expose signals to induce their degradation, target engagement and modification, where E3 ubiquitin ligases or autophagy receptors recognize substrates and modify them for the final commitment to a specific degradation pathway.

conjugating enzyme [4, 5]. Finally, it is the ubiquitin E3 ligase that mediates transfer of Ub to the substrate protein and thereby confers substrate selectivity to the system. Three major types of ubiquitin E3 ligases can be distinguished: HECT-type, RING/U-box-type, and RING-in-between-RING (RBR) E3 ligases [6, 7]. HECT-type E3 ligases form a thioester with Ub and directly transfer the modifier to the substrate protein. RING/U-box-type E3 ligases prime the E2~Ub thioester conjugate for nucleophilic attack by the target residue within the substrate protein [6, 8]. RBR ligases use one RING domain for E2~Ub conjugate priming, while the second RING domain contains an active site cysteine to form a thioester intermediate with Ub before substrate ubiquitination [6, 8]. Ub can be attached to the side chain of a lysine residue within the substrate or another Ub molecule to promote the formation of poly-Ub chains. Chain editing by Ub ligases and deubiquitination enzymes (DUBs) can further modulate downstream processing of the substrate [9]. The Ub chain type determines the fate of the substrate protein – a link referred to as the Ub code [10]. The proteasome primarily degrades proteins carrying K48-linked Ub chains but also K11- or K29-linked chains can induce protein degradation. Accordingly, the Ub code needs to be considered when choosing to hijack "writers" and "editors" of Ub signals for TPD strategies [10]. Substrate degradation is initiated at the 19S proteasome lid, where receptors recognize Ub signals, while a ring of AAA unfoldase in the 19S base engages an unstructured stretch of amino acids – known as the proteasome initiation site – within the substrate protein and starts pulling [11]. If substrates lack an unfolded stretch, an additional AAA protein, p97/VCP (Cdc48 in yeast), is required for unfolding [12, 13]. The Ub signal is removed, and the substrate is eventually proteolytically processed in the 20S proteasome core [11]. The detailed molecular understanding of substrate processing by the UPS stresses demands for efficient substrate targeting and degradation and thereby lays the groundwork for developing TPD strategies.

2.1.2 Lysosomal Targeting

Lysosomes are membrane-bounded organelles hosting (>50 different) hydrolases, which digest the incoming lumenal content. Substrates (cargo) for lysosomal degradation are delivered by the autophagy machinery or via vesicular transport from the plasma membrane (PM), the endoplasmic reticulum (ER), the Golgi apparatus, or the endosomal system (Figure 2.2).

Cytosolic content is targeted for lysosomal degradation by autophagy. Macroautophagy requires the nucleation and elongation of a double-membrane structure, the subsequent encapsulation of cargo, and finally closure of the double-membrane structure to form the autophagosome [14, 15]. The formation and maturation of the autophagosome involves the coordinated activity of six distinct protein complexes [15]. Critical for substrate targeting and therefore important in light of developing TPD strategies is the decoration of the autophagic membrane with LC3 proteins, which serve as interaction sites for autophagy receptors [16, 17]. LC3 proteins (six different LC3s or GABARAPs in mammalian cells) are ubiquitin-like proteins that are conjugated to phosphatidylethanolamine membrane lipids. This lipidation reaction is mediated by the E1 and E2 enzymes, ATG7 and ATG3, respectively [14]. The E3 enzyme catalyzing LC3 lipidation is a protein complex formed by another ubiquitin-like conjugate, ATG12-ATG5, and ATG16 [14]. Specialized autophagy receptors provide substrate selectivity by bridging cargo to the forming autophagosome [16, 17]. These receptors contain specific LC3 interacting regions (LIRs) or GABARAP interaction motifs (GIMs) and cargo recognition sites, which bind to sugar, lipid, or Ub signals displayed on autophagy substrates (Figure 2.2). The substrate spectrum of autophagy ranges from proteins and protein aggregates to entire damaged organelles and pathogens [18]. For a more detailed review on autophagy and selective receptors, we refer the reader to Refs. [16–18].

Selective substrate targeting of PM proteins to the lysosome can be regulated by ubiquitination. Ub signals are typically recognized by proteins of the vesicular transport machinery and the endosomal sorting complex required for transport (ESCRT) machinery [19–21]. Ub-dependent cargo sorting by ESCRT proteins promotes the generation of multi-vesicular bodies (MVBs) by forming intraluminal vesicles (ILVs), which can be entirely digested by lysosomal enzymes (Figure 2.2) [21]. The involvement of Ub signaling in proteoasomal and lysosomal targeting highlights the requirement to further dissect the Ub code. In addition to Ub signals, direct interaction with lysosome-targeting receptors (LTRs) can target proteins from the PM or the Golgi apparatus to lysosomes [22].

Irrespective of the delivery system (vesicular carriers or double-membrane-enclosed autophagosomes), lysosomal degradation finally requires the fusion with the delivery vehicle (Figure 2.2) to provide substrates access to the lysosomal lumen and enable digestion by lysosomal hydrolases. Although key molecular players supporting the process of lysosomal fusion including membrane-tethering complexes, SNAREs (soluble *N*-ethylmaleimide-sensitive factor attachment protein receptors), and Rab GTPases have been identified, our molecular understanding of lysosome fusion remains limited [23]. Finally, a specialized pathway, chaperone-mediated autophagy (CMA), bypasses the need for fusion and targets protein substrates directly into the lysosomal lumen via the LAMP-2A transporter [24].

The two cellular degradation systems, proteasome and lysosomes, show differences in their substrate spectrum and requirements for substrate delivery mechanisms. Yet, in this chapter, we want to highlight conceptual similarities of selective substrate targeting mechanisms as these represent excellent starting points for developing targeted degradation strategies. To this end, it is important to note that the substrate pool of both degradation systems needs to be tightly controlled to avoid unwanted accumulation or depletion of proteins. Misregulated protein levels can have deleterious effects and are the underlying cause of multiple diseases [25, 26]. Degradation pathways rely on elements conferring substrate selectivity and regulatory checkpoints to control substrate processing. The processes of (*) regulatory target recruitment by exposure of signals that indicate the need for degradation, (*) target engagement, for example, by ubiquitin E3 ligases or autophagy receptors and (reversible) target modification, and (*) the final commitment to degradation of the modified target protein (Figure 2.2) present opportunities to modulate the cellular system for research and even therapeutic purposes.

2.2 Targeted Protein Degradation from the Cytosol and the Nucleus

TPD strategies exert their biological effect by inducing POI degradation and thereby causing cellular perturbation. POIs in the cytosol and the nucleus span a wide variety of protein classes. In a clinical setting, the modulation of oncogenes, such as kinases, phosphatases, hormone receptors, and epigenetic readers, is of high priority [27–29]. These targets have traditionally been addressed with small-molecule approaches, such as the development of inhibitors, which now provide ideal starting points for developing pharmacological TPD strategies. In addition, TPD holds promise in addressing target proteins so far seen as undruggable, provided that ligands for inducing proximity to a biological effector are available. As an alternative to developing protein-specific ligands, cell biology research often resorts to established ligand-binding protein domains that can easily be fused to POIs and allow addressing cell biological questions as well as evaluating the TPD mode of action for therapeutic targets. For example, the HaloTag domain, which covalently conjugates to chloroalkenes and the FKBP12^{F36V}-domain (dTAG), which binds to multiple synthetic ligands, have proven to be valuable tools in developing and applying TPD strategies [30–33]. The auxin-inducible degron (AID) domain, which binds to derivatives of the plant hormone auxin, provides control over AID-fusion protein levels [34, 35]. The value of using protein domains for TPD approaches is also highlighted by the recent development of the aTAG system, based on proteins MTH1 and BRD9, and the BromoTag system, based on BRD4 [36, 37].

2.2.1 Targeting to the Proteasome

Conceptually, the proteasomal degradation of POIs from the cytosol and the nucleus of eukaryotic cells has been achieved by hijacking cellular pathways for regulatory target recruitment (2.2.1.1), target engagement by the ubiquitination machinery (2.2.1.2), and direct engagement of the proteasome (2.2.1.3).

2.2.1.1 Regulatory Target Recruitment

Regulatory recruitment of degradation targets typically depends on the conditional presentation of signals on a protein's surface that indicate the need for its degradation. Thus, changes in protein conformation, assembly state, and post-translational modifications can influence a protein's susceptibility to degradation and thereby affect its half-life [38]. Pharmacological tools that trigger or mimic these regulatory signals can provide the basis for targeted degradation of POIs [38, 39].

The conformational state of a protein is a key determinant of its susceptibility to degradation. Exposure of hydrophobic amino acids on the surface of proteins indicates misfolding and warrants the activity of the protein quality control (PQC) machinery to initiate refolding or degradation processes. With the goal of preventing the accumulation of potentially toxic, misfolded protein species, molecular chaperones shield hydrophobic patches and support proteins in (re)establishing their native fold [40]. In addition to refolding of quality control substrates, the collaboration of chaperones and the ubiquitination machinery promotes the degradation of terminally misfolded proteins or orphan subunits of protein complexes [40, 41]. Chaperones interfacing with ubiquitin E3 ligases are, for example, Hsp70 and Hsp90, which collaborate with the ligase CHIP to ubiquitinate unfolded protein substrates [42, 43]. Similarly, the UFD-2 E3 ligase uses the myosin chaperone UNC-45 to access unfolded myosin substrates [44]. Chemical genetics approaches have harnessed the cellular PQC machinery to promote protein degradation, with different degrees of precision. Inhibiting chaperone function, for example, has proven successful in shifting the equilibrium from attempts at protein refolding to degradation for certain substrates [45, 46]. In more targeted approaches, protein domains, whose folding state can be controlled with a small-molecule ligand, were developed to regulate the stability of POI fusions [39, 47]. These so-called destabilization domains, derived from dihydrofolate reductase (DHFR) and 12 kDa FK506-binding protein (FKPB12), remain properly folded in the presence of their respective small-molecule ligands trimethoprim (TMP) and Shield-1 [48–50]. Upon ligand washout, the POI fusions are recognized as misfolded by chaperones and degraded by the UPS [50]. Strategies exerting the opposite effect, where the ligand has a destabilizing effect on the protein domain or induces the exposure of hydrophobic residues on the surface, have also been established. A ligand for the HaloTag domain containing a hydrophobic moiety, such as an adamantly group, causes protein destabilization and thereby promotes interaction with chaperones and the UPS – a method referred to as hydrophobic tagging [32, 51, 52]. Protein destabilization is also explored as a therapeutic strategy. For example, selective estrogen receptor degraders (SERDs) are molecules that affect the levels of endogenous estrogen receptor, a target for breast cancer therapy [53].

In addition to surface hydrophobicity, specific amino acid motifs, at the N- or C-termini of proteins, can serve as the so-called degrons, i.e. signals for protein degradation [54]. N- or C-degrons are recognized by ubiquitin E3 ligases, N-recognins and specific cullin-RING ligases (CRLs), respectively, and thereby engage the UPS for their turnover [54]. Proteins can be inherently short-lived, harboring a destabilizing N-terminus upon synthesis or destabilizing residues can be exposed in a regulatory manner. For example, proteolytic processing can expose or remove degrons from proteins [55, 56]. Protein complex assembly can limit accessibility to degrons by burying them at interaction sites [57]. In other words, degrons can help distinguish excess, unassembled protein subunits or misassembled complexes that need to be removed from the cell. Moreover, premature termination of translation can result in the formation of C-degrons to ensure the removal of truncated, non-functional protein products [58, 59]. Genetic fusion of degron sequences to proteins can be used as a strategy to control protein turnover. Genetic strategies can be combined with chemical biology methods to exert temporal control over degron exposure. An engineered degron, also referred to as cryptic degron, that is exposed only upon binding the ligand Shield-1 was appended to the C-terminus of the FKBP domain, establishing the ligand-induced degradation (LID) system [60]. The opposite strategy was followed by establishing the small-molecule-assisted shutoff (SMASh) methodology, where ligand binding stops the self-removal of a degron and thereby induces POI degradation [61].

Another efficient way of generating degrons in cells is by post-translational modification of proteins. This strategy represents a fast and effective means of regulating protein levels, as compared to regulation at the transcriptional or translational level. Phosphodegrons, for example, are an integral part of cell cycle regulation, where progression from one stage to the next is dependent on the quantitative and acute degradation of select inhibitors [62, 63]. With the advent of phosphorylation-inducing chimeric small molecules (PHICs) [64] and phosphorylation targeting chimeras (PhosTACs) [65], it is conceivable to recruit kinases or phosphatases to POIs for the modulation of a phosphodegron, thereby affecting POI degradation.

The examples discussed here illustrate that hydrophobicity and degrons can serve as modulators of protein turnover when displayed on the surface of POIs. In addition, degrons have inspired the development of recruiting elements in heterobifunctional compounds inducing proximity between POIs and ubiquitin E3 ligases (see the following Section 2.2.1.2).

2.2.1.2 Target Engagement by the Ubiquitination Machinery

Target engagement by the ubiquitination machinery at the level of the E3 ligase is a step that has been largely exploited by chemical genetic and therapeutic approaches to induce TPD. E3 ligases bind to signals on the surface of their target proteins and thereby induce proximity between an E2 ~ Ub- or E3 ~ Ub-thioester conjugate and a lysine residue on the target to mediate target ubiquitination [8]. E3 ligases can directly interact with their targets or establish an interaction with the help of adaptor proteins. In multi-subunit E3 ligases, such as the large family of CRLs, core subunits collaborate with multiple substrate adaptors to access a wide variety of targets [66]. TPD approaches rely on the principle that inducing proximity between an E3 ligase and a POI results in POI polyubiquitination and subsequent degradation. To this end, proteolysis targeting chimeras (PROTACs) and molecular glues are prime examples of assuming the role of customizable substrate adaptors and promoting POI degradation [67, 68].

A PROTAC is a heterobifunctional molecule that consists of a POI-binding ligand conjugated via a linker to an E3 ligase ligand [68]. Ligands engaging E3 ligases come in different flavors [69]. Structural characterization of E3 ligase–degron pairs has provided key information for the design of peptidic or small-molecule-based E3 ligase ligands. Most prominently, the small-molecule ligand extensively used to engage the VHL E3 ligase complex was designed based on a substrate-derived peptide [70–72]. Other E3 ligase recruiting ligands that are routinely developed into PROTACs and PROTAC-type compounds, referred to as SNIPERs or degronimids, are small molecules that often stem from serendipitous discoveries [28, 73, 74]. Active development of E3 ligase ligands and the expected expansion of the small-molecule-accessible E3 ligase pool are of high importance for TPD [69, 75, 76], as the chosen E3 ligase can influence the ability to induce POI degradation and afford POI selectivity [77–79]. Moreover, engaging diverse E3 ligases may not only increase the substrate spectrum of PROTACs but also their specificity, considering the cell- and tissue-specific expression patterns of certain ubiquitin ligases. PROTACs targeting viral E3 ligases expressed in host cells may even provide an avenue to exclusively target infected cells.

Another class of proximity-inducing molecules that promote the E3 ligase-dependent ubiquitination of target proteins are molecular glues. Molecular glues bind to and alter the surface of E3 ligases and thereby change their substrate spectrum [67]. The auxin family of plant hormones – a family of molecular glues found in nature – induces the degradation of transcriptional repressors to regulate gene expression programs during plant development and growth. To do so, auxin family hormones modify the interface between the E3 ligase adaptor protein TIR1 and transcriptional repressors to produce an active, SCF-type ubiquitination complex [80]. On the basis of the IAA17 transcriptional repressor, the AID domain was developed [34]. AID (or AID2) fusion proteins are rapidly degraded in an SCF-TIR1- and proteasome-dependent manner [34, 35]. Synthetic molecular glues engaging substrate adaptors of E3 ligases were initially discovered by delineating the molecular target of the drug thalidomide [81]. Now commonly referred to as immune modulatory imide drugs (IMiDs), thalidomide and its glutarimide-containing derivatives are extensively used in TPD approaches [74]. IMiDs target the cereblon (CRBN) subunit of a CRL and promote the ubiquitination and degradation of the so-called neosubstrates [67]. The term neosubstrates refers to a substrate pool that is only accessible to the CRBN–IMiD complex. Modification of a surface-exposed moiety of IMiDs results in the recruitment of different neosubstrates [74]. IMiDs also serve as the E3 ligase recruiting ligands in a large number of PROTAC molecules. The second prominent scaffold for synthetic molecular glue degraders is indisulam, an aryl sulfonamide that engages the CRL subunit DCAF15 [82, 83]. Recently, the development of strategies to rationalize the discovery of molecular glue degraders has afforded a compound inducing the degradation of cyclin K by promoting an interaction with CDK12 and ubiquitination by a CRL [84]. Ongoing efforts in discovering molecular glues will certainly advance the TPD field and show great promise in identifying degraders for POIs that lack apparent tractable domains (see also Chapter 6 for more details).

2.2.1.3 Engaging the Proteasome

Downstream of the ubiquitination by E3 ligases, substrates engage the degradation machinery [85]. Certain ubiquitinated substrates require active extraction from their native environment and/or unfolding by the p97 AAA–ATPase before proteasomal degradation [12, 13]. With a detailed molecular understanding of p97 and its adaptor proteins, it is conceivable that inducing proximity between the unfoldase and POIs may be developed into an efficient TPD strategy. Notably, p97 can also recruit substrates in a ubiquitin-independent manner, mediated by specific adapters [86, 87], which may simplify such approaches. The detailed understanding of substrate recruitment to the proteasome has been applied to induce ubiquitin-independent TPD. At the 26S proteasome, the receptors Rpn1, Rpn10, and Rpn13 engage the Ub chain displayed on the substrate protein [11]. In addition to these receptors that are an integral part of the proteasome lid, the so-called adaptor or shuttling proteins play an important role in targeting ubiquitinated substrates for degradation [11, 85]. Adaptors such as RAD23A, RAD23B, or ubiquilins contain a ubiquitin-like (UbL) domain, which serves as the interaction site for proteasome receptors. Induced dimerization of POIs with the UbL domain of an adaptor protein, implemented with genetic fusion proteins, provided proof of concept that direct recruitment can be exploited for TPD in mammalian cells [88]. Direct recruitment to the proteasome with a small-molecule approach, relying on a modified proteasome inhibitor, was recently achieved by chemical knockdown with affinity and degradation dynamics (CANDDY) [89]. In this approach, a heterobifunctional molecule simultaneously interacting with the oncogene $KRAS^{G12D}$ and the proteasome induced oncogene degradation [89]. Future development of these approaches holds promise in promoting TPD strategies, which bypass the need for substrate modification.

2.2.2 Targeting to Lysosomes

Selective targeting of cytosolic and nuclear substrates (cargo) for lysosomal degradation is mediated by CMA and macroautophagy [18, 24].

Substrates that undergo CMA carry a pentapeptide motif (KFERQ) as the determining signal, which is bound by the Hsc70 chaperone [24]. The detailed molecular characterization of this selectivity-conferring chaperone–substrate interaction provided the basis for CMA-based TPD strategies [90, 91]. Specifically, a peptide that induces proximity between the mutant huntingtin protein and Hsc70 afforded CMA-dependent target degradation in cells and even mouse models [91]. Moreover, a KFERQ-based peptide motif in combination with a POI-targeting moiety and a cell membrane penetrating domain was used to target cytosolic proteins for lysosomal degradation in primary neuronal cultures [90].

Protein aggregates, pathogens, or damaged organelles that are cleared by selective macroautophagy typically expose specific sugar or lipid signals and are characterized by the accumulation of Ub signals [18]. These signals are recognized by autophagy receptors, which confer substrate selectivity to the system [16, 17]. Autophagy receptors bridge cargo to the forming autophagosome, primarily by direct interaction with LC3 proteins [16, 18]. The ability to simultaneously engage cargo and the autophagy machinery has been successfully co-opted by different methods to promote targeted lysosomal degradation. The broad substrate spectrum of macroautophagy, ranging from proteins to organelles and even intracellular pathogens, offers a variety of signals that can be mimicked in order to induce proximity between POIs and the autophagy machinery. The generation of molecules mimicking a modification initially found to promote the clearance of intracellular bacteria afforded selective autophagy-inducing compounds [92]. Modification of cytoplasmic group A streptococci with cGMP correlates with the formation of K63-linked ubiquitin modification, recruitment of the autophagy receptor p62, and subsequent clearance of the pathogen. In a proof-of-concept experiment, a cGMP derivative was displayed on the surface of the HaloTag domain, leading to its lysosomal degradation [92]. Heterobifunctional molecules, autophagy targeting chimeras (AUTACs), take advantage of this cGMP-based signal to recruit the autophagy machinery to POIs [92]. Targets of AUTACs include cytosolic proteins, and also nuclear proteins can be targeted for lysosomal degradation during mitosis and nuclear breakdown [92]. Additional heterobifunctional compounds that are explored for autophagy-based TPD access the autophagy receptor p62. Moreover, the molecular interaction between cargo and autophagy initiation complex may be amenable for TPD [93]. Finally, screening efforts lead to the development of autophagosome-tethering compounds (ATTECs) that link LC3 proteins, which decorate the autophagic membrane, to aggregates of mutant huntingtin protein [94, 95]. ATTECs serve as synthetic autophagy receptors, inducing proximity between the isolation membrane and select cargo, thereby inducing its degradation [94, 95]. Compelling concepts targeting POIs for autophagy are emerging; however, we still require an in-depth understanding of the molecular mechanisms underlying selective autophagy to enable future development of lysosome-based TPD approaches from the cytosol [16, 93].

In addition to targeting the POIs for autophagic degradation, the removal of entire damaged organelles is an attractive avenue for AUTACs and ATTECs. Notably, the sole recruitment of the autophagy machinery, specifically LC3 or the p62 autophagy receptor, to the Golgi apparatus was not sufficient to induce its autophagic degradation [96]. Similarly, decorating healthy mitochondria with AUTACs did not induce mitophagy [92]. Only damaged, fragmented mitochondria, created, for example, by cell treatment with the depolarizing agent carbonyl cyanide m-chlorophenylhydrazone (CCCP) or knockdown of select mitochondrial proteins, were subjected to AUTAC-induced degradation [92]. These observations may suggest that fragments of organelles are more amenable degradation targets than fully intact ones, or indicate the need for additional regulatory signals to induce the clearance of organelles. In general, these studies highlight the complexity of the autophagic process and point to possible additional requirements beyond proximity-inducing strategies. Current research suggests that the regulatory clearance of organelles starts with the display of signals that indicate organelle damage [97, 98]. The rupture of lysosomes, for example, leads to the exposure of otherwise lumenal sugar structures on glycosylated proteins to the cytosol. Galectins recognize these structures and recruit the ubiquitination machinery and autophagy receptors to coordinate clearance of damaged organelles [99, 100]. Moreover, damaged mitochondria display mitochondrial membrane protein prohibitin-2 and the PINK1 kinase on their surface [101, 102]. Mimicking these signals could serve to recruit the autophagy machinery. Both damaged lysosomes and mitochondria have further been shown to accumulate specific Ub signals [97, 98]. Further identification and molecular characterization of autophagy-specific E3 ligases and Ub signals would represent a major advance in the pursuit of lysosomal TPD approaches.

2.3 Targeted Degradation from Membrane-Enclosed Organelles and the Extracellular Space

Eukaryotic cells are characterized by subcellular compartments with distinct protein and lipid content. This compartmentalization poses a challenge for the protein degradation machineries in accessing substrate proteins. Yet, controlling the levels of proteins at the PM and the extracellular space such as immune checkpoint proteins, antibodies, growth factors, or cell surface receptors is critical for cellular health and development [103, 104]. Similarly, controlled protein degradation from the lumen or the membrane of the ER and the Golgi apparatus is critical. On the one hand, these compartments of the secretory pathway serve as a supply chain, determining PM protein composition; on the other, the levels of ER and Golgi resident proteins need to be regulated. In addition to regulatory proteolysis, misfolded or damaged organellar proteins need to access degradation pathways to maintain protein homeostasis [105]. Similar to the difficulties that cells have to overcome with respect to the membrane barrier between substrates and degradation machinery, challenges in developing TPD approaches in this space lie in ensuring efficient transport across membranes for proteasomal degradation and accurate targeting of vesicular content to lysosomes.

Proteins that can be engaged at the cytosolic face of the PM or at the surface of organelles have been targeted using chemical biology tools, which were initially established for soluble cytosolic targets [32, 106–108]. However, novel methods are required to expand the degradable target protein space to TM proteins that are not accessible from the cytosolic face as they lack tractable, ligandable cytosolic domains and to access extracellular and soluble, lumenal proteins (Figures 2.3–2.5). We believe that these methods can similarly be inspired by established cellular degradation pathways that work across membranes to eventually engage the proteasome or lysosomes. In the following Sections 2.3.1–2.3.3, we review degradation pathways from the PM, the ER, and the Golgi apparatus, which show potential for being hijacked with chemical biology tools and highlight examples of pathways that have successfully been co-opted for TPD.

2.3.1 Degradation from the Plasma Membrane (PM) and the Extracellular Space

The turnover of extracellular and TM proteins typically relies on their internalization at the PM in vesicular carriers, sorting-based transport through the endosomal system, and subsequent lysosomal degradation. On the extracellular face, constitutive endocytosis can be distinguished from ligand-triggered processes. With respect to the cytosolic face, the internalization at the PM is typically classified according to the type of machinery required for vesicle formation and scission and/or the involvement of the ubiquitination system.

2.3.1.1 Internalization at the PM and Endosomal Sorting

Endocytosis of extracellular and TM proteins can be mediated by the clathrin coat, caveolins, or occur independent of the two protein complexes [109–111]. Studies of select substrate proteins have led to the proposal that the type of endocytosis affects the fate of the internalized proteins [112]. Accordingly, further work on substrate-selective endocytic pathways is highly important to support efforts at co-opting endocytosis for TPD.

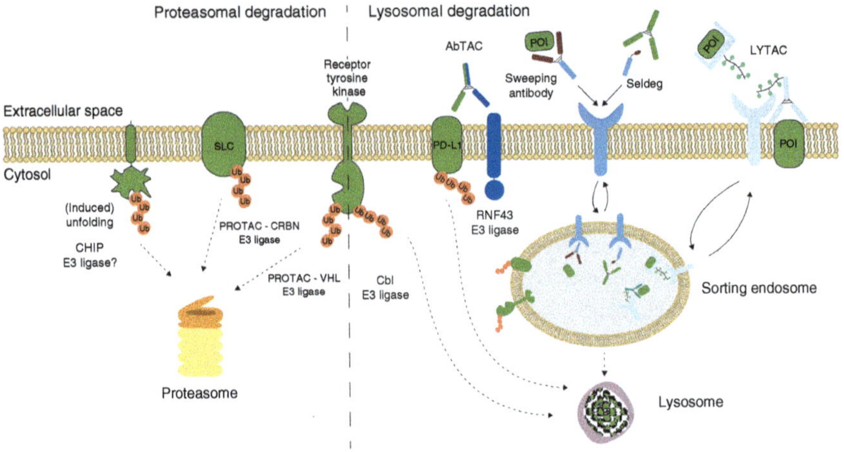

Figure 2.3 Degradation of proteins from the plasma membrane (PM). Degradation of PM proteins can be induced by using hydrophobic tagging or PROTACs to facilitate substrate ubiquitination and further proteasomal or lysosomal degradation. Lysosomal degradation can also be achieved from the extracellular space through AbTACs, which recruit the RNF43 E3 ubiquitin ligase, or by lysosome targeting chimeras (LYTACs), sweeping antibodies, and Seldegs, which rely on endocytic receptors.

The best characterized form of internalization at the PM is clathrin-mediated endocytosis [109]. It depends on the assembly of adaptor proteins at the membrane, which in turn recruit the clathrin coat to form a vesicle. AP2 is the major adaptor protein complex initiating clathrin-mediated endocytosis at the PM [109]. Hot-wired endocytosis, or chemically induced endocytosis, takes advantage of this interaction by recruiting the clathrin coat using a PM-anchored AP2-derived interaction peptide [113]. Research on this system has contributed to the molecular understanding of clathrin-mediated endocytosis, and revealed recycling of cargo to the PM, yet it may also represent a starting point for inducing POI degradation from the PM, when extended or combined with other chemical biology tools [113]. As illustrated by this example, endocytosis does not by default lead to lysosomal degradation of cargo. Sorting at the endosome is a key step that determines whether internalized cargo is targeted to lysosomes or recycled back to the PM, sparing proteins from degradation [114]. Extracellular, soluble cargo, which is internalized by interacting with PM receptors, needs to be released in endosomes for continued transport to lysosomes. TM cargo and the PM receptors themselves rely on the formation of ILVs for their lysosomal turnover [114]. Ubiquitination of TM proteins at the PM or at endosomes and the ESCRT machinery play a critical role in the formation of ILVs [20, 114]. Maturation of endosomes, i.e. the transition from early to late endosome and the final fusion of the late endosome with the lysosome, completes the degradation pathway.

The processes of cellular uptake, recycling, and degradation are well understood for antibodies and antibody–antigen complexes, a class of highly abundant extracellular proteins [115]. IgG proteins, a specific class of antibodies enter the cell by fluid phase pinocytosis, i.e. via vesicular uptake of bulk extracellular fluid, and reach the sorting endosome [115]. From there, they may be targeted for lysosomal degradation; however, in the endosome, at low pH (~6.0), they are also able to bind with high affinity to the FcRn receptor, which triggers their recycling to the cell surface [115]. On the basis of this molecular understanding, protein engineering has been employed to develop TPD strategies [104]. High-affinity FcRn interactors, the so-called Abdegs (antibodies that enhance IgG degradation), have successfully been employed to block the antibody recycling pathway and thereby promote IgG clearance [116]. An adapted version of this strategy is Seldegs, which promote the degradation of antigen-specific antibodies [117]. Seldegs are Fc-antigen fusions that strongly interact with FcRn and their antibody target at neutral and acidic pH, i.e. at the PM and in endosomes. In contrast to natural IgGs, these high-affinity protein complexes promote lysosomal delivery and accordingly antibody degradation (Figure 2.3) [117, 118]. Antibodies, natural and therapeutic variants, are not only taken up by themselves but as antibody–antigen complexes to achieve biological effects in immune reactions. Efficient lysosomal targeting and degradation of antigens requires their release in the sorting endosome. The so-called sweeping antibodies that promote antibody–antigen interaction at neutral pH (at the PM) and disfavor it at acidic pH (in the endolysosomal system) were used to induce lysosomal degradation of soluble extracellular targets [119]. Increased affinity of sweeping antibodies to FcRn at the PM afforded increased internalization rates.

Receptor-mediated endocytosis of extracellular proteins and subsequent targeting to lysosomes is not only relevant for antibody proteins but a process that also controls the levels of extracellular hormones, growth factors, secreted enzymes, and neurotransmitters. Receptor-mediated degradation of these targets shows great potential to be co-opted for TPD approaches. To date, the cation-independent mannose-6-phosphate receptor (CI-M6PR) and the liver-specific lysosome trafficking receptor, asialoglycoprotein receptor (ASGPR) have been exploited for targeting extracellular and cell surface targets for lysosomal degradation [120–123]. Both receptors bind to specific surface glycan structures on their substrates, a molecular interaction that provided the basis for generating lysosome-targeting compounds designated lysosome targeting chimeras (LYTACs) or molecular degrader of extracellular proteins through the ASGPR (MoDE–As) (Figure 2.3). These heterobifunctional compounds link lysosome-targeting receptors at the PM to soluble POIs and thereby promote POI uptake and subsequent lysosomal degradation. LYTACs have also been used to induce the degradation of TM proteins, demonstrating broad applicability of the targeting approach [121]. These first reports harnessing CI-M6PR and ASGPR show great potential, yet we still lack a detailed molecular understanding of how ligand binding triggers receptor internalization and degradation. A mechanistic insight into endocytosis and cellular transport of receptor–ligand pairs will create important reference points for developing and expanding LYTAC-type strategies.

2.3.1.2 Ubiquitination at the PM

Ubiquitination has emerged as a key cellular post-translational modification triggering internalization at the PM. Especially in yeast, endocytosis of most cell surface proteins relies on ubiquitination by the soluble E3 ligase Rsp5 [124]. Homologs of Rsp5 in mammalian cells belong to the NEDD4 ligase family and have been observed on different cellular organelles, yet their molecular role in endocytosis and membrane protein ubiquitination in general remains to be addressed [124]. In mammalian cells, the turnover of the receptor tyrosine kinase EGFR is a well-studied example of Ub-mediated endocytosis and degradation. EGFR is ubiquitinated by the cytosolic E3 ligase Cbl, which triggers clathrin-independent endocytosis and subsequent transport through the endosomal system to lysosomes for degradation [125] (Figure 2.3). Yet, endocytosis of EGFR can also proceed in a Ub-independent manner, pointing out that in mammalian cells, ubiquitination is sufficient but not necessary to trigger receptor internalization [125], a theme that has also been observed for other PM proteins [124].

Given the involvement of Ub signaling in PM protein turnover, PROTACs have been used to target POIs with accessible cytosolic domains for degradation. The substrate spectrum of PROTACs recruiting the VHL or CRBN E3 ligases includes single- and multi-pass PM proteins, such as receptor tyrosine kinases and solute carriers (SLCs), respectively [106, 107]. Interestingly, PROTACs induced the proteasome-dependent degradation of their TM targets, in contrast to what has been observed for the endogenous turnover [106, 107]. This finding once more stresses the importance of dissecting the Ub code. Hydrophobic tagging has also afforded the degradation of multi-pass TM proteins fused to a cytosolic HaloTag domain, illustrating that unfolded domains at the PM underlie quality control in mammalian cells [32]. The ubiquitination machinery involved in this process has not been identified; however, the QC E3 ligase CHIP localizes to the PM upon heat shock, suggesting an involvement in membrane-associated PQC [126]. Hydrophobic tagging and PROTACs provide valuable tools to study proteasomal degradation from the PM and shed light on so far elusive cellular PQC mechanisms [127].

As indicated by the examples discussed so far, ubiquitination at the PM is often mediated by soluble, cytosolic E3 ligases, which cannot be accessed directly by chemical tools from the extracellular space. However, TM ubiquitin ligases featuring extracellular domains also participate in targeting PM substrates for degradation. E3 ligase families with an important role in membrane protein turnover are RNF- (RING-type, TM domain), MARCH- (RING-type, TM domain), and ZNRF1/2-family (RING-type, N-myristyolyated, endosome- and lysosome-localized) E3 ligases [124]. Our current molecular understanding of these ligases is limited and certainly needs to be enhanced to put them to use in TPD strategies. A well-studied example however is RNF43, a single-pass TM E3 ligase that ubiquitinates the Wnt signaling receptor frizzled and targets it for lysosomal degradation [128]. This framework offers the possibility to control the cytosolic ubiquitination machinery from the extracellular space. An elegant way to promote communication across the PM to induce TPD was introduced with the development of antibody-based PROTACs (AbTACs) (Figure 2.3) [129]. AbTACs support the formation of a trimeric E3 ligase–AbTAC–POI complex on the extracellular face, while inducing target ubiquitination on the cytosolic face. Specifically, an AbTAC engaging RNF43 and the POI PD-L1, lacking any ligandable cytosolic domain, promotes target degradation [129]. This approach bypasses the need for a tractable cytosolic domain otherwise required for POI engagement.

Of note, the degradation of extracellular and cell surface proteins does not exclusively depend on the intracellular degradation machinery. In addition to the lysosome and the proteasome, secreted proteases play an important role in digesting extracellular targets. Recruitment of these proteases may represent an avenue for targeting POIs that are not amenable to internalization, such as large aggregates.

2.3.2 Degradation from the Endoplasmic Reticulum (ER)

The ER is the major site for secretory and TM protein biogenesis in eukaryotic cells [130]. Accordingly, ER-localized POIs for TPD approaches include proteins that are destined for downstream compartments such as the PM or the extracellular space but also ER-resident proteins that, for example, determine the organelle shape and function. Approximately, one-third of all newly synthesized proteins are co-translationally imported into the ER, where they associate with chaperones to assist their folding [105]. Considering its central role in protein synthesis, the ER is equipped with several PQC mechanisms including targeting aberrant proteins for proteasomal or lysosomal degradation [131–133]. The study of such PQC mechanisms has generated valuable knowledge on protein degradation and can provide the basis for designing strategies for TPD from the ER.

2.3.2.1 ER-Associated Protein Degradation (ERAD) – Proteoasomal Degradation from the ER

The proteasomal degradation of ER proteins involves a pathway known as ER-associated protein degradation (ERAD), where proteins with folding defects or degradation signals are ubiquitinated by ER membrane ubiquitin ligase complexes and retrotranslocated to the cytosol (Figure 2.4). ERAD was initially characterized in yeast, where distinct E3 ligases serve pathways defined by substrate protein characteristics: Hrd1 for ERAD-L and ERAD-M substrates (with folding lesions within the ER lumen and within the membrane, respectively) Doa10 for ERAD-C substrates (carrying cytosolic folding lesions) [134–137]. While the different types of PQC substrates may still be classified in mammalian cells, a higher degree of complexity is observed with respect to the ubiquitination system (Table 2.1). A recent in silico analysis identified 37 E3 ligases with RING-finger motifs and TM regions that are potentially involved in ERAD [138]. The currently best characterized ERAD E3 ligase is Hrd1 in yeast with the mammalian homologs, HRD1 and gp78 [139]. The cytosolic RING domain of Hrd1 promotes substrate ubiquitination in combination with the E2 enzyme Ubc7 (UBC6e in mammals), recruited to the ER membrane and activated by its cofactor Cue1 [140]. Considering the cytosolic localization of the ubiquitination machinery, ERAD-L substrates must be recruited to the Hrd1 complex and partially retrotranslocated to expose a segment to the cytosol, following recognition in the ER lumen [132]. Recognition of ERAD-L substrates depends primarily on their folding and glycosylation state. Folding and quality control of glycosylated proteins is mediated by the lectin chaperones calreticulin and calnexin,

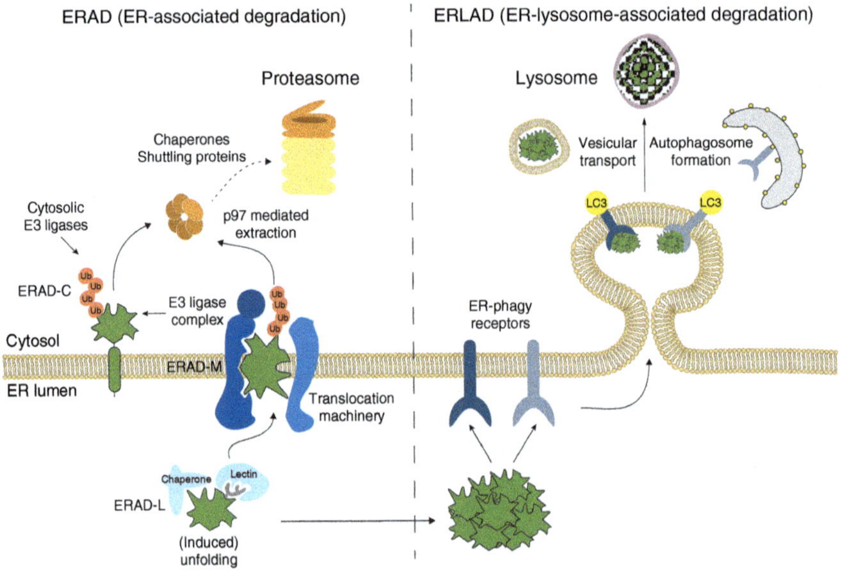

Figure 2.4 Degradation of proteins from the endoplasmic reticulum (ER). Two main degradation pathways operate at the ER: ER-associated degradation (ERAD) and ER-lysosome-associated degradation (ERLAD). ERAD mediates the proteasomal degradation of proteins with folding lesions or degradation signals located in the ER lumen (ERAD-L), the ER membrane (ERAD-M), or facing the cytosol (ERAD-C). ERLAD mediates the degradation of ERAD-resistant substrates through ER-phagy receptors, which mediate their delivery to lysosomes.

which bind to monoglucosylated N-glycans in proximity to unfolded regions [141]. If proper folding cannot be achieved, N-glycans are trimmed by the ER degradation-enhancing alpha-mannosidase-like proteins 1–3 (EDEMs 1–3) [142] to be further recognized by the lectins OS-9 and XTP-3B [143], which are responsible for the delivery of ERAD substrates to E3 ligase complexes [105, 141]. Accordingly, a potential recruiting element for TPD from the ER lumen could be based on N-glycan structures engaged by OS9 [144]. ERAD of non-glycosylated quality control substrates involves the ER-localized Hsp70 chaperone, BiP, and its cofactors [145]. BiP operates at the interface of protein folding and degradation. On the one hand, the chaperone promotes (re)folding of its substrates; on the other hand, it can also target terminally misfolded proteins for degradation. The precise molecular mechanism by which BiP "decides" to target terminally misfolded proteins for ERAD remains to be elucidated. Recent work points to an important role of the J-protein cofactors ERdj4 and ERdj5 [145, 146].

Recruitment of substrates bound to lumenal ER quality control factors to the HRD1 complex depends on their interaction with the Hrd3 subunit (SEL1L in mammals). Recruitment to a SEL1L fusion protein was used to induce degradation of POIs from the ER lumen [147]. Additionally, the Hrd1 complex requires the derlin Der1 (Derlin-1, -2, and -3 in mammals), a protein whose role remains elusive, but together with Hrd1, it has been proposed to mediate the retrotranslocation of

Table 2.1 Ubiquitin E3 ligases targeting Golgi or ER-localized substrate proteins.

Uniprot ID	Gene name	Protein name(s)	Type of E3 ligase	Localization	Reported ER and Golgi-localized substrates include	Comments
Q86TM6	SYVN1	HRD1/ Synoviolin 1	RING domain, TM domain	ER	CD147, NHK variant of α1-antitrypsin, Z variant of α1-antitrypsin, HGMR, TCR-α, CD3-δ, MHC, NS-1LC, p53, APP, gp78, CFTRΔF508, CD95/Fas, BLMP-1, PGC-1β, Nrf2, Neuroserpin, PMP22, LOX-1, Pael-R	Homolog of yeast Hrd1, integral ER membrane protein, ERAD of lumenal, TM, and cytosolic substrates
Q9UKV5	AMFR	gp78/AMFR/ RING finger protein 45	RING domain, TM domain	ER	Z variant of α1-antitrypsin, HGMR, TCR-α, CD3-δ, CFTRΔF508, apolipoprotein B100, CYP3A4, KAI1, HERP, DGAT2, mitofusins, HSPA5, huntingtin, SOD1, prion protein, neuroserpin, ataxin-3, PMP22, AMF	Homolog of yeast Hrd1, integral ER membrane protein, ERAD of lumenal, TM, and cytosolic substrates
O60337	MARCHF6	MARCH6/TEB4/ RING finger protein 176	RING domain, TM domain	ER	HMGR, type 2 iodothyronine deiodinase, SM, HO-1, NPC1, CL-1 degron	Homolog of yeast Doa10, integral ER membrane protein, ERAD of TM, and cytosolic substrates
Q8WU17	RNF139	Trc8/RNF139	RING domain, TM domain	ER	XBP1u, MHC-I, SREBP1, SREBP2, CL-1 degron, HO-1, integrin-α chains, CD112, interleukin-12 receptor, PTPRJ, thrombomodulin, HMGCR, HIV protein Gag, hERG potassium channels	Integral ER membrane protein, ERAD of lumenal, TM, and cytosolic substrates
Q96MT1	RNF145	Rnf145	RING domain, TM domain	ER	HMGCR	Integral ER membrane protein, ERAD of TM substrates
O60858	TRIM13	Rfn2/TRIM13/ Leu5/RING finger protein 77	RING domain, TM domain, B box	ER	CD3-δ, Cav1.2	Integral ER membrane protein, ERAD of TM substrates

(Continued)

Table 2.1 (Continued)

Uniprot ID	Gene name	Protein name(s)	Type of E3 ligase	Localization	Reported ER and Golgi-localized substrates include	Comments
Q96K19	RNF170	RNF17/putative LAG1-interacting protein	RING domain, TM domain	ER	IP3, TLR3	Integral ER membrane, ERAD of lumenal and TM substrates
A0AVI4	TMEM129	TMEM129	RING domain, TM domain	ER	MHC-I	Integral ER membrane E3 protein, ERAD of TM substrates
Q8WWF5	ZNRF4	ZNRF4/Nixin/RING finger protein 204/RING finger protein 4	RING domain, TM domain,	ER	Calnexin, RIP2	Integral ER membrane protein, ERAD of lumenal substrates
O00237	RNF103	RNF130/KF-1/Zfp-103	RING domain, TM domain	ER	Autoubiquitination	Integral ER membrane protein, possibly involved in ERAD
Q5M7Z0	RNFT1	RNFT1/PTD016	RING domain, TM domain	ER	Autophagic degradation of PDCD10	Integral ER membrane protein, possibly involved in ERAD, upregulated upon ER stress
Q99942	RNF5	RNF5/Rma1/Protein G16	RING domain, TM domain	ER and mitochondria	CFTRΔF508, STING, MAVS	Integral ER membrane E3 protein, ERAD of cytosolic substrates in cooperation with gp78, regulation of antiviral responses
Q96GF1	RNF185	RNF185	RING domain, TM domain	ER and mitochondria	CFTRΔF508, CYP51A1TM	Integral ER membrane protein, ERAD of TM and cytosolic substrates
Q96D59	RNF183	RNF183	RING domain, TM domain	ER, Golgi and lysosomes	Bcl-xL	Integral ER membrane protein, ERAD of cytosolic substrates

Q9H4P4	RNF41	Nrdp1/Rnf41	RING domain, SIAH domain	cytosol and ER	ErbB3	Cytosolic E3 ligase
P78317	RNF4	RFN4/SNURF	RING domain	Nucleus and cytosol	CFTRΔF508	Cytosolic E3 ligase, ERAD of cytosolic substrates
O60260	PRKN	Parkin	RING domain	ER, nucleus, mitochondria and cytosol	Pael-R, mutant GCase variants	Mainly cytosolic E3 ligase, ERAD of lumenal and cytosolic substrates
Q9UNE7	STUB1	CHIP/Antigen NY-CO-7 / CLL-associated antigen KW-8 / Carboxy terminus of Hsp70-interacting protein /STIP1 homology and U box-containing protein 1	U-box	Nucleus and cytosol, PM after heat shock	CFTRΔF508, CYP51A4, Pael-R, NCC	Cytosolic E3 ligase, ERAD of cytosolic substrates
Q9HCE7	SMURF1	Smurf1	HECT domain	cytosol and PM	WFS1	Cytosolic E3 ligase, ERAD of lumenal substrates

(Continued)

Table 2.1 (Continued)

Uniprot ID	Gene name	Protein name(s)	Type of E3 ligase	Localization	Reported ER and Golgi-localized substrates include	Comments
Q9UK22	FBXO2	Fbx2	Substrate adaptor of an SCF-type (Skp, cullin, F-box) E3 ligase complex	ER and cytosol	CFTRΔF508, pre-integrin β1, TCR-α, APP, ADAM10, BACE1	Cytosolic and ER membrane-associated protein. ERAD of lumenal, TM, and cytosolic substrates, recognition of sugar chains
Q9NRD1	FBXO6	Fbx6/Fbs2		Cytosol	TCR-α	Cytosolic protein, ERAD of lumenal substrates, recognition of sugar chains
Q9Y297	BTRC	β−TrCP/ mE3RS-IkappaB/ HOS/FWD1		Nucleus and cytosol	CD4, Tetherin	Cytosolic E3 protein, ERAD of TM, and cytosolic substrates, hijacked by HIV
Q96SW2	CRBLN	Cereblon	Substrate adaptor of CRL complex	Nucleus and cytosol	ER- and Golgi-resident SLCs fused to dTAG	Cytosolic protein hijacked by dTAG system
Q9Y4X5	ARIH1	Ariadne RBR E3 ubiquitin protein ligase 1	RBR	Golgi and nucleus		Works together with SCF complex
Q8N9I9	DTX3	Deltex E3 ubiquitin ligase 3	RING domain	Golgi and nucleus		
Q9H0M0	WWP1	WW domain containing E3 ubiquitin protein ligase 1	HECT domain	Golgi		
Q9P2E8	MARCH4		RING domain, TM domain	Golgi		

ERAD-L substrates [148]. ERAD-M substrates, which are characterized by hydrophilic and charged residues within their TM region, are also targeted by the Hrd1 complex; however, the lumenal factors Yos9 and Kar2p (OS-9 and BiP in mammals) and Der1 are dispensable for this ERAD pathway [134, 149]. Instead, it requires the derlin Dfm1, which has a central role in the ERAD-M retrotranslocation machinery [150]. Interestingly, Dfm1 was also shown to be required for the translocation of ERAD-L substrates with folded domains [151]. ERAD-C in yeast is mediated by the Doa10 complex, where the Doa10 E3 ubiquitin ligase (MARCH6/TEB4 in mammals), in concert with the E2 enzymes Ubc6 (Ube2j1 and Ube2j2 in mammals) and Ubc7, ubiquitinates substrates with cytosolic folding lesions [134, 152]. Similar to ERAD-M, Dfm1 was also reported to play a role in the Doa10 complex [150].

All ERAD pathways converge on the extraction of the ubiquitinated substrate from the ER membrane in a process mediated by the AAA protein p97 (Figure 2.4) [153]. p97 is recruited to the ER membrane by the ERAD factors UBXD2, UBXD8, and VIMP and by the Derlins-1 and -2, also involved in substrate retrotranslocation [132, 154]. p97 forms a complex with the heterodimeric substrate adaptor Ufd1-Npl4, which contains Ub-binding domains, and recognizes the polyubiquitinated ERAD substrates [153]. Once extracted, ERAD substrates must be quickly degraded to prevent hydrophobic misfolded domains exposed to the cytosol from aggregating. This is achieved through the action of the cytosolic chaperones Hsc70 and Bag6, which also assist in proteasomal targeting [155, 156]. Additionally, shuttling proteins, including ubiquilins, RAD23A, RAD23B, DNAJB2, Ubl4A, and Trc35, deliver ERAD substrates from p97 to the proteasome [132].

Viruses provide valuable examples of how to hijack the ERAD machinery for TPD. To this end, targeting newly synthesized major histocompatibility class I (MHC-I) complex for degradation to evade the immune system is a common strategy, followed by several intracellular pathogens. The human cytomegalovirus, specifically, viral protein US2 induces the degradation of MHC I via the ER-localized multi-pass TM E3 ligase Trc8 [157] and viral protein US11 by recruiting the E3 ligase TMEM129 via Derlin-1 [158]. Similarly, the human immunodeficiency virus type 1 encodes a transmembrane protein, Vpu, which is able to induce the degradation of CD4, a glycoprotein involved in antigen recognition. Vpu interacts with the cytosolic and TM domain of CD4 and at the same time recruits an atypical, cytosolic E3 ligase, SCF$\beta^{-\text{TrCP}}$ [159]. Chemical biology tools, such as PROTACs, can elicit a similar outcome. For example, ER-resident SLCs were successfully degraded using the dTAG system by hijacking the cytosolic CRBN E3 ligase [106]. It will be interesting to expand this approach to ER-resident TM E3 ligases. As an alternative to hijacking endogenous ubiquitin ligases, the mouse gammaherpesvirus 68 encodes an E3 enzyme, mK3 that is recruited to the ER membrane to ubiquitinate MHC-I [160, 161]. In turn, using viral E3 ligases for the development of PROTACs may present a strategy to specifically induce degradation of essential proteins in virus-infected cells.

Interestingly, the lumenal ERAD machinery can also be hijacked by bacterial AB toxins, such as the cholera or Shiga toxin, to achieve retrotranslocation from the ER lumen to the cytosol. Following cellular uptake and transport through the endocytic system, these toxins rely on the activity of several members of the protein disulfide isomerase family to unfold their enzymatically active subunits and the chaperone BiP to be delivered to the retrotranslocation machinery. Once in the cytosol, instead of being degraded by the proteasome, the active subunit of these toxins is released, refolds, and exerts its biological activity [162], highlighting the importance of proteasome shuttling proteins for productive ERAD. In analogy to AB toxins, TPD approaches can be designed to take advantage of the recognition machinery of physiological ERAD-L substrates to translocate proteins to the cytosol. Recruitment of ER chaperones can be controlled by the folding state of the POI. This is the rationale underlying destabilization domains and hydrophobic tagging (see also Section 2.2.1.1). In fact, hydrophobic tagging was used to generate a misfolded ER lumenal HaloTag fusion protein, which engaged the chaperone BiP and was eventually degraded by the proteasome in a p97-dependent manner [163]. This study established that chemical biology-based destabilization strategies can be used to control the levels of ER proteins. Fusion proteins with other destabilizing domains, such as DHFR- or FKBP-based domains, may also be employed to induce ERAD.

2.3.2.2 ER Lysosome-Associated Degradation (ERLAD)

In addition to ERAD, the ER has evolved mechanisms to eliminate terminally misfolded proteins, which are resistant to ERAD, by ER-to-lysosome-associated degradation (ERLAD) pathways [164] (Figure 2.4). Failure to undergo ERAD can be due to the lack of recognition by lumenal ERAD factors or by virtue of large substrate size and high propensity to form aggregates, preventing retrotranslocation to the cytosol [133]. This effect is exemplified by serpins, such as α1-antitrypsin Z (ATZ), where monomers are degraded via ERAD, but ATZ polymers or aggregates are subject to ERLAD [165]. Recent studies support a model where ERAD-resistant misfolded proteins are segregated into ER subdomains, engaged by the autophagy machinery and targeted for lysosomal degradation, in a process that involves decoration with lipidated LC3 and, in certain situations, autophagosome biogenesis [166]. Accordingly, ERLAD pathways can be categorized as autophagic and non-autophagic [166]. In the case of ATZ, calnexin segregates polymers into ER subdomains, from where they are engulfed in ER-derived vesicles by the action of the ER-phagy receptor, FAM134B (Figure 2.4). This pathway does not require autophagosome formation but instead involves the delivery of ATZ polymers via vesicular traffic to the endolysosomal system [165]. A different type of ERLAD was observed for the degradation of misfolded procollagen, which also includes calnexin and FAM134B but requires autophagosome biogenesis [167], revealing that the same ER-phagy receptor can induce distinct degradation pathways. In addition to FAM134B, the ER-phagy receptor CCPG1 was shown to protect against ER luminal protein aggregation [168]. Whether other ER-phagy receptors are also involved in ERLAD is still not clear. Given the successful hijacking of the cytosolic autophagy machinery, we anticipate that the identification and molecular characterization of additional ER-phagy receptors will eventually enable co-opting ERLAD pathways for TPD approaches. Additionally, work on ERAD pathways highlights the power of studying different types of (model) substrates in identifying molecular mechanisms of degradation pathways. Accordingly, characterizing different substrates and substrate-specific features that are engaged by the ERLAD machinery should point out opportunities for recruiting the degradation machinery to POIs.

2.3.3 Degradation from the Golgi

The Golgi apparatus is the major site for protein maturation, sorting, and transport in mammalian cells [169–172]. TM- and secreted proteins received from the ER, traverse the Golgi, acquire post-translational modifications, and are finally delivered to downstream compartments, such as the PM and the endolysosomal system. To achieve gradual modification and sorting of protein substrates, the Golgi apparatus consists of a polarized stack of membrane-enclosed compartments, the so-called cisternae, laterally linked to form the Golgi ribbon in mammalian cells [173]. This characteristic morphology is maintained by a rich matrix of structural proteins and tethers on the cytosolic face of the organelle [174, 175].

Proteins destined for degradation from the Golgi apparatus can be extracted for subsequent proteasomal degradation, transported to the lysosome, or retrieved to the ER via retrograde trafficking to eventually undergo ERAD [105].

Proteasomal degradation of matrix proteins from the cytosolic face of the Golgi was reported in the context of Golgi stress [176]. Treating cells with an ionophore, such as monensin, induces the p97-dependent extraction of matrix proteins, e.g. GM130, and subsequent proteasomal degradation, eventually leading to structural changes of the Golgi (Figure 2.5) [176]. Elements of the ubiquitination machinery that support this

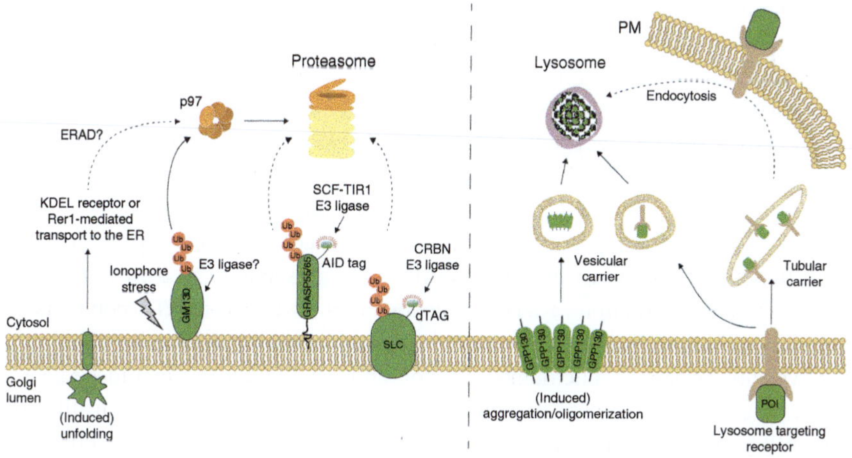

Figure 2.5 Degradation of proteins from the Golgi apparatus. Proteasomal degradation of Golgi proteins can be induced by Golgi stress and by the recruitment of ubiquitin E3 ligases through the dTAG and the auxin-inducible degron (AID) systems. Misfolded proteins are retrieved to the endoplasmic reticulum (ER) and may undergo ER-associated degradation (ERAD). Lysosomal degradation can be achieved through induction of protein aggregation or recognition by lysosomal targeting receptors. Golgi-to-lysosome transport may involve transient localization to the plasma membrane (PM) and endocytosis.

process remain yet to be identified. Cellular fractionation experiments suggest the recruitment of the proteasome to the Golgi membrane. Targeted degradation from the cytosolic face of the Golgi using the AID system demonstrated that the recruitment of soluble cytosolic E3 ligases, such as the SCF-TIR1 ligase, can be used to degrade matrix proteins and thereby regulate Golgi morphology [177]. The induced degradation of Golgi matrix proteins GRASP55-AID and GRASP65-AID not only defined their role in maintaining the Golgi ribbon structure but it also provides a tool to acutely interfere with the integrity and therefore functionality of the organelle [177]. The dTAG system, which recruits the cytosolic CRBN E3 ligase complex, also enabled the degradation of multi-pass TM Golgi-resident proteins and TM proteins that pass through the Golgi en route to the PM (Figure 2.5) [106]. Natural ubiquitin E3 ligases targeting Golgi proteins in mammalian cells remain largely elusive. Only a handful of E3 ligases were shown to localize to the Golgi apparatus (Table 2.1), with some of them showing a dynamic localization between cytosol and Golgi. Future work on defining their substrate pool and molecular details of ligase–substrate interactions is required for a better understanding of Golgi-related degradation pathways, which could help generate novel TPD strategies. In addition to proteasomal degradation from the Golgi membrane, evidence for ubiquitin-dependent lysosomal targeting comes from studies in yeast, where a TM E3 ligase complex targets orphaned protein subunits and misfolded TM proteins for degradation [178–180]. The role of mammalian homologs of the complex remains to be determined, and importantly a subunit with E3 ligase activity remains yet to be identified [178].

Studies on protein degradation from the Golgi lumen have largely focused on the mechanisms of lysosomal targeting. The Golgi apparatus interfaces with the secretory and endocytic pathways. Accordingly, the organelle is in constant flux, managing incoming and outgoing protein traffic from the ER and the endolysosomal system [169, 170]. The molecular mechanism of cargo selection and sorting at the Golgi is still subject to ongoing research [172]. To date, a few receptors that mediate transport from the Golgi to lysosomes have been characterized [22]. Two types of mannose-6-phosphate receptors (M6PR – CD-MPR and CI-MPR) bind to M6P signals on lysosomal hydrolases, escort them to the lysosome, and upon cargo release the receptors return to the Golgi. In addition to trafficking folded proteins to lysosomes, the sortilin receptor has been studied in the context of Golgi protein quality control. Similar to its yeast homolog, Vps10, sortilin is able to recognize misfolded proteins and target them for lysosomal degradation [181]. To achieve correct targeting of transport carriers, the processes of lumenal cargo sorting and the assembly of the cytosolic transport machinery, adaptor, and coat proteins, need to be coordinated [22, 182]. On the cytosolic face, the transport of CD-MPR and sortilin from the Golgi to lysosomes depends on the adaptor GGA and the clathrin coat [182]. The resultant carriers cycle between the Golgi and lysosomes, providing constant and direct access to the degradation machinery. In an approach conceptually similar to LYTACs [121], which target CI-MPR and POIs at the PM, lysosome-targeting receptors could be hijacked at the Golgi. Lysosomal targeting from the Golgi can also involve an intermediate step at the PM [22]. Tubular carriers initially transport LAMP1, a lysosomal resident protein, and the transferrin receptor to the PM [182].

Upon AP2-dependent endocytosis, they reach the lysosome [182]. In the context of TPD, proteins that only transiently reside at the PM could serve as vehicle for Golgi- or PM-to-lysosome transport. An in-depth understanding of trafficking from the Golgi (via the PM) to lysosomes would certainly give rise to ideas of how POIs can piggy-back on proteins and by extension carriers targeted to lysosomes.

The oligomerization or aggregation state of proteins has emerged as an important signal for sorting into carriers targeted from the Golgi to lysosomes. For instance, aggregation of the Golgi protease Furin leads to its lysosomal degradation [183]. The Golgi-resident protein GPP130 forms large oligomers upon binding to Mn^{2+} and is also transported to the lysosome for degradation, in a pathway that depends on sortilin [184, 185]. A similar strategy is applied by the U21 glycoprotein of the human herpesvirus-7, in which U21 clusters MHC-I molecules targeting them for lysosomal degradation to evade the immune system [186]. Notably, induced protein oligomerization using the $FKBP12^{F36M}$ domain afforded controlled lysosomal degradation of POI fusions [187]. However, this process is not dependent on the sortilin receptor [185]. While the molecular mechanism of lysosomal targeting remains elusive, $FKBP12^{F36M}$ domain fusion proteins, U21, and MHC-I are found in the same carriers [186], providing a starting point for the molecular dissection of the transport and degradation pathway. An alternative pathway for lysosomal targeting of proteins that accumulate at the Golgi, e.g. upon inhibition of secretion, is Golgi membrane-associated degradation (GOMED) [188]. Proteins such as pro-insulin (a precursor of insulin secreted by pancreatic β-cells), which en route to the PM, can be targeted for degradation in double-membrane-enclosed Golgi-derived compartments that fuse with lysosomes [188]. The detailed molecular mechanism of this clearance pathway has yet to be elucidated but was shown to be independent of the autophagy machinery, as it also proceeds in ATG5-deficient cells [188]. In addition to protein aggregation, conformation-dependent protein sorting defines a quality control checkpoint at the Golgi. To this end, misfolded proteins can be targeted from the Golgi back to the ER via chaperone interaction and the KDEL receptor or the Rer1 receptor [189–192]. By returning proteins to the ER, the Golgi leverages the extensive ER quality control network and substrates can gain access to ER degradation pathways [105]. Modulating the folding state of Golgi proteins using hydrophobic tagging or the DHFR destabilization domain induces their retrieval to the ER [193]. While these Golgi model proteins interact with ER chaperones, demonstrating their recognition as PQC substrates, further processing steps at the ER remain to be elucidated [193].

In addition to strategies that harness the active export of Golgi proteins, it may be possible to target Golgi resident proteins for degradation by counteracting their retention in the organelle. Retention of proteins in the Golgi was shown to depend, for example, on adaptor proteins, oligomerization (kin-recognition), or lipid-mediated partitioning [194]. Interfering with these molecular mechanisms could provide a means to initiate protein export. A challenge with this approach is however to ensure the correct targeting from the Golgi to lysosomes, again requiring a more detailed understanding of post-Golgi vesicular transport.

2.4 Concluding Remarks

In recent years, the development of TPD systems has attracted considerable interest for clinical application and use in cell biology research. Prime examples of successful TPD strategies are PROTACs and molecular glues, which link POIs and ubiquitin E3 ligases to induce POI ubiquitination and proteasomal degradation. POI modification with Ub can have different downstream effects, and future work unraveling the Ub code will certainly make an important contribution to modulating POI degradation and function. To further configure PROTAC- and molecular glue-based strategies, expanding the set of molecules engaging E3 ligases will be important. In addition to substrate recognition and ubiquitination, we want to stress the benefits of strategies that harness substrate processing by the proteasome or by p97 and its adaptor proteins.

A major challenge for TPD strategies remains targeting TM and secretory proteins, which are not accessible from the cytosol. These include PM proteins facing the extracellular space or TM proteins facing the lumen of membrane-enclosed organelles, such as the ER or the Golgi, locations that are not directly accessible to the major cellular degradation systems. In these cases, TPD strategies must contemplate protein internalization at PM or extraction from the membrane to the cytosol. Approaches targeting proteins for lysosomal degradation, via endocytosis (e.g. LYTACs) or autophagy (e.g. AUTACs and ATTECs), highlight the power of coopting different types of cellular degradation pathways to access "difficult protein targets" and possibly entire organelles. While accessing extracellular and PM proteins can be achieved through endocytic pathways, the TPD of ER proteins may rely on PQC mechanisms such as ERAD or ERLAD. This highlights the need for a detailed molecular understanding of ERQC mechanisms. Similarly, Golgi PQC research, which is still in its infancy, requires further study for future design of TPD. Unraveling the molecular mechanisms underlying PQC and related degradation pathways will pave the way to developing and expanding TPD strategies in this space.

Acknowledgments

We thank Hemmo Meyer, Mariell Pettersson, and Stacey Paiva for critical reading of the manuscript. This work was funded by the Deutsche Forschungsgemeinschaft (DFG, German Research Foundation) – SFB1430 – Project-ID 424228829 and the Sofja Kovaleveskaja Award by the Alexander von Humboldt Foundation.

References

1 Cohen-Kaplan, V., Livneh, I., Avni, N. et al. (2016). The ubiquitin-proteasome system and autophagy: coordinated and independent activities. *Int. J. Biochem. Cell Biol.* 79: 403–418.

2 Harper, J.W. and Bennett, E.J. (2016). Proteome complexity and the forces that drive proteome imbalance. *Nature* 537 (7620): 328–338.
3 Bard, J.A.M., Goodall, E.A., Greene, E.R. et al. (2018). Structure and function of the 26S proteasome. *Annu. Rev. Biochem.* 87: 697–724.
4 Schulman, B.A. and Harper, J.W. (2009). Ubiquitin-like protein activation by E1 enzymes: the apex for downstream signalling pathways. *Nat. Rev. Mol. Cell Biol.* 10 (5): 319–331.
5 Ye, Y. and Rape, M. (2009). Building ubiquitin chains: E2 enzymes at work. *Nat. Rev. Mol. Cell Biol.* 10 (11): 755–764.
6 Berndsen, C.E. and Wolberger, C. (2014). New insights into ubiquitin E3 ligase mechanism. *Nat. Struct. Mol. Biol.* 21 (4): 301–307.
7 Morreale, F.E. and Walden, H. (2016). Types of ubiquitin ligases. *Cell* 165 (1): 248–e1.
8 Zheng, N. and Shabek, N. (2017). Ubiquitin ligases: structure, function, and regulation. *Annu. Rev. Biochem.* 86: 129–157.
9 Clague, M.J., Urbe, S., and Komander, D. (2019). Breaking the chains: deubiquitylating enzyme specificity begets function. *Nat. Rev. Mol. Cell Biol.* 20 (6): 338–352.
10 Komander, D. and Rape, M. (2012). The ubiquitin code. *Annu. Rev. Biochem.* 81: 203–229.
11 Chen, X., Htet, Z.M., Lopez-Alfonzo, E. et al. (2021). Proteasome interaction with ubiquitinated substrates: from mechanisms to therapies. *FEBS J.* 288 (18): 5231–5251.
12 Meyer, H., Bug, M., and Bremer, S. (2012). Emerging functions of the VCP/p97 AAA-ATPase in the ubiquitin system. *Nat. Cell Biol.* 14 (2): 117–123.
13 Stolz, A., Hilt, W., Buchberger, A., and Wolf, D.H. (2011). Cdc48: a power machine in protein degradation. *Trends Biochem. Sci.* 36 (10): 515–523.
14 Nakatogawa, H., Suzuki, K., Kamada, Y., and Ohsumi, Y. (2009). Dynamics and diversity in autophagy mechanisms: lessons from yeast. *Nat. Rev. Mol. Cell Biol.* 10 (7): 458–467.
15 Soreng, K., Neufeld, T.P., and Simonsen, A. (2018). Membrane trafficking in autophagy. *Int. Rev. Cell Mol. Biol.* 336: 1–92.
16 Gubas, A. and Dikic, I. (2021). A guide to the regulation of selective autophagy receptors. *FEBS J.* 289 (1): 75–89.
17 Stolz, A., Ernst, A., and Dikic, I. (2014). Cargo recognition and trafficking in selective autophagy. *Nat. Cell Biol.* 16 (6): 495–501.
18 Kirkin, V. (2020). History of the selective autophagy research: how did it begin and where does it stand today? *J. Mol. Biol.* 432 (1): 3–27.
19 MacGurn, J.A., Hsu, P.C., and Emr, S.D. (2012). Ubiquitin and membrane protein turnover: from cradle to grave. *Annu. Rev. Biochem.* 81: 231–259.
20 Henne, W.M., Buchkovich, N.J., and Emr, S.D. (2011). The ESCRT pathway. *Dev. Cell* 21 (1): 77–91.
21 Migliano, S.M. and Teis, D. (2018). ESCRT and membrane protein ubiquitination. *Prog. Mol. Subcell. Biol.* 57: 107–135.

22 Braulke, T. and Bonifacino, J.S. (2009). Sorting of lysosomal proteins. *Biochim. Biophys. Acta* 1793 (4): 605–614.

23 Nakamura, S. and Yoshimori, T. (2017). New insights into autophagosome-lysosome fusion. *J. Cell Sci.* 130 (7): 1209–1216.

24 Kaushik, S. and Cuervo, A.M. (2012). Chaperone-mediated autophagy: a unique way to enter the lysosome world. *Trends Cell Biol.* 22 (8): 407–417.

25 Hipp, M.S., Kasturi, P., and Hartl, F.U. (2019). The proteostasis network and its decline in ageing. *Nat. Rev. Mol. Cell Biol.* 20 (7): 421–435.

26 Valastyan, J.S. and Lindquist, S. (2014). Mechanisms of protein-folding diseases at a glance. *Dis. Model. Mech.* 7 (1): 9–14.

27 Mullard, A. (2021). Targeted protein degraders crowd into the clinic. *Nat. Rev. Drug Discov.* 20 (4): 247–250.

28 Pettersson, M. and Crews, C.M. (2019). PROteolysis TArgeting chimeras (PROTACs) - past, present and future. *Drug Discov. Today Technol.* 31: 15–27.

29 Cromm, P.M., Crews, C.M., and Weinmann, H. (2020). *Chapter 1 PROTAC-mediated Target Degradation: A Paradigm Changer in Drug Discovery? Protein Degradation with New Chemical Modalities: Successful Strategies in Drug Discovery and Chemical Biology*, 1–13. The Royal Society of Chemistry.

30 Nabet, B., Roberts, J.M., Buckley, D.L. et al. (2018). The dTAG system for immediate and target-specific protein degradation. *Nat. Chem. Biol.* 14 (5): 431–441.

31 Buckley, D.L., Raina, K., Darricarrere, N. et al. (2015). HaloPROTACS: use of small molecule PROTACs to induce degradation of HaloTag fusion proteins. *ACS Chem. Biol.* 10 (8): 1831–1837.

32 Neklesa, T.K., Tae, H.S., Schneekloth, A.R. et al. (2011). Small-molecule hydrophobic tagging-induced degradation of HaloTag fusion proteins. *Nat. Chem. Biol.* 7 (8): 538–543.

33 Winter, G.E., Buckley, D.L., Paulk, J. et al. (2015). Phthalimide conjugation as a strategy for *in vivo* target protein degradation. *Science* 348 (6241): 1376–1381.

34 Nishimura, K., Fukagawa, T., Takisawa, H. et al. (2009). An auxin-based degron system for the rapid depletion of proteins in nonplant cells. *Nat. Methods* 6 (12): 917–922.

35 Yesbolatova, A., Saito, Y., Kitamoto, N. et al. (2020). The auxin-inducible degron 2 technology provides sharp degradation control in yeast, mammalian cells, and mice. *Nat. Commun.* 11 (1): 5701.

36 Bond, A.G., Craigon, C., Chan, K.H. et al. (2021). Development of BromoTag: a "bump-and-hole"-PROTAC system to induce potent, rapid, and selective degradation of tagged target proteins. *J. Med. Chem.* 64 (20): 15477–15502.

37 C4Therapeutics-team. Development of AchillesTAGdegradation systems and their application to control CAR-T activity 2021. Available from: http://c4therapeutics.com/wp-content/uploads/2020/07/aTAG-Poster.pdf.

38 Faust, T.B., Donovan, K.A., Yue, H. et al. (2021). Small-molecule approaches to targeted protein degradation. *Ann. Rev. Cancer Biol.* 5 (1): 181–201.

39 Burslem, G.M. and Crews, C.M. (2017). Small-molecule modulation of protein homeostasis. *Chem. Rev.* 117 (17): 11269–11301.

40 Kim, Y.E., Hipp, M.S., Bracher, A. et al. (2013). Molecular chaperone functions in protein folding and proteostasis. *Annu. Rev. Biochem.* 82: 323–355.

41 Arndt, V., Rogon, C., and Hohfeld, J. (2007). To be, or not to be–molecular chaperones in protein degradation. *Cell. Mol. Life Sci.* 64 (19–20): 2525–2541.

42 Murata, S., Minami, Y., Minami, M. et al. (2001). CHIP is a chaperone-dependent E3 ligase that ubiquitylates unfolded protein. *EMBO Rep.* 2 (12): 1133–1138.

43 Connell, P., Ballinger, C.A., Jiang, J. et al. (2001). The co-chaperone CHIP regulates protein triage decisions mediated by heat-shock proteins. *Nat. Cell Biol.* 3 (1): 93–96.

44 Hellerschmied, D., Roessler, M., Lehner, A. et al. (2018). UFD-2 is an adaptor-assisted E3 ligase targeting unfolded proteins. *Nat. Commun.* 9 (1): 484.

45 Patel, P.D., Yan, P., Seidler, P.M. et al. (2013). Paralog-selective Hsp90 inhibitors define tumor-specific regulation of HER2. *Nat. Chem. Biol.* 9 (11): 677–684.

46 Zavareh, R.B., Spangenberg, S.H., Woods, A. et al. (2021). HSP90 inhibition enhances cancer immunotherapy by modulating the surface expression of multiple immune checkpoint proteins. *Cell. Chem. Biol.* 28 (2): 158–68 e5.

47 Sebastian, R.M. and Shoulders, M.D. (2020). Chemical biology framework to illuminate proteostasis. *Annu. Rev. Biochem.* 89: 529–555.

48 Iwamoto, M., Bjorklund, T., Lundberg, C. et al. (2010). A general chemical method to regulate protein stability in the mammalian central nervous system. *Chem. Biol.* 17 (9): 981–988.

49 Banaszynski, L.A., Chen, L.C., Maynard-Smith, L.A. et al. (2006). A rapid, reversible, and tunable method to regulate protein function in living cells using synthetic small molecules. *Cell* 126 (5): 995–1004.

50 Egeler, E.L., Urner, L.M., Rakhit, R. et al. (2011). Ligand-switchable substrates for a ubiquitin-proteasome system. *J. Biol. Chem.* 286 (36): 31328–31336.

51 Tae, H.S., Sundberg, T.B., Neklesa, T.K. et al. (2012). Identification of hydrophobic tags for the degradation of stabilized proteins. *Chembiochem* 13 (4): 538–541.

52 Neklesa, T.K., Noblin, D.J., Kuzin, A.P. et al. (2013). A bidirectional system for the dynamic small molecule control of intracellular fusion proteins. *ACS Chem. Biol.* 8 (10): 2293–2300.

53 Patel, H.K. and Bihani, T. (2018). Selective estrogen receptor modulators (SERMs) and selective estrogen receptor degraders (SERDs) in cancer treatment. *Pharmacol. Ther.* 186: 1–24.

54 Varshavsky, A. (2019). N-degron and C-degron pathways of protein degradation. *Proc. Natl. Acad. Sci. U. S. A.* 116 (2): 358–366.

55 Piatkov, K.I., Oh, J.H., Liu, Y., and Varshavsky, A. (2014). Calpain-generated natural protein fragments as short-lived substrates of the N-end rule pathway. *Proc. Natl. Acad. Sci. U. S. A.* 111 (9): E817–E826.

56 Piatkov, K.I., Brower, C.S., and Varshavsky, A. (2012). The N-end rule pathway counteracts cell death by destroying proapoptotic protein fragments. *Proc. Natl. Acad. Sci. U. S. A.* 109 (27): E1839–E1847.

57 Mena, E.L., Jevtic, P., Greber, B.J. et al. (2020). Structural basis for dimerization quality control. *Nature* 586 (7829): 452–456.

58 Koren, I., Timms, R.T., Kula, T. et al. (2018). The eukaryotic proteome is shaped by E3 ubiquitin ligases targeting C-terminal degrons. *Cell* 173 (7): 1622–35 e14.

59 Lin, H.C., Yeh, C.W., Chen, Y.F. et al. (2018). C-terminal end-directed protein elimination by CRL2 ubiquitin ligases. *Mol. Cell* 70 (4): 602–13 e3.

60 Bonger, K.M., Chen, L.C., Liu, C.W., and Wandless, T.J. (2011). Small-molecule displacement of a cryptic degron causes conditional protein degradation. *Nat. Chem. Biol.* 7 (8): 531–537.

61 Chung, H.K., Jacobs, C.L., Huo, Y. et al. (2015). Tunable and reversible drug control of protein production via a self-excising degron. *Nat. Chem. Biol.* 11 (9): 713–720.

62 Ang, X.L. and Wade, H.J. (2005). SCF-mediated protein degradation and cell cycle control. *Oncogene* 24 (17): 2860–2870.

63 Bassermann, F., Eichner, R., and Pagano, M. (2014). The ubiquitin proteasome system - implications for cell cycle control and the targeted treatment of cancer. *Biochim. Biophys. Acta* 1843 (1): 150–162.

64 Siriwardena, S.U., Munkanatta Godage, D.N.P., Shoba, V.M. et al. (2020). Phosphorylation-inducing chimeric small molecules. *J. Am. Chem. Soc.* 142 (33): 14052–14057.

65 Chen, P.H., Hu, Z., An, E. et al. (2021). Modulation of phosphoprotein activity by phosphorylation targeting chimeras (PhosTACs). *ACS Chem. Biol.*

66 Harper, J.W. and Schulman, B.A. (2021). Cullin-RING ubiquitin ligase regulatory circuits: a quarter century beyond the F-box hypothesis. *Annu. Rev. Biochem.* 90: 403–429.

67 Kozicka, Z. and Thoma, N.H. (2021). Haven't got a glue: protein surface variation for the design of molecular glue degraders. *Cell Chem. Biol.* 28 (7): 1032–1047.

68 Coleman, K.G. and Crews, C.M. (2018). Proteolysis-targeting chimeras: harnessing the ubiquitin-proteasome system to induce degradation of specific target proteins. *Ann. Rev. Cancer Biol.* 2 (1): 41–58.

69 Ishida, T. and Ciulli, A. (2021). E3 ligase ligands for PROTACs: how they were found and how to discover new ones. *SLAS Discov.* 26 (4): 484–502.

70 Buckley, D.L., Gustafson, J.L., Van Molle, I. et al. (2012). Small-molecule inhibitors of the interaction between the E3 ligase VHL and HIF1alpha. *Angew. Chem. Int. Ed. Engl.* 51 (46): 11463–11467.

71 Buckley, D.L., Van Molle, I., Gareiss, P.C. et al. (2012). Targeting the von Hippel-Lindau E3 ubiquitin ligase using small molecules to disrupt the VHL/HIF-1alpha interaction. *J. Am. Chem. Soc.* 134 (10): 4465–4468.

72 Min, J.H., Yang, H., Ivan, M. et al. (2002). Structure of an HIF-1alpha -pVHL complex: hydroxyproline recognition in signaling. *Science* 296 (5574): 1886–1889.

73 Naito, M., Ohoka, N., Shibata, N., and Tsukumo, Y. (2019). Targeted protein degradation by chimeric small molecules, PROTACs and SNIPERs. *Front. Chem.* 7: 849.

74 Ito, T., Yamaguchi, Y., and Handa, H. (2021). Exploiting ubiquitin ligase cereblon as a target for small-molecule compounds in medicine and chemical biology. *Cell Chem. Biol.* 28 (7): 987–999.

75 Jevtic, P., Haakonsen, D.L., and Rape, M. (2021). An E3 ligase guide to the galaxy of small-molecule-induced protein degradation. *Cell Chem. Biol.* 28 (7): 1000–1013.

76 Kannt, A. and Dikic, I. (2021). Expanding the arsenal of E3 ubiquitin ligases for proximity-induced protein degradation. *Cell Chem. Biol.* 28 (7): 1014–1031.

77 Lai, A.C., Toure, M., Hellerschmied, D. et al. (2016). Modular PROTAC design for the degradation of oncogenic BCR-ABL. *Angew. Chem. Int. Ed. Engl.* 55 (2): 807–810.

78 Ottis, P., Toure, M., Cromm, P.M. et al. (2017). Assessing different E3 ligases for small molecule induced protein ubiquitination and degradation. *ACS Chem. Biol.* 12 (10): 2570–2578.

79 Bondeson, D.P., Smith, B.E., Burslem, G.M. et al. (2018). Lessons in PROTAC design from selective degradation with a promiscuous warhead. *Cell. Chem. Biol.* 25 (1): 78–87 e5.

80 Tan, X., Calderon-Villalobos, L.I., Sharon, M. et al. (2007). Mechanism of auxin perception by the TIR1 ubiquitin ligase. *Nature* 446 (7136): 640–645.

81 Ito, T., Ando, H., Suzuki, T. et al. (2010). Identification of a primary target of thalidomide teratogenicity. *Science* 327 (5971): 1345–1350.

82 Bussiere, D.E., Xie, L., Srinivas, H. et al. (2020). Structural basis of indisulam-mediated RBM39 recruitment to DCAF15 E3 ligase complex. *Nat. Chem. Biol.* 16 (1): 15–23.

83 Faust, T.B., Yoon, H., Nowak, R.P. et al. (2020). Structural complementarity facilitates E7820-mediated degradation of RBM39 by DCAF15. *Nat. Chem. Biol.* 16 (1): 7–14.

84 Mayor-Ruiz, C., Bauer, S., Brand, M. et al. (2020). Rational discovery of molecular glue degraders via scalable chemical profiling. *Nat. Chem. Biol.* 16 (11): 1199–1207.

85 Livneh, I., Cohen-Kaplan, V., Cohen-Rosenzweig, C. et al. (2016). The life cycle of the 26S proteasome: from birth, through regulation and function, and onto its death. *Cell Res.* 26 (8): 869–885.

86 Kracht, M., van den Boom, J., Seiler, J. et al. (2020). Protein phosphatase-1 complex disassembly by p97 is initiated through multivalent recognition of catalytic and regulatory subunits by the p97 SEP-domain adapters. *J. Mol. Biol.* 432 (23): 6061–6074.

87 Weith, M., Seiler, J., van den Boom, J. et al. (2018). Ubiquitin-independent disassembly by a p97 AAA-ATPase complex drives PP1 holoenzyme formation. *Mol. Cell* 72 (4): 766–77 e6.

88 Wilmington, S.R. and Matouschek, A. (2016). An inducible system for rapid degradation of specific cellular proteins using proteasome adaptors. *PLoS One* 11 (4): e0152679.

89 Imanishi S, Huang L, Itakura S, Ishizaka M, Tsukamoto M, Saito M, et al. (2021) *in vivo* KRAS G12D/V Degradation Mediated by CANDDY Using a Modified Proteasome Inhibitor. bioRxiv. 2021, https://doi.org/10.1101/2021.04.23.441075.

90 Fan, X., Jin, W.Y., Lu, J. et al. (2014). Rapid and reversible knockdown of endogenous proteins by peptide-directed lysosomal degradation. *Nat. Neurosci.* 17 (3): 471–480.

91 Bauer, P.O., Goswami, A., Wong, H.K. et al. (2010). Harnessing chaperone-mediated autophagy for the selective degradation of mutant huntingtin protein. *Nat. Biotechnol.* 28 (3): 256–263.

92 Takahashi, D., Moriyama, J., Nakamura, T. et al. (2019). AUTACs: cargo-specific degraders using selective autophagy. *Mol. Cell* 76 (5): 797–810 e10.

93 Takahashi, D. and Arimoto, H. (2021). Selective autophagy as the basis of autophagy-based degraders. *Cell Chem. Biol.* 28 (7): 1061–1071.

94 Li, Z., Wang, C., Wang, Z. et al. (2019). Allele-selective lowering of mutant HTT protein by HTT-LC3 linker compounds. *Nature* 575 (7781): 203–209.

95 Li, Z., Zhu, C., Ding, Y. et al. (2020). ATTEC: a potential new approach to target proteinopathies. *Autophagy* 16 (1): 185–187.

96 Loos, F., Xie, W., Sica, V. et al. (2019). Artificial tethering of LC3 or p62 to organelles is not sufficient to trigger autophagy. *Cell Death Dis.* 10 (10): 771.

97 Papadopoulos, C. and Meyer, H. (2017). Detection and clearance of damaged lysosomes by the endo-lysosomal damage response and lysophagy. *Curr. Biol.* 27 (24): R1330–R1341.

98 Harper, J.W., Ordureau, A., and Heo, J.M. (2018). Building and decoding ubiquitin chains for mitophagy. *Nat. Rev. Mol. Cell Biol.* 19 (2): 93–108.

99 Chauhan, S., Kumar, S., Jain, A. et al. (2016). TRIMs and galectins globally cooperate and TRIM16 and galectin-3 co-direct autophagy in endomembrane damage homeostasis. *Dev. Cell* 39 (1): 13–27.

100 Thurston, T.L., Wandel, M.P., von Muhlinen, N. et al. (2012). Galectin 8 targets damaged vesicles for autophagy to defend cells against bacterial invasion. *Nature* 482 (7385): 414–418.

101 Wei, Y., Chiang, W.C., Sumpter, R. Jr. et al. (2017). Prohibitin 2 is an inner mitochondrial membrane mitophagy receptor. *Cell* 168 (1–2): 224–38 e10.

102 Lazarou, M., Sliter, D.A., Kane, L.A. et al. (2015). The ubiquitin kinase PINK1 recruits autophagy receptors to induce mitophagy. *Nature* 524 (7565): 309–314.

103 Di Fiore, P.P. and von Zastrow, M. (2014). Endocytosis, signaling, and beyond. *Cold Spring Harb. Perspect. Biol.* 6 (8): a016865.

104 Ahn, G., Banik, S.M., and Bertozzi, C.R. (2021). Degradation from the outside in: targeting extracellular and membrane proteins for degradation through the endolysosomal pathway. *Cell Chem. Biol.* 28 (7): 1072–1080.

105 Sun, Z. and Brodsky, J.L. (2019). Protein quality control in the secretory pathway. *J. Cell Biol.* 218 (10): 3171–3187.

106 Bensimon, A., Pizzagalli, M.D., Kartnig, F. et al. (2020). Targeted degradation of SLC transporters reveals amenability of multi-pass transmembrane proteins to ligand-induced proteolysis. *Cell. Chem. Biol.* 27 (6): 728–39 e9.

107 Burslem, G.M., Smith, B.E., Lai, A.C. et al. (2018). The advantages of targeted protein degradation over inhibition: an RTK case study. *Cell. Chem. Biol.* 25 (1): 67–77 e3.

108 Xie, T., Lim, S.M., Westover, K.D. et al. (2014). Pharmacological targeting of the pseudokinase Her3. *Nat. Chem. Biol.* 10 (12): 1006–1012.

109 Robinson, M.S. (2015). Forty years of clathrin-coated vesicles. *Traffic* 16 (12): 1210–1238.

110 Muriel, O., Sanchez-Alvarez, M., Strippoli, R., and Del Pozo, M.A. (2018). Role of the endocytosis of caveolae in intracellular signaling and metabolism. *Prog. Mol. Subcell. Biol.* 57: 203–234.

111 Mayor, S. and Pagano, R.E. (2007). Pathways of clathrin-independent endocytosis. *Nat. Rev. Mol. Cell Biol.* 8 (8): 603–612.

112 Mosesson, Y., Mills, G.B., and Yarden, Y. (2008). Derailed endocytosis: an emerging feature of cancer. *Nat. Rev. Cancer* 8 (11): 835–850.

113 Wood, L.A., Larocque, G., Clarke, N.I. et al. (2017). New tools for "hot-wiring" clathrin-mediated endocytosis with temporal and spatial precision. *J. Cell Biol.* 216 (12): 4351–4365.

114 Raiborg, C. and Stenmark, H. (2009). The ESCRT machinery in endosomal sorting of ubiquitylated membrane proteins. *Nature* 458 (7237): 445–452.

115 Roopenian, D.C. and Akilesh, S. (2007). FcRn: the neonatal Fc receptor comes of age. *Nat. Rev. Immunol.* 7 (9): 715–725.

116 Vaccaro, C., Zhou, J., Ober, R.J., and Ward, E.S. (2005). Engineering the Fc region of immunoglobulin G to modulate *in vivo* antibody levels. *Nat. Biotechnol.* 23 (10): 1283–1288.

117 Devanaboyina, S.C., Khare, P., Challa, D.K. et al. (2017). Engineered clearing agents for the selective depletion of antigen-specific antibodies. *Nat. Commun.* 8: 15314.

118 Gan, Z., Ram, S., Vaccaro, C. et al. (2009). Analyses of the recycling receptor, FcRn, in live cells reveal novel pathways for lysosomal delivery. *Traffic* 10 (5): 600–614.

119 Igawa, T., Ishii, S., Tachibana, T. et al. (2010). Antibody recycling by engineered pH-dependent antigen binding improves the duration of antigen neutralization. *Nat. Biotechnol.* 28 (11): 1203–1207.

120 Ahn, G., Banik, S.M., Miller, C.L. et al. (2021). LYTACs that engage the asialoglycoprotein receptor for targeted protein degradation. *Nat. Chem. Biol.* 17 (9): 937–946.

121 Banik, S.M., Pedram, K., Wisnovsky, S. et al. (2020). Lysosome-targeting chimaeras for degradation of extracellular proteins. *Nature* 584 (7820): 291–297.

122 Caianiello, D.F., Zhang, M., Ray, J.D. et al. (2021). Bifunctional small molecules that mediate the degradation of extracellular proteins. *Nat. Chem. Biol.* 17 (9): 947–953.

123 Zhou, Y., Teng, P., Montgomery, N.T. et al. (2021). Development of triantennary N-acetylgalactosamine conjugates as degraders for extracellular proteins. *ACS Cent. Sci.* 7 (3): 499–506.

124 Sardana, R. and Emr, S.D. (2021). Membrane protein quality control mechanisms in the endo-lysosome system. *Trends Cell Biol.* 31 (4): 269–283.

125 Caldieri, G., Malabarba, M.G., Di Fiore, P.P., and Sigismund, S. (2018). EGFR trafficking in physiology and cancer. *Prog. Mol. Subcell. Biol.* 57: 235–272.

126 Kopp, Y., Lang, W.H., Schuster, T.B. et al. (2017). CHIP as a membrane-shuttling proteostasis sensor. *eLife* 6.

127 Babst, M. (2014). Quality control: quality control at the plasma membrane: one mechanism does not fit all. *J. Cell Biol.* 205 (1): 11–20.

128 Koo, B.K., Spit, M., Jordens, I. et al. (2012). Tumour suppressor RNF43 is a stem-cell E3 ligase that induces endocytosis of Wnt receptors. *Nature* 488 (7413): 665–669.

129 Cotton, A.D., Nguyen, D.P., Gramespacher, J.A. et al. (2021). Development of antibody-based PROTACs for the degradation of the cell-surface immune checkpoint protein PD-L1. *J. Am. Chem. Soc.* 143 (2): 593–598.

130 Schwarz, D.S. and Blower, M.D. (2016). The endoplasmic reticulum: structure, function and response to cellular signaling. *Cell. Mol. Life Sci.* 73 (1): 79–94.

131 Phillips, B.P., Gomez-Navarro, N., and Miller, E.A. (2020). Protein quality control in the endoplasmic reticulum. *Curr. Opin. Cell Biol.* 65: 96–102.

132 Christianson, J.C. and Ye, Y. (2014). Cleaning up in the endoplasmic reticulum: ubiquitin in charge. *Nat. Struct. Mol. Biol.* 21 (4): 325–335.

133 Fregno, I. and Molinari, M. (2019). Proteasomal and lysosomal clearance of faulty secretory proteins: ER-associated degradation (ERAD) and ER-to-lysosome-associated degradation (ERLAD) pathways. *Crit. Rev. Biochem. Mol. Biol.* 54 (2): 153–163.

134 Carvalho, P., Goder, V., and Rapoport, T.A. (2006). Distinct ubiquitin-ligase complexes define convergent pathways for the degradation of ER proteins. *Cell* 126 (2): 361–373.

135 Carvalho, P., Stanley, A.M., and Rapoport, T.A. (2010). Retrotranslocation of a misfolded luminal ER protein by the ubiquitin-ligase Hrd1p. *Cell* 143 (4): 579–591.

136 Huyer, G., Piluek, W.F., Fansler, Z. et al. (2004). Distinct machinery is required in Saccharomyces cerevisiae for the endoplasmic reticulum-associated degradation of a multispanning membrane protein and a soluble luminal protein. *J. Biol. Chem.* 279 (37): 38369–38378.

137 Vashist, S. and Ng, D.T. (2004). Misfolded proteins are sorted by a sequential checkpoint mechanism of ER quality control. *J. Cell Biol.* 165 (1): 41–52.

138 Kaneko, M., Iwase, I., Yamasaki, Y. et al. (2016). Genome-wide identification and gene expression profiling of ubiquitin ligases for endoplasmic reticulum protein degradation. *Sci. Rep.* 6: 30955.

139 Schoebel, S., Mi, W., Stein, A. et al. (2017). Cryo-EM structure of the protein-conducting ERAD channel Hrd1 in complex with Hrd3. *Nature* 548 (7667): 352–355.

140 Biederer, T., Volkwein, C., and Sommer, T. (1997). Role of Cue1p in ubiquitination and degradation at the ER surface. *Science* 278 (5344): 1806–1809.

141 Araki, K. and Nagata, K. (2011). Protein folding and quality control in the ER. *Cold Spring Harb. Perspect. Biol.* 3 (11): a007526.

142 Shenkman, M., Groisman, B., Ron, E. et al. (2013). A shared endoplasmic reticulum-associated degradation pathway involving the EDEM1 protein for glycosylated and nonglycosylated proteins. *J. Biol. Chem.* 288 (4): 2167–2178.

143 van der Goot, A.T., Pearce, M.M.P., Leto, D.E. et al. (2018). Redundant and antagonistic roles of XTP3B and OS9 in decoding glycan and non-glycan degrons in ER-associated degradation. *Mol. Cell* 70 (3): 516–30 e6.

144 Satoh, T., Chen, Y., Hu, D. et al. (2010). Structural basis for oligosaccharide recognition of misfolded glycoproteins by OS-9 in ER-associated degradation. *Mol. Cell* 40 (6): 905–916.

145 Pobre, K.F.R., Poet, G.J., and Hendershot, L.M. (2019). The endoplasmic reticulum (ER) chaperone BiP is a master regulator of ER functions: getting by with a little help from ERdj friends. *J. Biol. Chem.* 294 (6): 2098–2108.

146 Ushioda, R., Hoseki, J., Araki, K. et al. (2008). ERdj5 is required as a disulfide reductase for degradation of misfolded proteins in the ER. *Science* 321 (5888): 569–572.

147 Vecchi, L., Petris, G., Bestagno, M., and Burrone, O.R. (2012). Selective targeting of proteins within secretory pathway for endoplasmic reticulum-associated degradation. *J. Biol. Chem.* 287 (24): 20007–20015.

148 Wu, X., Siggel, M., Ovchinnikov, S. et al. (2020). Structural basis of ER-associated protein degradation mediated by the Hrd1 ubiquitin ligase complex. *Science* 368 (6489): eaaz2449.

149 Mehrtash, A.B. and Hochstrasser, M. (2019). Ubiquitin-dependent protein degradation at the endoplasmic reticulum and nuclear envelope. *Semin. Cell Dev. Biol.* 93: 111–124.

150 Neal, S., Jaeger, P.A., Duttke, S.H. et al. (2018). The Dfm1 derlin is required for ERAD retrotranslocation of integral membrane proteins. *Mol. Cell* 69 (2): 306–20 e4.

151 Fonseca D, Carvalho P (2020). The derlin Dfm1 promotes retrotranslocation of folded protein domains from the endoplasmic reticulum. bioRxiv 2020, https://doi.org/10.1101/2020.06.02.131128.

152 Zattas, D., Berk, J.M., Kreft, S.G., and Hochstrasser, M. (2016). A conserved C-terminal element in the yeast Doa10 and human MARCH6 ubiquitin ligases required for selective substrate degradation. *J. Biol. Chem.* 291 (23): 12105–12118.

153 Ye, Y., Meyer, H.H., and Rapoport, T.A. (2001). The AAA ATPase Cdc48/p97 and its partners transport proteins from the ER into the cytosol. *Nature* 414 (6864): 652–656.

154 Lemberg, M.K. and Strisovsky, K. (2021). Maintenance of organellar protein homeostasis by ER-associated degradation and related mechanisms. *Mol. Cell* 81 (12): 2507–2519.

155 Claessen, J.H., Sanyal, S., and Ploegh, H.L. (2014). The chaperone BAG6 captures dislocated glycoproteins in the cytosol. *PLoS One* 9 (3): e90204.

156 Matsumura, Y., David, L.L., and Skach, W.R. (2011). Role of Hsc70 binding cycle in CFTR folding and endoplasmic reticulum-associated degradation. *Mol. Biol. Cell* 22 (16): 2797–2809.

157 Stagg, H.R., Thomas, M., van den Boomen, D. et al. (2009). The TRC8 E3 ligase ubiquitinates MHC class I molecules before dislocation from the ER. *J. Cell Biol.* 186 (5): 685–692.

158 van den Boomen, D.J., Timms, R.T., Grice, G.L. et al. (2014). TMEM129 is a Derlin-1 associated ERAD E3 ligase essential for virus-induced degradation of MHC-I. *Proc. Natl. Acad. Sci. U. S. A.* 111 (31): 11425–11430.

159 Magadan, J.G., Perez-Victoria, F.J., Sougrat, R. et al. (2010). Multilayered mechanism of CD4 downregulation by HIV-1 Vpu involving distinct ER retention and ERAD targeting steps. *PLoS Pathog.* 6 (4): e1000869.

160 Boname, J.M. and Stevenson, P.G. (2001). MHC class I ubiquitination by a viral PHD/LAP finger protein. *Immunity* 15 (4): 627–636.

161 Wang, X., Herr, R.A., Chua, W.J. et al. (2007). Ubiquitination of serine, threonine, or lysine residues on the cytoplasmic tail can induce ERAD of MHC-I by viral E3 ligase mK3. *J. Cell Biol.* 177 (4): 613–624.

162 Nowakowska-Golacka, J., Sominka, H., Sowa-Rogozinska, N., and Slominska-Wojewodzka, M. (2019). Toxins utilize the endoplasmic reticulum-associated protein degradation pathway in their intoxication process. *Int. J. Mol. Sci.* 20 (6): 1307.

163 Raina, K., Noblin, D.J., Serebrenik, Y.V. et al. (2014). Targeted protein destabilization reveals an estrogen-mediated ER stress response. *Nat. Chem. Biol.* 10 (11): 957–962.

164 Oikonomou, C. and Hendershot, L.M. (2020). Disposing of misfolded ER proteins: a troubled substrate's way out of the ER. *Mol. Cell. Endocrinol.* 500: 110630.

165 Fregno, I., Fasana, E., Bergmann, T.J. et al. (2018). ER-to-lysosome-associated degradation of proteasome-resistant ATZ polymers occurs via receptor-mediated vesicular transport. *EMBO J.* 37 (17): e99259.

166 Molinari, M. (2021). ER-phagy responses in yeast, plants, and mammalian cells and their crosstalk with UPR and ERAD. *Dev. Cell* 56 (7): 949–966.

167 Forrester, A., De Leonibus, C., Grumati, P. et al. (2019). A selective ER-phagy exerts procollagen quality control via a Calnexin-FAM134B complex. *EMBO J.* 38 (2): e99847.

168 Smith, M.D., Harley, M.E., Kemp, A.J. et al. (2018). CCPG1 is a non-canonical autophagy cargo receptor essential for ER-phagy and pancreatic ER proteostasis. *Dev. Cell* 44 (2): 217–32 e11.

169 Progida, C. and Bakke, O. (2016). Bidirectional traffic between the Golgi and the endosomes - machineries and regulation. *J. Cell Sci.* 129 (21): 3971–3982.

170 Barlowe, C.K. and Miller, E.A. (2013). Secretory protein biogenesis and traffic in the early secretory pathway. *Genetics* 193 (2): 383–410.

171 Moremen, K.W., Tiemeyer, M., and Nairn, A.V. (2012). Vertebrate protein glycosylation: diversity, synthesis and function. *Nat. Rev. Mol. Cell Biol.* 13 (7): 448–462.

172 Ramazanov, B.R., Tran, M.L., and von Blume, J. (2021). Sending out molecules from the TGN. *Curr. Opin. Cell Biol.* 71: 55–62.

173 Klumperman, J. (2011). Architecture of the mammalian Golgi. *Cold Spring Harb. Perspect. Biol.* 3 (7): a005181.

174 Gillingham, A.K. and Munro, S. (2003). Long coiled-coil proteins and membrane traffic. *Biochim. Biophys. Acta* 1641 (2–3): 71–85.

175 Zhang, X. and Wang, Y. (2020). Nonredundant roles of GRASP55 and GRASP65 in the Golgi apparatus and beyond. *Trends Biochem. Sci.* 45 (12): 1065–1079.

176 Eisenberg-Lerner, A., Benyair, R., Hizkiahou, N. et al. (2020). Golgi organization is regulated by proteasomal degradation. *Nat. Commun.* 11 (1): 409.

177 Zhang, Y. and Seemann, J. (2021). Rapid degradation of GRASP55 and GRASP65 reveals their immediate impact on the Golgi structure. *J. Cell Biol.* 220 (1).

178 Schmidt, O., Weyer, Y., Baumann, V. et al. (2019). Endosome and Golgi-associated degradation (EGAD) of membrane proteins regulates sphingolipid metabolism. *EMBO J.* 38 (15): e101433.

179 Dobzinski, N., Chuartzman, S.G., Kama, R. et al. (2015). Starvation-dependent regulation of Golgi quality control links the TOR signaling and vacuolar protein sorting pathways. *Cell Rep.* 12 (11): 1876–1886.

180 Reggiori, F. and Pelham, H.R. (2002). A transmembrane ubiquitin ligase required to sort membrane proteins into multivesicular bodies. *Nat. Cell Biol.* 4 (2): 117–123.

181 Gelling, C.L., Dawes, I.W., Perlmutter, D.H. et al. (2012). The endosomal protein-sorting receptor sortilin has a role in trafficking alpha-1 antitrypsin. *Genetics* 192 (3): 889–903.

182 Chen, Y., Gershlick, D.C., Park, S.Y., and Bonifacino, J.S. (2017). Segregation in the Golgi complex precedes export of endolysosomal proteins in distinct transport carriers. *J. Cell Biol.* 216 (12): 4141–4151.

183 Wolins, N., Bosshart, H., Kuster, H., and Bonifacino, J.S. (1997). Aggregation as a determinant of protein fate in post-Golgi compartments: role of the luminal domain of furin in lysosomal targeting. *J. Cell Biol.* 139 (7): 1735–1745.

184 Mukhopadhyay, S., Bachert, C., Smith, D.R., and Linstedt, A.D. (2010). Manganese-induced trafficking and turnover of the cis-Golgi glycoprotein GPP130. *Mol. Biol. Cell* 21 (7): 1282–1292.

185 Venkat, S. and Linstedt, A.D. (2017). Manganese-induced trafficking and turnover of GPP130 is mediated by sortilin. *Mol. Biol. Cell* 28 (19): 2569–2578.

186 Dirck, A.T., Whyte, M.L., and Hudson, A.W. (2020). HHV-7 U21 exploits Golgi quality control carriers to reroute class I MHC molecules to lysosomes. *Mol. Biol. Cell* 31 (3): 196–208.

187 Tewari, R., Bachert, C., and Linstedt, A.D. (2015). Induced oligomerization targets Golgi proteins for degradation in lysosomes. *Mol. Biol. Cell* 26 (24): 4427–4437.

188 Yamaguchi, H., Arakawa, S., Kanaseki, T. et al. (2016). Golgi membrane-associated degradation pathway in yeast and mammals. *EMBO J.* 35 (18): 1991–2007.

189 Yamamoto, K., Fujii, R., Toyofuku, Y. et al. (2001). The KDEL receptor mediates a retrieval mechanism that contributes to quality control at the endoplasmic reticulum. *EMBO J.* 20 (12): 3082–3091.

190 Hara, T., Hashimoto, Y., Akuzawa, T. et al. (2014). Rer1 and calnexin regulate endoplasmic reticulum retention of a peripheral myelin protein 22 mutant that causes type 1A Charcot-Marie-tooth disease. *Sci. Rep.* 4: 6992.

191 Yamasaki, A., Hara, T., Maejima, I. et al. (2014). Rer1p regulates the ER retention of immature rhodopsin and modulates its intracellular trafficking. *Sci. Rep.* 4: 5973.

192 Briant, K., Johnson, N., and Swanton, E. (2017). Transmembrane domain quality control systems operate at the endoplasmic reticulum and Golgi apparatus. *PLoS One* 12 (4): e0173924.

193 Hellerschmied, D., Serebrenik, Y.V., Shao, L. et al. (2019). Protein folding state-dependent sorting at the Golgi apparatus. *Mol. Biol. Cell* 30 (17): 2296–2308.

194 Lujan, P. and Campelo, F. (2021). Should I stay or should I go? Golgi membrane spatial organization for protein sorting and retention. *Arch. Biochem. Biophys.* 707: 108921.

3

E3 Ubiquitin Ligases as Molecular Machines and Platforms for Drug Development

Rafael M. Ioris, Katherine Ferris and Vincenzo D'Angiolella

University of Oxford, Medical Research Council Institute for Radiation Oncology, Department of Oncology, Old Road Campus Research Building, Roosevelt Drive, Oxford, OX3 7DQ, UK

3.1 Introduction

3.1.1 Ubiquitin Code and Targeted Protein Degradation

Ubiquitylation entails a cascade of enzymatic reactions where multiples of ubiquitin molecules are covalently attached to a target protein. Polyubiquitylation of proteins acts as a signaling mechanism for protein degradation by the proteasome in most cases [1, 2]. The process is initiated when a ubiquitin molecule is activated by an E1-activating enzyme (E1), in an ATP-dependent reaction [3], and transferred to an E2-conjugating (E2) enzyme. An E3-ligase (E3) enzyme is the third gear of the reaction and responsible for the recognition of target substrates, favoring ubiquitin transfer from the E2-conjugating enzyme directly to the substrates or through an intermediate step [4, 5].

The human genome codes for two E1 enzymes [6, 7], ~38 E2s and ~700 E3s [4]. The hierarchical organization ensures selectivity in substrate targeting and, at the same time, diversity in ubiquitin chain elongation. E3 ligases can be divided into three main groups named after their characteristic domains for E2s recruitment: Ring (Really Interesting New Gene), HECT (homologous to the E6AP carboxyl terminus), and RBR (RING-in-Between-RING) (Figure 3.1a).

E3s represent a large and diverse family of enzymes with significantly different mechanisms of action and recognition. Indeed, ubiquitylation is not a binary signal like phosphorylation, and ubiquitin molecules can be linked to substrates in monomeric forms (monoubiquitylation) or in chains (polyubiquitylation). Polyubiquitylation chains can be formed by the sequential addition of ubiquitin molecules through covalent linkage on the K48 residue of ubiquitin itself. While K48 linkages are the most common in cells, ubiquitin chains can be formed through linkages with all other

Inducing Targeted Protein Degradation: From Chemical Biology to Drug Discovery and Clinical Applications, First Edition. Edited by Philipp Cromm.

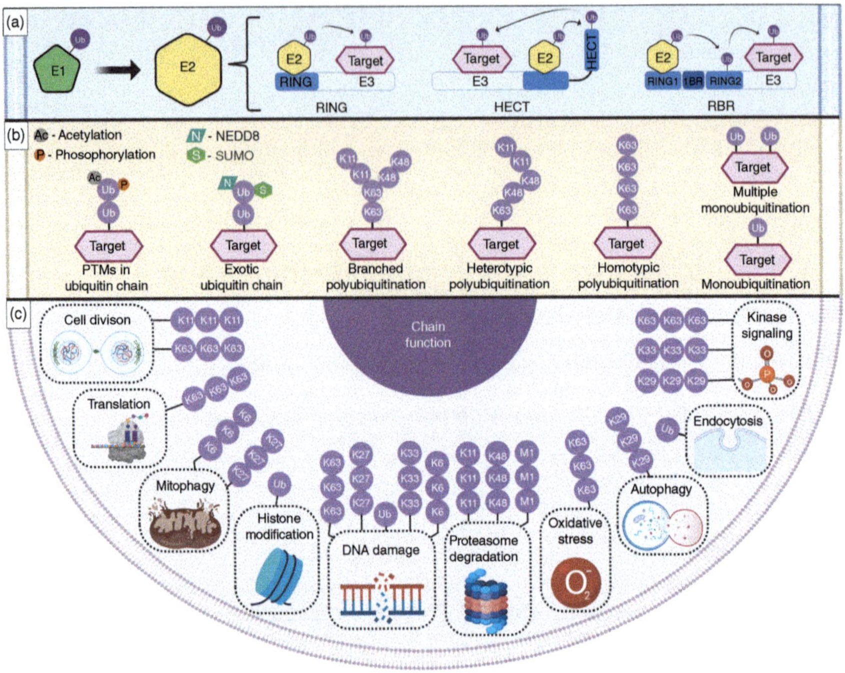

Figure 3.1 (a) Ubiquitylation cascade and main type of E3 ligases. (b) Type of ubiquitin chains. (c) Main type of ubiquitin chains and suggested functions.

available lysines on ubiquitin (K6, K11, K27, K29, K33, K48, and K63) and/or on the initiating methionine (M1). In addition to forming homotypic chains with a single linkage type, E3s can also produce heterotypic or mixed chains containing two or more linkage types. The topologies of the mixed chains are important for signaling, and mixed or branched chain topologies have been identified (Figure 3.1b) [2]. In addition to chains composed of ubiquitin, other ubiquitin-like molecules (such as SUMO and NEDD8) have been detected linked to ubiquitin chains to generate polymorphic chains. Finally, the ubiquitin molecule can be modified by acetylation and phosphorylation as a further signaling event. Such a diversity of chain composition underlies a ubiquitin "code" where substrates modified by ubiquitin chains can be channeled to different fates according to the type and class of ubiquitin chains generated (Figure 3.1c) [2].

Ubiquitylation modulates protein interaction, activity, localization, and degradation [2, 8–10]. Mass spectrometry (MS)-based approaches identified ubiquitylation in all subcellular locations and involved in virtually all essential cellular process, vastly influencing cell physiology and pathophysiology, including cancer [2, 9, 11]. Nevertheless, we are still at the very beginning of deciphering the ubiquitin code. Techniques to assess the diversity of chain topology/architecture and the mechanisms used by E3s to shape such chains are just emerging [12], and few studies have addressed functional roles for non-canonical ubiquitin chains.

Novel drug modalities hijack E3s to promote the degradation of neosubstrates only in the presence of the drug. These are divided generally into molecular glues (small molecules) and proteolysis targeting chimeras (PROTACs). Both drug modalities promote the formation of a ternary complex (E3–small molecule–neosubstrate) to direct degradation of selected proteins in the cellular milieu. PROTACs and molecular glues open a new frontier in drug design as they allow the targeting of proteins lacking enzymatic functions, significantly expanding the druggable space. However, much is still unknown in the ubiquitin field, and understanding E3 function and mechanisms of action could facilitate and diversify modalities of targeted degradation.

3.1.2 General Concepts of E3 Ligase Mechanism and Regulation

Protein ubiquitylation associated with degradation represents a crucial mechanism that allows irreversible state transitions to adapt quickly in changing environmental conditions. The assumptions for such systems are that E3 ligases must be specific in recognizing modified substrates, and controlled, to avoid unwanted protein degradation. In this section, we introduce two general concepts that form the basis of E3 ligase function: substrate recruitment and regulation of ligase activity. Specific examples will be described in the sections dedicated to each E3 ligase group.

3.2 Substrate Recruitment and Degron Recognition

An attribute of E3 ligases is that they recognize individual proteins using specific interaction domains to select targets for ubiquitylation from among thousands of proteins. The protein interaction domains can recognize specific amino acid sequences called "degrons" (including linear degrons, N-degron, and C-degron) [13], structural motifs (degron-independent interactions) [14], or specific small molecules that bridge two proteins [15–17].

Degrons are short, unique, and linear amino acid sequences present in the substrates. Many degrons have been described, and some of them require further post-translational modifications (PTMs) to prime them for interaction with E3s. For example, phosphorylation of both serine residues within the linear sequence DSGXXS allows recognition by the E3 ligase β-TrCP [18]. Other, analogous phosphodegrons have been identified as well [19–21]. Organisms, over thousands of years, have evolved incredibly clever strategies to sense metabolite levels and trigger sudden changes in protein levels through ubiquitylation and subsequent degradation. This is exemplified by the transcription factor hypoxia-inducible factor 1α (HIF1α), which, in the presence of oxygen, exposes hydroxylated prolines recognized by the E3 ligase Von Hippel–Lindau tumor suppressor (VHL). In this way, HIF1α is rapidly degraded in normoxia. In hypoxia, prolyl hydroxylation of HIF1α is hampered, thus preventing recognition by VHL and favoring a sudden increase of HIF1α to start a transcriptional response to limiting oxygen levels [22, 23].

N-terminal or C-terminal parts of proteins are also recognized for degradation via specialized pathways of recognition executed by multiple E3 ubiquitin ligases. Specialized pathways have been described for recognition of N- and C-degrons, with the first N-degron described in 1986 [24] and multiple C-degrons described only since 2018 [25]. N-degrons are characterized by a destabilizing N-terminal residue modified by acetylation and other modifications and by the presence of nearby lysines acting as ubiquitin acceptors residues [26]. The destabilizing modification of the N-terminus can be generated during translation (constitutive) or by the action of specific enzymes (conditional). Some of these enzymes are able to modify α-amino groups (through acetylation, formylation, leucylation, arginylation, and deamidation) and cleave N-terminal peptides (exopeptidases) or large fragments (endopeptidases) to expose the so-called N-end degrons [26, 27]. The C-terminal degradation pathway has been identified in a single elegant screen in human cells where several degrons have been described with paired E3 ligases [25]. There is evidence that C-terminal degradation represents a crucial mechanism of co-translational protein quality control [28] but the full scope of C-terminal degradation will require many years to come to light. Initial evidence is pointing to analogous N-degron and C-degron quality control mechanisms [27] in clearing unfolded [29, 30] and/or mislocalized proteins [31, 32].

Many protein–protein interactions do not involve linear motifs but rather the structural ones [33, 34]. Unsurprisingly, E3 ligases and substrates can also interact through specific structural motifs induced by metabolites or other factors [35, 36]. An example is found in control of cholesterol synthesis by the endoplasmic reticulum (ER). When cholesterol levels are elevated, the excess of lipid causes a structural change in HMG-CoA reductase, a rate-limiting enzyme in cholesterol production. This structural change activates the protein quality control system, targeting HMG-CoA reductase for degradation through the ER-associated degradation (ERAD) machinery [37, 38]. Some E3 ligases have been reported to recognize non-protein substrates and protein substrates bridged by small molecules such as zinc [15, 16], further increasing the complexity of degron signals. The possibility that small molecules participate in E3-subtrate recognition was first discovered in plants and opened a completely novel concept in the ubiquitin field. The plant hormone auxin was shown to bridge the E3 ligase TIR1 and the indole-3-acetic acid (IAA) transcriptional repressors to promote their degradation [39]. This discovery represented the first example of "molecular glues" that paved the way to a plethora of studies to use the auxin system in heterologous organisms to trigger protein degradation. The study also spurred interest in identifying artificial and physiological molecular glues in other organisms.

3.2.1 Regulating E3 Ligases Activity

The activity of E3 ubiquitin ligases is strictly controlled to prevent unwanted protein degradation [21, 40]. Ubiquitylation, phosphorylation, ADP-ribosylation, and modification via other ubiquitin-like molecules (Ubl) are all PTMs contributing to regulation of E3 activity [13].

There are several examples of phosphorylation activating E3 ligases, including some HECT and RING E3s, and multisubunit complexes such as the anaphase promoting complex/cyclosome (APC/C) [21, 40, 41]. In the case of APC/C, phosphorylation of the core subunits is necessary for activity of the complex while phosphorylation of the coactivator, Cdh1, prevents the activity of APC/C^{Cdh1} specifically [40]. APC/C activity is also directly inhibited by two proteins, namely, Emi1 and Mad2, to ensure strict regulation of APC/C activity.

Modification of cullins by Ubl, NEDD8, is essential for the activity of the E3 ligases that use cullins as scaffolds [42]. In these multisubunit complexes, ubiquitin transfer occurs only when NEDD8 is covalently attached to the cullin. The neddylation of cullins triggers a conformational change, which positions the E2 into close proximity of the substrates to allow ubiquitin transfer [43].

Polymeric chains of ADP-ribose, also known as poly(ADP-ribosylation) or PARylation, is another PTM that regulates ubiquitylation [44–47]. Substrate PARylation has been shown to prime for ubiquitylation, while ubiquitin PARylation has been proposed as a mechanism to prevent ubiquitin transfer to a substrate [45, 47]. The E3 ligase RNF146 binds to tankyrase (TNKS), a poly(ADP-ribosylation) polymerase, which in turn binds and PARylates a specific substrate [45]. The interaction between E3 ligase and PARylated substrate primes ubiquitylation by changing the E3 conformation and exposing the E2 binding site [45]. Other modes of regulation exist, such as the presence of cofactors, direct inhibition of E3s, and the possibility to alternate E2s on the same E3 scaffold. We envision that there will be intense investigation in this area as understanding the regulation of E3 ubiquitin ligase activity will be crucial for optimal targeting using PROTACs and molecular glues.

3.3 RING E3 Ligases

3.3.1 Definition and Discovery

The RING domain was described in 1991 with the discovery of Ring1 (Really Interesting New Gene 1) as a cysteine-rich sequence motif with a central conserved histidine binding two zinc cations [48]. Initially, it was believed to represent a new structural class of zinc-finger DNA binding motifs. The authors also suggested the possibility that the zinc motif could form a structure involved in protein–protein interactions. Later, in 1994, structural work demonstrated that the zinc atoms bound to cysteines and one histidine at the domain's core help to maintain a rigid and circular structure, resembling a ring, allowing protein–protein interactions [49].

In their original description of the Ring1 motif, Freemont et al. reported seven proteins containing a related motif [48], including the yeast RAD18, which was the first example linking the RING motif to ubiquitination [50]. Currently, several variations to the canonical RING domain are described, including variants where the position of conserved zinc binding cysteines and the histidine are inverted or replaced (e.g. aspartic acid in RBX1/ROC1). RBX1 is an example of the canonical

RING domain variation, where the motif contains a 20-amino-acid insertion that can accommodate a third zinc binding site [51]. Another domain, called U-Box, is also a variant adopting a ring-shaped domain stabilized by hydrophilic amino acids, forming hydrogen bonds rather than binding to zinc atoms [52–54].

It is now established that these domains are required to recruit E2s for protein ubiquitylation. Indeed, publications from several independent laboratories reported initial findings on the function of the RING domains in ubiquitylation [55–64]. Together, those results established the essentiality of the RING motif and its zinc binding ability to bind and activate the E2 enzyme, promoting direct transfer of ubiquitin to substrate. These results paved the way to the identification of a much larger group of E3s (RING E3s), currently estimated at ~700 genes [65].

3.3.2 Subgroups

RING-type E3 ubiquitin ligase has a common feature: the RING domain works as a docking site for the ubiquitin-charged E2, putting it in close proximity to the substrate to allow direct ubiquitin transfer onto the target protein [66]. Although there is a common feature, the RING domain identifies a vast collection of different proteins and E3 ligases with substantially diverse characteristics. Most proteins containing RING domains also contain additional domains and properties, leading to subgroup classifications [66]. Among the RING-type E3 ubiquitin ligases, we distinguish two main subtypes: monomeric and oligomeric E3s. Cullin ring ubiquitin ligases (CRLs), which account for almost half of the E3s (~270 CRLS) [66], are prototypical multi-subunit (oligomeric) enzymes that use cullins (Cul1, Cul2/5, Cul3, Cul4A/B, and Cul7) as scaffolds to bridge a variable substrate receptor and a RING domain-containing protein (RBX1 and RBX2) for ubiquitin transfer [66, 67]. Cullin1-based E3s assemble a complex composed of Skp1, Cul1, and an F-box protein (SCF) [68]. In this particular E3 machinery, the Cul1 N-terminus binds to Skp1 (adaptor subunit), which in turn binds to a variable F-box protein (substrate receptor). Another member of the complex, RBX1, contains the RING domain responsible for binding to the E2 conjugating enzyme [68]. The other cullin complexes function similarly, with variations in adaptors, substrate receptors, and RING domain proteins (summarized in Figure 3.2).

Cul2 and Cul5 are the most structurally related among the cullins and use elongin B and C as adaptors to engage a variable substrate recruitment protein [69]. In Cul3 complexes, several BTB domain-containing proteins assemble directly with Cul3 and act as both an adaptor and a substrate recognition subunit. The BTB domain-containing proteins recognize substrates with their MATH (Meprin and TRAF homology) motif and Kelch beta-propeller repeats [70]. Cul4 machineries, which comprise Cul4A and Cul4B, use Ddb1 as an adapter. Ddb1 assembles with a large family of DCAF (Ddb1- and Cul4-associated factor) proteins using a WDXR motif within the substrate recruitment factors [71]. Cul7 is similar to Cul1 in using Skp1 as an adaptor and recruiting Fbxw8 as a substrate receptor [72], but it can only assemble complexes with Fbxw8 and no other F-box proteins [67]. Cul9 is less well

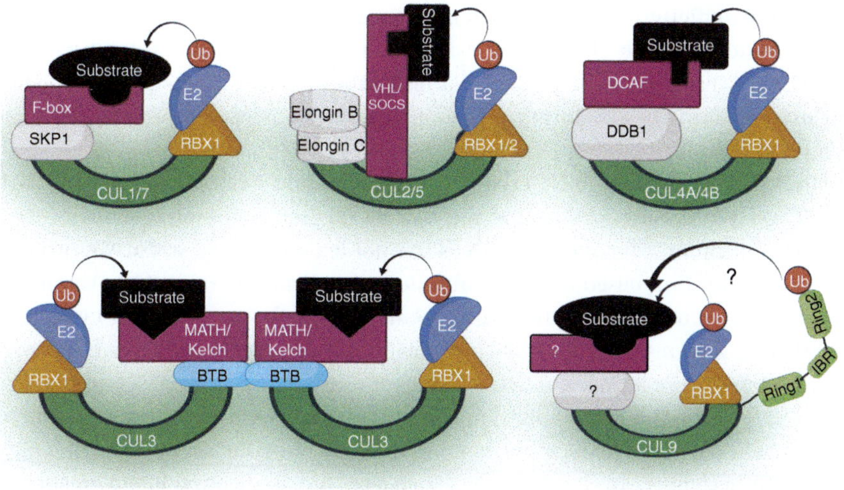

Figure 3.2 The cullin ring ubiquitin ligases (CRLs). The picture presents canonical assembly for Cul1, Cul2/5, Cul3, and Cul4A/4B. Cul9 assembly is less well established and a potential functional organization is depicted.

understood, and it contains an RBR domain in its sequence, which could be used to transfer ubiquitin to the substrate in a non-canonical manner (Figure 3.2).

A common feature of CRL complexes is their activation by a ubiquitin-like protein called NEDD8 (neuronal precursor cell-expressed developmentally down-regulated protein 8) [73]. Recently, the initial IκBα ubiquitylation steps by the CRL1/β-TRCP/UBE2D complex were captured using cryo-EM, suggesting a NEDD8-dependent model for substrate priming [74]. This study suggests a dynamic and mobile link among NEDD8, CUL1 WHB domains, and RBX1 RING domains, narrowing the gap between E2-Ub-charged UBE2D and IκBα substrate, and allowing ubiquitin transfer [74].

Among the best studied and physiologically relevant multimeric RING E3s, it is important to mention the APC/C. This large multimeric enzyme accommodates more than 15 proteins in its catalytic core, including two substrate adaptors, Cdc20 and Cdh1, and it works with two different E2s. Such complexity allows for multiple control mechanisms that facilitate irreversible cell cycle transitions, preventing errors that could result in cell death or transformation. Indeed, APC/C^{Cdc20} activation is crucial to control the rapid chromosome division at the metaphase/anaphase transition to prevent chromosome mis-segregation [75]. The prompt and correct activation of APC/C at anaphase is controlled by a titration mechanism operated by an inhibitor of APC/C^{Cdc20}, Mad2, which is required to sense chromosome alignment. Once the initial degradation events are triggered and the cyclin dependent kinase (CDK) activity, which marks the beginning of mitosis, is reduced, APC/C^{Cdc20} switches adaptor to operate as APC/C^{Cdh1}. The degrons recognized by APC/C^{Cdc20} and APC/C^{Cdh1} are RxxL, and RxxL and KEN, respectively, allowing Cdh1 to maintain the APC/C activity on Cdc20 substrates while also broadening the substrate specificity. The APC/C has the capacity to generate different ubiquitin linkages and branched chains. The catalytic process is operated by multiple E2s, with (UbcH10-aka Ube2C) and UbcH5 priming the substrate for ubiquitylation, and the extension E2 Ube2S forming long K11-linked chains for protein degradation [76, 77].

RING-type zinc-finger (RNF) domain, in supposedly monomeric E3, occurs in ~72 RING E3 ligases, constituting the second biggest family of E3s after CRLs. A subclassification of monomeric RNFs has not been proposed so far. We propose here a classification based on their subcellular localization (Table 3.1). Among 72 RNFs, 30 are nuclear, including 16 present in both the nucleus and cytoplasm (another 11 are present only in the cytoplasm). The endoplasmatic reticulum harbors 14 RNFs, 2 are found in mitochondria and 2 are found in the Golgi apparatus. Seven RNFs have unknown subcellular location to date. However, the presence of transmembrane domains suggests membrane localization for 28 RNF E3s, of which at least 10 have been localized at the cell surface. A classification based on subcellular localization might help efforts aimed at developing binders targeting E3s with different properties.

Table 3.1 Monomeric RING E3 ubiquitin ligases.

Name	Subcellular localization	TM domain	Cell surface	References
RNF1/Ring1	Nucleus			[78]
RNF2/Ring1B/Ring2	Nucleus			[79]
RNF12/RLIM	Nucleus			[80]
RNF20	Nucleus			[81, 82]
RNF38	Nucleus			[83]
RNF40	Nucleus			[82]
RNF113A	Nucleus			[84–86]
RNF165	Nucleus			[87]
RNF168	Nucleus			[88–91]
RNF169	Nucleus			[92–94]
RNF184/MSL2/MSL2L1	Nucleus			[95]
RNF138	Nucleus (chromosome)			[96–98]
RNF219/OBI1	Nucleus (chromosome)			[99]
RNF113B	Possibly nucleus			[100]
RNF4	Nucleus and cytoplasm			[101–105]
RNF6	Nucleus and cytoplasm			[106, 107]
RNF8	Nucleus and cytoplasm			[91, 108–110]

(*Continued*)

Table 3.1 (Continued)

Name	Subcellular localization	TM domain	Cell surface	References
RNF10	Nucleus and cytoplasm			[111–113]
RNF17/TDRD4	Nucleus and cytoplasm			[114, 115]
RNF25	Nucleus and cytoplasm			[116]
RNF111	Nucleus and cytoplasm			[117–119]
RNF114	Nucleus and cytoplasm			[120]
RNF123	Nucleus and cytoplasm			[121, 122]
RNF126	Nucleus and cytoplasm			[123]
RNF146	Nucleus and cytoplasm			[46, 124, 125]
RNF151	Nucleus and cytoplasm			[126]
RNF187	Nucleus and cytoplasm			[127]
RNF208	Nucleus and cytoplasm			[128]
RNF34	Nucleus, cytoplasm, and cell membrane		X	[129–132]
RNF11	Nucleus, cytoplasm, early endosomes			[133, 134]
RNF43	Nucleus, ER, and cell membrane		X	[135]
RNF32	Cytoplasm			[136]
RNF39	Cytoplasm			[137]
RNF130/GOLI	Cytoplasm		X	[138]
RNF157	Cytoplasm			[139, 140]
RNF166	Cytoplasm			[141]
RNF167/RING105	Cytoplasm	X	X	[142]
RNF181	Cytoplasm			[143]
RNF182	Cytoplasm	X		[144, 145]
RNF207	Cytoplasm			[146]
RNF213	Cytoplasm			[147, 148]
RNF220	Cytoplasm			[149]
RNF135	Cytoplasm and stress granule			[150–152]
RNF41/FLRF/Nrdp1	Cytoplasm and ER			[153–156]
RNF13	ER		X	[157, 158]
RNF103	ER			[159]
RNF133	ER		X	[160]
RNF139/TRC8	ER	X		[161–165]
RNF145	ER	X		[166, 167]

(*Continued*)

Table 3.1 (Continued)

Name	Subcellular localization	TM domain	Cell surface	References
RNF148	ER	X	X	[168]
RNF170	ER	X		[169, 170]
RNF186	ER	X		[171]
RNF26	ER	X		[172, 173]
RNF121	Possibly ER	X		[100]
RNF5	ER membrane and mitochondrion membrane	X		[174–178]
RNF185	ER membrane and mitochondrion outer membrane	X		[179, 180]
RNF122	ER and Golgi	X		[181]
RNF183	ER, Golgi, and lysosome	X		[182]
RNF128/GRAIL	Cytoskeleton	X	X	[183, 184]
RNF24	Golgi	X		[185]
RNF125	Golgi			[186–189]
RNF152	Lysosome	X		[190, 191]
RNF44	Unknown			[192]
RNF190/MARCH10	Unknown			—
RNF214	Unknown			—
RNF224	Unknown			—
RNF149/DNAPTP2	Unknown	X	X	[193]
RNF150	Unknown	X	X	—
RNF175	Unknown	X		[194, 195]

In the table, we highlight monomeric RINGs and their subcellular localization. TM, transmembrane domain, and cell surface are also indicated.
TM, transmembrane domain; ER, endoplasmic reticulum.

In addition to canonical RNFs, a variation of the RING domain (U-box) identified seven E3s in humans and ~60 in plants. The U-Box is a 75-amino acid motif that lacks the cysteine residues for Zn^{2+} coordination and uses a characteristic network of hydrogen bonds to stabilize the circular structure of the domain [52]. Besides the functional domain, U-Box members lack common features and possess diverse functions ranging from protein quality control to DNA damage and repair [53].

3.3.3 Insights into RINGs Regulation and Function

Discussing the function of all RNFs is beyond the scope of this chapter, but we highlight below a few examples of reciprocal regulation and non-canonical ubiquitylation.

An example of a CRL-type Cul1 (also called SCF) is constituted by $SCF^{Cyclin\ F}$, which interplays with APC/C^{Cdh1} to regulate the cell cycle events occurring in G2 and M phases [21, 40, 196, 197]. $SCF^{Cyclin\ F}$ controls the production of deoxyribonucleotide triphosphates (dNTPs) during the cell cycle by regulating the stability of RRM2, a subunit of ribonucleotide reductase, which converts NTPs to dNTPs. $SCF^{Cyclin\ F}$ recognizes an RxI motif in RRM2 and ubiquitylates it for degradation. The recognition of the RxI only occurs after phosphorylation on T33 by CDK1/cyclin A at the completion of S phase to restrict dNTP production in the S phase [21]. To reset of the cell cycle and further control the cyclin F activity, cyclin F itself is recognized by β-TrCP and APC/C [196, 198]. Thus, a concerted action of E3 ubiquitin ligases controls accurate and irreversible cell cycle phase transitions.

It is important to mention that ubiquitylation also plays a crucial role during pathogen–host interactions. In some instances, viruses exploit endogenous E3 ligases to prevent virus recognition by the immune system and to facilitate viral replication [199, 200]. In other instances, ubiquitylation represents an important intracellular defense mechanism for pathogen clearance. For example, it has been recently observed that RNF213 coats invasive bacteria with ubiquitin molecules, restricting bacterial proliferation [148]. The mechanism of bacterial ubiquitylation by RNF213 uncovers the first non-proteinaceous ubiquitylation dock, the lipopolysaccharides (LPS) surrounding the bacteria *Salmonella*. Additionally, LPS ubiquitylation is independent of the RNF213's Ring domain, relying, instead, on the dynein-like core and the RZ finger domain [148]. These results open the possibility that, firstly, many more non-proteinaceous ubiquitin acceptors could exist and, secondly, entire classes of E3 ligases that do not possess the classical RING domains might be operating.

3.4 HECT E3 Ubiquitin Ligases

3.4.1 Definition and Discovery

The first human E3 ubiquitin ligase to be cloned was E6-AP (E6-associated protein), one of the proteins hijacked during a human papilloma virus (HPV) infection, and sequence analysis identified a ~350-residue carboxy-terminal domain that was conserved in 14 proteins [201]. This domain was labeled "homologous to E6-AP carboxy-terminus" and identifies the 28 HECT family members in the human genome [202]. It also contains the catalytic cysteine residue that forms a thioester bond with ubiquitin during its transfer from E2 to the substrate, and formation of this covalent intermediate is the other distinguishing feature of the HECT family [201].

3.4.2 Subgroups

While all E3 ligases in the HECT family share a common carboxyl-terminal domain, variation in the remainder of their sequences splits them into three groups [202–204].

- NEDD4 family: a C2 and three to four WW domains [205]
- Domain containing E3 ubiquitin protein ligase family (HERC): one or more RCC1 like domains (RLDs) (small and large subfamilies) [206]
- Other family: contain a HECT domain but not a C2, WW, or RLD region [203]

The HECT domain provides a common starting point for the mechanism of ubiquitin transfer, and the variation in its sequence contributes to E2 specificity, while the upstream domains regulate enzyme activity and determine substrate selection [203].

3.4.3 Structure and Mechanism

HECT E3 ligases are split into amino-terminal regulatory modules and a carboxyl-terminal catalytic HECT domain, providing the basis for their categorization [203]. Until recently, structures were only available for fragments of these proteins, showing the structures of individual or a few domains but failing to explore the conformation of the whole ligase. Two structures are now available for full-length HUWE1, providing the first insight into the overall structure of HECT enzymes [207, 208]. The protein coils round on itself, bringing the carboxyl-terminal HECT domain close to the amino-terminal substrate recruitment region. Ring closure is required to stabilize the protein, but there is also enough flexibility in the structure for the HECT domain to reach the various substrate binding domains embedded in the rest of the protein [207, 208]. It is, however, unclear if other HECT ligases adopt this conformation, especially as many of them are less than half the size of HUWE1. Further work on full-length structures is required to provide a more physiological context for previous studies that focus on isolated domains, as detailed below.

Detailed analysis of the N-terminal domains is beyond the scope of this chapter, for which it is sufficient to note that the structural variety of these domains facilitates selective recruitment of a range of substrates and that some of the domains have additional functions, such as the guanine nucleotide exchange activity of the RLD domains of HERC1 [209].

The C-terminal HECT domain is split into two lobes, amino (N)- and carboxyl (C)-terminal, which are responsible for E2 recruitment and catalysis, respectively [210]. Flexibility at the interface between the lobes permits the multiple conformations observed in structural studies of different HECT domains [211–214]. The N-terminal lobe is further subdivided into two subdomains, whose interactions also accommodate conformational flexibility [210, 215]. This flexibility is likely essential to the catalytic activity of the domain [215]. The first HECT domain structure to be solved placed the E2 and E3 catalytic cysteines 41 Å apart, significantly outside the range needed for ubiquitin transfer. In this model, the C-lobe is positioned at one end of the N-lobe, forming an L-shaped structure [210]. A subsequent study of a different HECT domain identified an inverted T shape, with the C-lobe arranged more centrally over the N-lobe. This brought the catalytic cysteines closer, but at 16.5 Å, the distance separating them still prevented transfer [211]. The same study showed, however, that rotation around the three-residue hinge connecting the two lobes reduced this to 5 Å and suggested that "inherent flexibility" within the model would allow the cysteines to come within 2.5 Å of each other, the distance required for catalysis. Notably, mutation of any two of the hinge residues to proline to restrict conformational flexibility prevented ubiquitin transfer, highlighting the catalytic importance of a flexible interface between the two lobes [211].

The need for conformational flexibility is currently the clearest aspect of the HECT E3 catalytic mechanism. By contrast, the process by which incoming ubiquitin and substrate molecules are aligned and the mechanism for chain elongation are poorly understood. Several structural features have been identified as relevant to one or more steps of the ubiquitination process, such as β-strand augmentation between the C-terminal tails of the HECT domain and incoming ubiquitin molecules [204, 213], but a full, detailed mechanism has yet to be characterized. The current model describes the binding of a ubiquitin-conjugated E2 to a site on the small N-lobe subdomain, whose poor sequence conservation may facilitate E2 selectivity. The C-lobe then rotates by more than 100° [211, 213] to face the substrate at the other end of the complex where the HECT domain C-terminal tail may orient the ubiquitin molecule or activate the target lysine on the substrate to facilitate ligation, as well as potentially influencing linkage specificity [213, 214, 216]. In addition, most HECT E3s have a non-covalent ubiquitin binding site in the N-lobe, whose interaction with ubiquitin is thought to promote chain elongation [217, 218]. Several chain elongation models have been proposed, primarily sequential addition and indexation [211, 219]. In the former, the HECT domain rotates between the substrate and E2 for each round of ubiquitination, and each ubiquitin molecule forms a thioester intermediate with the E3 catalytic cysteine. The indexation mechanism, however, suggests that smaller movements occur in each round, repositioning the cysteine-bound ubiquitin chain just enough to expose a lysine on the C-terminal molecule to an incoming, E2-bound ubiquitin that is then added to the chain. Only the initial ubiquitin molecule forms a thioester bond with the E3 cysteine, and this bond remains intact until the chain is transferred as a unit to the substrate. This mechanism is consistent with the substrate-independent chain assembly seen in HECT E3s, but neither model has been proved conclusively, and it remains possible that both are used (Figure 3.3) [211].

3.4.4 Regulation

3.4.4.1 Intramolecular Interactions

Conformational flexibility also contributes to regulation of some HECTs, particularly the NEDD4 group, many of which adopt closed conformations to block the catalytic activity. In Itchy E3 ubiquitin protein ligase homolog (ITCH), for example, it is the WW domains that bind to the HECT domain, whereas in SMURF2, both the C2 and WW1 domains are required [224, 225]. The importance of conformational flexibility is highlighted by the inability of the highly similar but shorter SMURF1 protein to use the same mechanism *in cis* [226]. Its C2 domain still binds to the catalytic region of the protein, but the absence of the WW1 domain found in SMURF2 means that the domains must be on separate peptides, requiring homodimerization [227]. It should be noted, however, that the WW1 domain has been

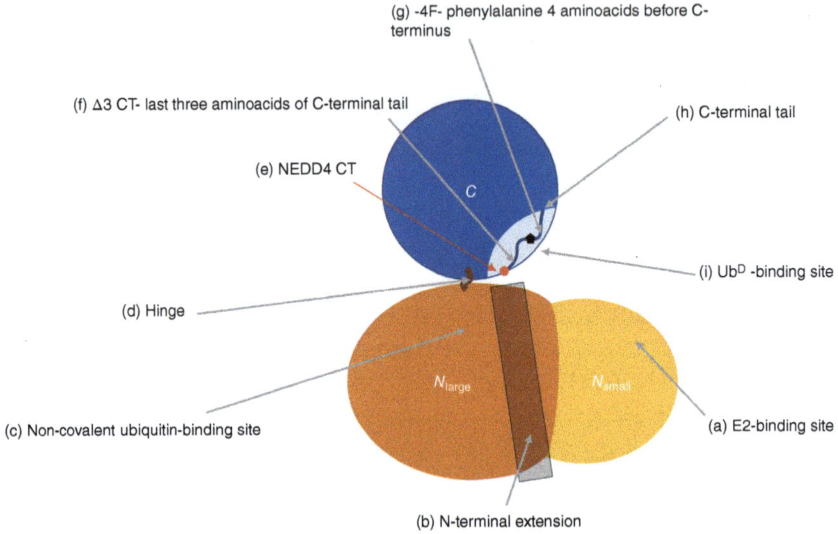

Figure 3.3 Features of HECT E3s based on position in the E3 scaffold. (a) **E2 binding site.** Small domain of N-lobe has low sequence conservation, potentially to accommodate selection from multiple E2s. Differences in the residues that interact with the key Phe residue in loop 4 of the E2 may dictate specificity [212]. (b) **N-terminal extension.** Important for stability [220, 221]. (c) **Non-covalent ubiquitin binding site.** N-lobe binds to L8-I44-V70 surface of ubiquitin, positioning it away from the catalytic and E2 binding sites [217]. This site may bind substrate-bound ubiquitin, holding substrate in place for chain elongation [214, 217, 218]. Includes residues from both N-lobe subdomains [218]. (d) **Hinge** 3 residues – mutation of any two to proline inhibits ubiquitin transfer [211]. (e) **NEDD4 CT.** C terminus of HECT proteins in NEDD4 subgroup has conserved acidic residue required for substrate ubiquitination but not transthiolation. This residue is not conserved in other HECT subfamilies [214]. (f) **Δ-3 CT.** Last three residues are catalytically important in some HECT domains but the exact role is unclear. These residues could be involved in linkage specificity. For example, replacing the last four residues of NEDD4 with the last three from E6AP alters the ratio of K63 and K48 linkages produced by NEDD4 [214]. In AREL1, deletion fully inhibits autoubiquitination and impairs substrate ubiquitination [218, 221]. In Rsp5, deletion inhibits ligation, but mutation of all three residues to alanine, or the last one to arginine does not affect the catalytic activity [213]. (g) **-4F.** Could be involved in interactions between the C-terminal tail and the N-lobe [213, 216]. Important for ligation but not for transthiolation [213, 222]. Position four residues from C-terminus is important – mutating or moving the phenylalanine impairs substrate ubiquitination [222]. (h) **C-terminal tail.** Flexible in most conformations, hence missing from most structures of active domain. Catalytically important, possibly by stabilizing structure, orienting ubiquitin lysine for nucleophilic attack or by contributing to reaction itself [214, 216]. During isopeptide bond formation, tail is sandwiched between N-lobe and ubiquitin [216]. Interaction with ubiquitin results in β-strand augmentation that is needed for thioester formation [204, 214]. Subsequent conformational changes in the C-terminal tail are required for isopeptide bond formation, but not transthiolation [204]. (i) **Ub^{D} binding site.** Hydrophobic patch on C-lobe interacts with hydrophobic region of ubiquitin [223].

shown to contribute directly to interactions with the HECT domain, and the linker sequence is also important, so it is not simply the additional flexibility of the extra length that drives the difference in inactive structures [225]. Disruption of the interactions between the N-terminal and HECT domains releases the ligase from its inhibited conformation. In HECTs with C2 domains, this can be achieved by the binding of these regions to Ca^{2+} ions, disrupting the electrostatic interactions with the HECT domain to allow the enzyme to adopt its active conformation and also mediating new interactions with IP3 and PIP_2 to regulate E3 localization [228, 229]. Alternatively, interactions with other proteins or the addition of post-translational modifications (PTMs) can be used to block the intramolecular interactions that hold HECT E3s in their inactive conformations. These are discussed further below.

Intramolecular interactions are also sometimes required for the active conformation of a HECT E3 ligase. HUWE1 demonstrates this with its activation segment, whose interactions with the dimerization surface of the same polypeptide prevents formation of an inactive, asymmetric homodimer [230].

3.4.4.2 Intermolecular Interactions

As mentioned above, dimerization and higher order oligomerization also contribute to HECT regulation. HUWE1 dimers are inactive, although their asymmetric structure may permit the activity of one monomer while the other is inhibited [230]. In contrast, E6AP activity is increased by homotrimerization [231], and the role of intermolecular interactions in HECT regulation is extended further by the formation of heterogeneous complexes. Additional proteins can disrupt intramolecular interactions to inhibit or activate E3. When p14ARF binds to HUWE1, it releases the activation segment, exposing the surface needed to form inactive dimers [230]. Binding of NDFIP1 to the WW domains of NEDD4, however, disrupts the inhibitory interactions between the WW and HECT domains, releasing the catalytic site into its active conformation [232, 233]. NDFIP1 also acts as an adaptor protein, recruiting phosphatase and tensin homolog (PTEN) to NEDD4 for modification with a ubiquitin signal that will induce translocation to the nucleus [234, 235]. Interestingly, the same adaptor and substrate bound to WWP2 results in ubiquitin-induced proteasomal degradation of PTEN, which can also be induced by NEDD4 if an alternative adaptor protein, NUMB endocytic adaptor protein (NUMB), is used [236, 237]. This highlights the importance of adaptor proteins not just in regulating E3 conformations but also in determining target substrates and the types of ubiquitin signal added to them. For some ligases, the adaptor protein is also required for E2 recruitment. SMURF2, for example, cannot bind to UbcH7, its cognate E2, with sufficient affinity without first binding SMAD7 [215]. In other cases, E2–E3 interactions are disrupted to regulate the ligase activity, as demonstrated by ISG15 blocking E2 recruitment when bound non-covalently to the HECT domain of NEDD4 [238].

Another interaction partner involved in regulating ubiquitylation patterns is ubiquitin itself. Some HECT E3s contain an additional ubiquitin binding site in the N-lobe of the HECT domain, away from the catalytic surface, and non-covalent binding of ubiquitin to this site increases enzyme processivity and hence the length of the ubiquitin chain added to the substrate [218]. Ubiquitin variants (UbVs) and small-molecule inhibitors may allow artificial manipulation of this site to bias E3s toward processive polyubiquitination or toward distributive monoubiquitination, in which a greater number of substrate proteins are modified, but only with a single ubiquitin moiety [239].

3.4.4.3 Post-translational Modifications

As well as binding ubiquitin non-covalently in the N-lobe and for catalysis in the C-lobe of the HECT domain, HECT E3s can themselves be modified with ubiquitin chains, often in an autocatalytic manner. This typically results in proteasomal degradation of the enzyme to reduce its overall activity in the cell, a mechanism balanced out by changes at the transcriptional and translational level [240–242]. Deubiquitinases (DUBs) also counteract this mechanism, removing ubiquitin moieties to stabilize the ligase, and where the DUB is also a substrate for its cognate E3, this forms a regulatory feedback loop, as shown by TRIP12 and its DUB, USP17, and UBR5 with deubiquitinating enzyme A (DUBA) [243, 244]. DUB activity may also be involved in the regulation of adaptor protein turnover. A model of adaptor switching has been demonstrated in yeast HECT protein Rsp5p, which binds to an adaptor and ubiquitinates it to facilitate substrate recruitment [245]. The bound adaptor is then released in favor of a competing adaptor when deubiquitinated by its respective DUB. It is plausible that a similar model exists in mammalian systems to provide another control mechanism for directing HECT activity.

Just as ubiquitination does not always result in substrate degradation, nor does ligase ubiquitination always direct E3s to the proteasome. Ubiquitination of K525 in NEDD4 induces interactions between the HECT domain and the α1 helix N-terminal to it. These interactions provide the energy to pull the helix away from a surface that is then exposed for trimerization, resulting in complexes that inhibit ubiquitination activity [246].

Phosphorylation can alter interactions in a similar manner, with c-Src-mediated phosphorylation of the C2 or HECT domain of NEDD4 disrupting interaction of the two regions to favor the active conformation of the enzyme [247]. In HUWE1, phosphorylation by spleen associated tyrosine kinase (SYK) prevents binding of p14ARF that would otherwise block the intramolecular interactions needed to maintain HUWE1 in its active conformation [248]. NEDD4-2 phosphorylation, however, provides a binding site for 14-3-3, which then blocks substrate binding, while phosphorylation of E6AP inhibits formation of the active trimer, depending on the modification site [249, 250].

Relevant sites for phosphorylation-mediated regulation are not confined to the E3 itself, but also include those on substrates and ubiquitin itself. UBE3C catalyzes the formation of both K29- and K48-linked ubiquitin chains, but phosphorylation of S20 in ubiquitin increases catalytic preference for K48 linkages [251]. In substrates, the role of phosphorylation is predominantly degron formation for those ligases that recognize phosphorylated motifs, such as HUWE1 binding to transcription factor Miz1 and HECTD2 to anti-inflammatory PIAS1 [252, 253].

Although not as extensively characterized, other PTMs also contribute to HECT regulation. Neddylation of SMURF2, for instance, increases its auto-ubiquitination rate to promote its degradation [254], but SMURF1 auto-neddylation stimulates activity of this E3 [255], as does non-covalent binding of Nedd8 to the HECT domains of both enzymes [256]. SUMOylation has also been described as a stimulatory mechanism for SMURF2, further diversifying the list of PTMs used in HECT regulation [257].

3.4.5 Insights into Hect Functions

An exhaustive analysis of the functions of the HECT family is beyond the scope of this chapter, which instead outlines a few examples to illustrate the main mechanisms behind their roles which are summarized in Table 3.2. The reader is directed to the references therein for a more comprehensive description of the roles played by HECT E3s.

3.4.5.1 Growth Signaling

A common role of HECT E3s in cell signaling pathways is regulation of pathway component abundance as a way of switching signaling pathways on and off. The importance of this role is highlighted by HUWE1-mediated degradation of β-catenin in the context of Wnt pathway hyperactivation, preventing aberrant transcription of the effector genes and limiting the phenotypic effects of excessive pathway activity. This provides an important safety mechanism against the development of colon cancer for example as functional APC, which is normally involved in restricting β-catenin activity, is often lost in this tumor type [306].

Beyond inducing proteasomal degradation, HECT E3 activity can influence the localization of pathway components. Following K27-linked polyubiquitylation by WWP1, PTEN is unable to move to the plasma membrane where it would normally catalyze the conversion of PIP_3 to PIP_2 to facilitate signal transduction. Alternatively, PTEN monoubiquitylation by NEDD4-1 induces nuclear translocation, giving the phosphatase access to a different set of substrates [235].

In some cases, HECT E3 function is independent of ligase activity. ITCH catalyzes multiubiquitylation of PI4KIIα to mediate recruitment of downstream signaling factors, but PI4KIIα activity is regulated by the interaction with ITCH, not the ubiquitin modifications. Similarly, TSC2 is excluded from the TSC1–TSC2 that inhibits downstream mTORC1 activity by ligase-independent interaction with HERC1. In the case of SMURF2 binding to NEDD9, the interaction protects the target against ubiquitin-induced degradation. This increases the levels of NEDD9 available to stimulate Aurora A, a crucial step in progression through the G_2-M phase of the cell cycle [298].

3.4.5.2 Immunity

HECT involvement in the immune system is a key example of non-ubiquitylation functions of these E3s. HERC5 also catalyzes the addition of ISG15, a ubiquitin-like protein, to substrates. Following viral infection, HERC5-mediated ISGylation of IRF3 stabilizes and activates the transcription factor to upregulate the interferon response, while modification of the viral protein NS1A prevents its interaction with host protein importin-α, excluding it from the nucleus and thereby preventing viral replication [271].

The canonical, degradative effects of ubiquitylation also play an essential role in immunity and can be directed toward invading pathogens, as demonstrated by SMURF1-induced autophagolysomal removal of *Mycobacterium tuberculosis* cells and by proteasomal degradation of the hepatitis C virus (HCV) core protein

Table 3.2 A brief outline of HECT E3 ligase functions and their implication in diseases.

Ligase	Target	Effect	Outcome	Cellular function	Disease	References
HERC1	c-RAF	Polyubiquitination (K48)	Proteasomal degradation[a]	Cell migration	Not reported	[258] [259]
	TSC2	Interaction	Target activity (inhibited)	Cell signaling Myelination	Peripheral neuropathies Acute lymphoblastic leukemia	[260, 261]
	ARF1/Rab proteins	Guanine nucleotide exchange/release	Target activity	Cytoskeleton and intracellular transport	Not reported	[262] [209] [263]
HERC2	BRCA1[a]	Polyubiquitination	Proteasomal degradation	Cell cycle *G_2-M checkpoint*	Breast cancer	[264]
	FBXO5			Metabolism	Not reported	[265]
	RNF8	Interaction	E2 recruitment	DNA damage response	Not reported	[266]
	RNF168		Stabilization		Not reported	
	p53		Promotes target oligomerization (stimulatory)	Transcription	Not reported	[267] [268]
HERC3	SMAD7	Polyubiquitination	Autolysosomal degradation	Cell signaling TGF-β pathway	Glioblastoma	[269]
HERC5	IRF3	ISGylation	Target stabilization and activation	Immune response Anti-viral gene transcription	Viral infection (Sendai virus)	[270]
	NS1A		Target inactivation	Immune response Viral gene replication	Viral infection (Influenza)	[271]

ITCH	Dvl	Polyubiquitination (K48)	Proteasomal degradation	Cell signaling	Heart disease	[272]
				Wnt pathway	Cardiac hypertrophy	[273]
	PI4KIIα	Multiubiquitination	Frotein recruitment		Not reported	[274]
		Interaction	Target activation	Intracellular transport (endosomes)		
WWP1	PTEN	Polyubiquitination (K27)	Target oligomerization	Cell signaling	Prostate cancer	[275]
			Target localization	*Cell proliferation*	Cancer risk	[276]
WWP2	PTEN	Polyubiquitination	Degradation	Apoptosis	Gastric cancer	[236]
						[277]
UBE3A	Ephexin5	Ubiquitination	Proteasomal degradation	Brain and CNS activity	Angelman syndrome	[278]
					Alzheimer's disease	[279]
						[280]
E6AP	HCV core protein	Polyubiquitylation	Proteasomal degradation	Immune response	Hepatitis C virus infection	[281]
UBE3A	Arc	Ubiquitination	Proteasomal degradation	Brain and CNS activity	Angelman's syndrome	[282]
SMURF1	MEKK2	Ubiquitination	Proteasomal degradation	Differentiation (osteoblasts)	Bone inflammation disorders	[283]
						[284]
	Insulin receptor (INSR)			Metabolism	Not reported	[285]
						[286]
	RUNX2			Differentiation (osteoblasts)	Not reported	[287]
						[288]
	Id1			Cell signaling	Not reported	[289]
				Senescence		
	M. tuberculosis-associated structures	Polyubiquitination (K48)	Autophagolysosomal degradation	Immune response (anti-bacterial)	*M. tuberculosis* infection	[290]

(*Continued*)

Table 3.2 (Continued)

Ligase	Target	Effect	Outcome	Cellular function	Disease	References
SMURF2	Smad1/2	Polyubiquitination	Proteasomal degradation	Cell signaling (TGF-β pathway)	Esophageal squamous cell carcinoma	[291–294]
				Embryogenesis		
	SIRT1			Chromatin remodeling	Colorectal cancer	[295]
				Cell cycle and migration genes		
	SnoN			Transcription	Not reported	[296]
	β-TrCP1		Degradation	Cell signaling (KRAS)	Lung adenocarcinoma	[297]
	UBCH5	Monoubiquitination	Interaction	E3 activity		
			Stabilizes E2-E3 complex			
	NEDD9	Interaction	Target stability	Cell cycle	Not reported	[298]
				Mitotic entry		
HACE1	RAC1	Ubiquitination[a]	Degradation	Inflammation	Parkinson's disease	[299]
						[300]
	Ubiquitinated proteins	Interaction	Protein recruitment	Autophagy	Heart disease	[301]
HECTD3	STAT3	Polyubiquitination	Target activation	Differentiation	Autoimmunity	[302]
		(K27)	Promotes activating phosphorylation	Th17 cells		
	MALT1	Polyubiquitination (K27 and K29)	Unknown			
	TRAF3	Polyubiquitination (K63)	Protein recruitment	Immune response	Bacterial infection	[303]

HUWE1	N-myc	Ubiquitination	Froteasomal degradation	Transcription	Glioblastoma	[304]
				Differentiation HSCs	Tumor suppressor	[305]
	β-catenin			Cell signaling Wnt pathway	Intestinal cancer	[306]
	HDAC2			Chromatin remodeling	Not reported	[289]
	MYST2			Differentiation		[307]
	TGF-βR2[a]			Cell signaling	Gastric cancer	[294]
				Embryogenesis		[308]
	EGFR[a]			Cell signaling	Renal tubulointerstitial fibrosis	[309]
	Mcl-1	Polyubiquitination		Apoptosis	ID	[310]
						[311]
	p53			Cell growth and survival	Lung cancer	[312]
					ID	[313]
						[314]
						[311]

(*Continued*)

Table 3.2 (Continued)

Ligase	Target	Effect	Outcome	Cellular function	Disease	References
	H1, H2A, H2B, H3, and H4			Chromatin remodeling Spermatogenesis	Not reported	[315]
	Miz1	Polyubiquitination (K48)		Cell signaling TNFα pathway *Pro-apoptotic*	Cancer No specific type identified in humans; skin tumors used in mouse models	[252, 316]
	TIAM1			Cytoskeleton (cell-cell adhesion)	Lung cancer	[317]
	ATOH1			Transcription Differentiation Cochlear development	Not reported	[318]
	c-Myc	Polyubiquitination (K63)	Target activity regulation	Cell proliferation Transcription	Not reported	[319]
	Dvl		Prevents target oligomerization (inhibitory – oligomer required for activity)	Cell signaling Wnt pathway	Colon cancer[a] ID	[320] [321]
	HAUSP/USP7		Protein recruitment	Hypoxia response	Cancer (epithelial-mesenchymal transition [EMT] and metastasis)	[322]
	DNA Pol β	Monoubiquitination	Polyubiquitylation by CHIP	DNA repair (base excision)	Not reported	[323]
	γH2AX		Protein recruitment	DNA repair (replication stress)	Not reported	[324]

[a] Putative connection.

following polyubiquitylation by E6AP [281, 290]. E6AP is itself a viral target, with HCV protein E6 binding to it and redirecting its activity toward p53 to protect infected cells from apoptosis. In addition to their involvement with external pathogens, HECT E3s are also implicated in internal disease mechanisms. HACE1, for example, protects against the neuroinflammation seen in Parkinson's disease, while HECTD3 activity is linked with pathogenic Th17 cell differentiation in autoimmune conditions [299, 302].

Although these limited examples provide only a superficial insight into the functions fulfilled by HECT E3s, they serve to highlight the range of mechanisms used by the HECT ligases and the breadth of responses that could be influenced by targeting HECTs.

3.5 RING–IBR–RING (RBR)

3.5.1 Structure and Mechanism

RBR-type E3 ubiquitin ligases have been described recently. Three characteristic domains define RBR E3 ligases: RING1, IBR (in-between RING), and RING2 [325, 326]. Because of the presence of RING domains, RBRs were initially classified as RING-type E3 ligases [327, 328]. IBR and RING2 domains fold in a ring shape, but only RING1 is a canonical RING domain able to bind to a ubiquitin-charged E2 [325, 326]. RING2 is instead able to accept the ubiquitin molecule from the E2 because of the presence of an essential catalytic cysteine residue [329]. Thus, RBRs possess characteristics of both RING and HECT E3 ligases. They have a RING domain but, similarly to HECTs, use an E3–Ub intermediate before substrate ubiquitylation [329].

The 14 proteins containing an RBR domain vary significantly in the number and types of other domains in their N- and C-termini and thus their functions [330].The known RBRs are the following: Heme-oxidized IRP2 ubiquitin ligase 1L (HOIL-1L), HOIL-1 interaction protein (HOIP), RNF14, RNF19A, RNF19B, RNF144A, RNF144B, RNF216, RNF217, Ariadne homologue 1 (ARIH1), ARIH2, ankyrin repeat, and IBR domain-containing protein 1 (Ankib1), Parkinson protein 2 (PARK2), and Parkin-like cytoplasmic protein (PARC) [330, 331].

3.5.2 Insights into Their Regulation and Function

Although it is a small family of E3 ligases, RBRs have unique properties. For instance, HOIP (HOIL-1L interacting protein) is the catalytic member of the LUBAC (linear ubiquitin chain assembly complex), which is the only E3 ligase able to build linear ubiquitin chains (Met1 linkage) [332]. Another RBR, HOIL-1, is also part of the LUBAC but its role in linear ubiquitin chain assembly is not yet clear. HOIL-1 was also reported to catalyze the bond between the C-terminal Gly76 of a ubiquitin molecule to serine and threonine residues of target proteins, revealing novel examples of non-canonical lysine ubiquitylation of target substrates [333]. Other RBRs have been shown to catalyze non-K48 ubiquitylation, including a rather rare K6 linkage. However, more studies are needed to define whether the RBR conformation helps these enzymes shape non-canonical ubiquitin chains.

3.6 Conclusion and Insights into Drug Development

In this chapter, we attempt to provide a comprehensive overview of the known classes of E3s. Using selected examples, we highlight several mechanisms of recognition and action of E3s. The emerging picture is quite complex with multiple layers of regulation, highlighting that, to exploit the full potential of E3 targeting, it is necessary to have a thorough understanding of this class of enzymes.

There are multiple areas requiring further investigation. For instance, very little is known on how canonical and non-canonical ubiquitin chains are extended by E3s. Few E3 ligases have been shown to generate non-canonical ubiquitin chains compared to the complexity of the ubiquitin code identified through large-scale proteomic studies [334]. While diversification could be achieved through diverse E2–E3 combinations, ubiquitin chain diversification and extension would require specialized protein complexes. Based on the current data, it is possible to envision that more E3s are present in the genome besides the ones currently classified.

Further investigations are also necessary on the identification of linear and structural degrons. Our laboratory has revealed the first example of neomorphic mutations in E3s. In this case, we observe that cancer-associated mutations in the KBTBD4 CRL3 ubiquitin ligase drive the recognition of substrates not normally recognized by the KBTBD4 WT. Specifically, inframe insertion mutations in the Kelch domain of KBTBD4 alter substrate recognition, inducing the mutated E3 to ubiquitylate and degrade the chromatin remodeling CoREST complex [335]. While it is unclear whether this represents an oddity or a common feature of E3s, it expands the degron repertoire and paves the way to the generation of targeted PROTACs. The example above suggests that E3s have significant plasticity and adaptation properties (which might include redundancy). However, few studies have specifically addressed the mechanistic details that might drive this plasticity [336].

It is tantalizing to speculate that, like the plant auxin system, mammalian cells have developed similar processes where small molecules act as molecular glues to trigger trimolecular complex formation and targeted degradation. However, difficulties in identifying protein–molecule interactions have hampered progress in identifying degrons formed by small molecules. While PROTAC research has provided exciting developments and expansion in hijacking E3s to target neosubstrates, only a handful of molecular glues have been identified.

CRLs assemble multimeric complexes with good flexibility that might favor neosubstrate recognition. Studies on the mechanisms of resistance to PROTACs targeting CRLs revealed that the entire cullin system could be hampered [337, 338]. This observation implies that the effectiveness of all CRL-based PROTACs could be suppressed *via* a single resistance mutation. Thus, more efforts should be considered in developing drugs targeting non-CRL complexes, and more studies are necessary to establish the adaptability of non-CRL PROTACs to different substrates.

E3 ubiquitin ligases can employ a code to direct protein fates in a specific manner. The next frontier in targeted E3-based therapy may be to use the ubiquitin code with small molecules to shape protein localization and/or the recruitment of selected protein complexes.

Most drug development efforts are currently focusing on linker optimization between the molecule recruiting the E3 and the molecule recruiting the substrates to allow enough flexibility for ubiquitylation of the neosubstrate. However, we believe that once multiple E3s have their own cognate small molecules, chemical optimization can be diverted toward E3 ligases. In other words, molecules interacting with specific substrates can be optimized for degradation by selecting the most suitable E3 ligase (based on degradation profiles) rather than the linker. It is worth mentioning that E3 ligases could be chosen based on tissue and disease specificity in addition to degradation profiles. Overall, targeting E3 ubiquitin ligases is opening a new frontier in chemical targeting, but to obtain molecules with selected profiles, more studies are necessary to establish E3 substrates, catalytic mechanisms, and the regulation of E3s at cellular and tissue levels.

References

1 Hershko, A. and Ciechanover, A. (1998). The ubiquitin system. *Annu. Rev. Biochem.* 67: 425–479.

2 Komander, D. and Rape, M. (2012). The ubiquitin code. *Annu. Rev. Biochem.* 81: 203–229.

3 Wilkinson, K.D., Urban, M.K., and Haas, A.L. (1980). Ubiquitin is the ATP-dependent proteolysis factor I of rabbit reticulocytes. *J. Biol. Chem.* 255: 7529–7532.

4 Morreale, F.E. and Walden, H. (2016). Types of ubiquitin ligases. *Cell* 165: 248–248.e241.

5 Deshaies, R.J. and Joazeiro, C.A. (2009). RING domain E3 ubiquitin ligases. *Annu. Rev. Biochem.* 78: 399–434.

6 Jin, J., Li, X., Gygi, S.P., and Harper, J.W. (2007). Dual E1 activation systems for ubiquitin differentially regulate E2 enzyme charging. *Nature* 447: 1135–1138.

7 Ciechanover, A., Heller, H., Katz-Etzion, R., and Hershko, A. (1981). Activation of the heat-stable polypeptide of the ATP-dependent proteolytic system. *Proc. Natl. Acad. Sci. U.S.A.* 78: 761–765.

8 Emanuele, M.J. et al. (2011). Global identification of modular cullin-RING ligase substrates. *Cell* 147: 459–474.

9 Kim, W. et al. (2011). Systematic and quantitative assessment of the ubiquitin-modified proteome. *Mol. Cell* 44: 325–340.

10 Infante, P. et al. (2018). Itch/beta-arrestin2-dependent non-proteolytic ubiquitylation of SuFu controls Hedgehog signalling and medulloblastoma tumorigenesis. *Nat. Commun.* 9: 976.
11 Ge, Z. et al. (2018). Integrated genomic analysis of the ubiquitin pathway across cancer types. *Cell Rep.* 23: 213–226.e213.
12 Swatek, K.N. et al. (2019). Insights into ubiquitin chain architecture using Ub-clipping. *Nature* 572: 533–537.
13 Zheng, N. and Shabek, N. (2017). Ubiquitin ligases: structure, function, and regulation. *Annu. Rev. Biochem.* 86: 129–157.
14 Ravid, T. and Hochstrasser, M. (2008). Diversity of degradation signals in the ubiquitin–proteasome system. *Nat. Rev. Mol. Cell Biol.* 9: 679–690.
15 Yoshida, Y. et al. (2003). Fbs2 is a new member of the E3 ubiquitin ligase family that recognizes sugar chains. *J. Biol. Chem.* 278: 43877–43884.
16 Yoshida, Y. et al. (2002). E3 ubiquitin ligase that recognizes sugar chains. *Nature* 418: 438–442.
17 Manford, A.G. et al. (2021). Structural basis and regulation of the reductive stress response. *Cell* 184: 5375–5390.e5316.
18 Guardavaccaro, D. et al. (2003). Control of meiotic and mitotic progression by the F box protein beta-Trcp1 *in vivo*. *Dev. Cell* 4: 799–812.
19 Hao, B., Oehlmann, S., Sowa, M.E. et al. (2007). Structure of a Fbw7-Skp1-cyclin E complex: multisite-phosphorylated substrate recognition by SCF ubiquitin ligases. *Mol. Cell* 26: 131–143.
20 Wu, G. et al. (2003). Structure of a beta-TrCP1-Skp1-beta-catenin complex: destruction motif binding and lysine specificity of the SCF(beta-TrCP1) ubiquitin ligase. *Mol. Cell* 11: 1445–1456.
21 D'Angiolella, V. et al. (2012). Cyclin F-mediated degradation of ribonucleotide reductase M2 controls genome integrity and DNA repair. *Cell* 149: 1023–1034.
22 Ivan, M. et al. (2001). HIFalpha targeted for VHL-mediated destruction by proline hydroxylation: implications for O_2 sensing. *Science* 292: 464–468.
23 Jaakkola, P. et al. (2001). Targeting of HIF-alpha to the von Hippel-Lindau ubiquitylation complex by O_2-regulated prolyl hydroxylation. *Science* 292: 468–472.
24 Bachmair, A., Finley, D., and Varshavsky, A. (1986). *in vivo* half-life of a protein is a function of its amino-terminal residue. *Science* 234: 179–186.
25 Lin, H.C. et al. (2018). C-terminal end-directed protein elimination by CRL2 ubiquitin ligases. *Mol. Cell* 70: 602–613.e603.
26 Varshavsky, A. (2019). N-degron and C-degron pathways of protein degradation. *Proc. Natl. Acad. Sci. U.S.A.* 116: 358–366.
27 Timms, R.T. and Koren, I. (2020). Tying up loose ends: the N-degron and C-degron pathways of protein degradation. *Biochem. Soc. Trans.* 48: 1557–1567.
28 Koren, I. et al. (2018). The eukaryotic proteome is shaped by E3 ubiquitin ligases targeting C-terminal degrons. *Cell* 173: 1622–1635.e1614.
29 Ravalin, M. et al. (2019). Specificity for latent C termini links the E3 ubiquitin ligase CHIP to caspases. *Nat. Chem. Biol.* 15: 786–794.

30 Timms, R.T. et al. (2019). A glycine-specific N-degron pathway mediates the quality control of protein N-myristoylation. *Science* 365: eaaw4912. https://doi.org/10.1126/science.aaw4912.

31 Yeh, C.W. et al. (2021). The C-degron pathway eliminates mislocalized proteins and products of deubiquitinating enzymes. *EMBO J.* 40: e105846.

32 Tran, A. (2019). The N-end rule pathway and Ubr1 enforce protein compartmentalization via P2-encoded cellular location signals. *J. Cell Sci.* 132.

33 Alborzi, S.Z., Ahmed Nacer, A., Najjar, H. et al. (2021). PPIDomainMiner: inferring domain-domain interactions from multiple sources of protein-protein interactions. *PLoS Comput. Biol.* 17: e1008844.

34 Stelzl, U. et al. (2005). A human protein-protein interaction network: a resource for annotating the proteome. *Cell* 122: 957–968.

35 Xing, W. et al. (2013). SCF(FBXL3) ubiquitin ligase targets cryptochromes at their cofactor pocket. *Nature* 496: 64–68.

36 Zeng, Z. et al. (2010). Structural basis of selective ubiquitination of TRF1 by SCFFbx4. *Dev. Cell* 18: 214–225.

37 Shearer, A.G. and Hampton, R.Y. (2005). Lipid-mediated, reversible misfolding of a sterol-sensing domain protein. *EMBO J.* 24: 149–159.

38 Song, B.L., Sever, N., and DeBose-Boyd, R.A. (2005). Gp78, a membrane-anchored ubiquitin ligase, associates with Insig-1 and couples sterol-regulated ubiquitination to degradation of HMG CoA reductase. *Mol. Cell* 19: 829–840.

39 Tan, X. et al. (2007). Mechanism of auxin perception by the TIR1 ubiquitin ligase. *Nature* 446: 640–645.

40 Zhang, S. et al. (2016). Molecular mechanism of APC/C activation by mitotic phosphorylation. *Nature* 533: 260–264.

41 Debonneville, C. et al. (2001). Phosphorylation of Nedd4-2 by Sgk1 regulates epithelial Na(+) channel cell surface expression. *EMBO J.* 20: 7052–7059.

42 Duda, D.M. et al. (2008). Structural insights into NEDD8 activation of cullin-RING ligases: conformational control of conjugation. *Cell* 134: 995–1006.

43 Baek, K., Scott, D.C., and Schulman, B.A. (2021). NEDD8 and ubiquitin ligation by cullin-RING E3 ligases. *Curr. Opin. Struct. Biol.* 67: 101–109.

44 Wang, Z. et al. (2012). Recognition of the iso-ADP-ribose moiety in poly(ADP-ribose) by WWE domains suggests a general mechanism for poly(ADP-ribosyl)ation-dependent ubiquitination. *Genes Dev.* 26: 235–240.

45 DaRosa, P.A. et al. (2015). Allosteric activation of the RNF146 ubiquitin ligase by a poly(ADP-ribosyl)ation signal. *Nature* 517: 223–226.

46 Zhang, Y. et al. (2011). RNF146 is a poly(ADP-ribose)-directed E3 ligase that regulates axin degradation and Wnt signalling. *Nat. Cell Biol.* 13: 623–629.

47 Chatrin, C. et al. (2020). Structural insights into ADP-ribosylation of ubiquitin by Deltex family E3 ubiquitin ligases. *Sci. Adv.* 6.

48 Freemont, P.S., Hanson, I.M., and Trowsdale, J. (1991). A novel cysteine-rich sequence motif. *Cell* 64: 483–484.

49 Barlow, P.N., Luisi, B., Milner, A. et al. (1994). Structure of the C_3HC_4 domain by ^{1}H-nuclear magnetic resonance spectroscopy. A new structural class of zinc-finger. *J. Mol. Biol.* 237: 201–211.

50 Bailly, V., Lauder, S., Prakash, S., and Prakash, L. (1997). Yeast DNA repair proteins Rad6 and Rad18 form a heterodimer that has ubiquitin conjugating, DNA binding, and ATP hydrolytic activities. *J. Biol. Chem.* 272: 23360–23365.

51 Zheng, N. et al. (2002). Structure of the Cul1-Rbx1-Skp1-F boxSkp2 SCF ubiquitin ligase complex. *Nature* 416: 703–709.

52 Aravind, L. and Koonin, E.V. (2000). The U box is a modified RING finger - a common domain in ubiquitination. *Curr. Biol.* 10: R132–R134.

53 Hatakeyama, S. and Nakayama, K.I. (2003). U-box proteins as a new family of ubiquitin ligases. *Biochem. Biophys. Res. Commun.* 302: 635–645.

54 Vander Kooi, C.W. et al. (2006). The Prp19 U-box crystal structure suggests a common dimeric architecture for a class of oligomeric E3 ubiquitin ligases. *Biochemistry* 45: 121–130.

55 Joazeiro, C.A. et al. (1999). The tyrosine kinase negative regulator c-Cbl as a RING-type, E2-dependent ubiquitin-protein ligase. *Science* 286: 309–312.

56 Kamura, T. et al. (1999). Rbx1, a component of the VHL tumor suppressor complex and SCF ubiquitin ligase. *Science* 284: 657–661.

57 Levkowitz, G. et al. (1999). Ubiquitin ligase activity and tyrosine phosphorylation underlie suppression of growth factor signaling by c-Cbl/Sli-1. *Mol. Cell* 4: 1029–1040.

58 Lorick, K.L. et al. (1999). RING fingers mediate ubiquitin-conjugating enzyme (E2)-dependent ubiquitination. *Proc. Natl. Acad. Sci. U.S.A.* 96: 11364–11369.

59 Ohta, T., Michel, J.J., Schottelius, A.J., and Xiong, Y. (1999). ROC1, a homolog of APC11, represents a family of cullin partners with an associated ubiquitin ligase activity. *Mol. Cell* 3: 535–541.

60 Seol, J.H. et al. (1999). Cdc53/cullin and the essential Hrt1 RING-H2 subunit of SCF define a ubiquitin ligase module that activates the E2 enzyme Cdc34. *Genes Dev.* 13: 1614–1626.

61 Skowyra, D. et al. (1999). Reconstitution of G1 cyclin ubiquitination with complexes containing SCFGrr1 and Rbx1. *Science* 284: 662–665.

62 Tan, P. et al. (1999). Recruitment of a ROC1-CUL1 ubiquitin ligase by Skp1 and HOS to catalyze the ubiquitination of I kappa B alpha. *Mol. Cell* 3: 527–533.

63 Xie, Y. and Varshavsky, A. (1999). The E2-E3 interaction in the N-end rule pathway: the RING-H2 finger of E3 is required for the synthesis of multiubiquitin chain. *EMBO J.* 18: 6832–6844.

64 Yokouchi, M. et al. (1999). Ligand-induced ubiquitination of the epidermal growth factor receptor involves the interaction of the c-Cbl RING finger and UbcH7. *J. Biol. Chem.* 274: 31707–31712.

65 Hundley, F.V. et al. (2021). A comprehensive phenotypic CRISPR-Cas9 screen of the ubiquitin pathway uncovers roles of ubiquitin ligases in mitosis. *Mol. Cell* 81: 1319–1336.e1319.

66 Sun, Y., Wei, W., and Jin, J. (2020). *Cullin-RING Ligases and Protein Neddylation.* Springer.

67 Fouad, S., Wells, O.S., Hill, M.A., and D'Angiolella, V. (2019). Cullin ring ubiquitin ligases (CRLs) in cancer: responses to ionizing radiation (IR) treatment. *Front. Physiol.* 10: 1144.

68 Jin, J. et al. (2004). Systematic analysis and nomenclature of mammalian F-box proteins. *Genes Dev.* 18: 2573–2580.

69 Linossi, E.M. and Nicholson, S.E. (2012). The SOCS box-adapting proteins for ubiquitination and proteasomal degradation. *IUBMB Life* 64: 316–323.

70 Stogios, P.J., Downs, G.S., Jauhal, J.J. et al. (2005). Sequence and structural analysis of BTB domain proteins. *Genome Biol.* 6: R82.

71 He, Y.J., McCall, C.M., Hu, J. et al. (2006). DDB1 functions as a linker to recruit receptor WD40 proteins to CUL4-ROC1 ubiquitin ligases. *Genes Dev.* 20: 2949–2954.

72 Scheufele, F. et al. (2014). Evidence for a regulatory role of cullin-RING E3 ubiquitin ligase 7 in insulin signaling. *Cell Signal.* 26: 233–239.

73 Read, M.A. et al. (2000). Nedd8 modification of cul-1 activates SCF(beta(TrCP))-dependent ubiquitination of IkappaBalpha. *Mol. Cell. Biol.* 20: 2326–2333.

74 Baek, K. et al. (2020). NEDD8 nucleates a multivalent cullin-RING-UBE2D ubiquitin ligation assembly. *Nature* 578: 461–466.

75 Serpico, A.F. and Grieco, D. (2020). Recent advances in understanding the role of Cdk1 in the Spindle Assembly Checkpoint. *F1000Res* 9.

76 Watson, E.R., Brown, N.G., Peters, J.M. et al. (2019). Posing the APC/C E3 ubiquitin ligase to orchestrate cell division. *Trends Cell Biol.* 29: 117–134.

77 Barford, D. (2020). Structural interconversions of the anaphase-promoting complex/cyclosome (APC/C) regulate cell cycle transitions. *Curr. Opin. Struct. Biol.* 61: 86–97.

78 Shen, J. et al. (2018). The E3 ligase RING1 targets p53 for degradation and promotes cancer cell proliferation and survival. *Cancer Res.* 78: 359–371.

79 Scelfo, A. et al. (2019). Functional landscape of PCGF proteins reveals both RING1A/B-dependent-and RING1A/B-independent-specific activities. *Mol. Cell* 74: 1037–1052.e1037.

80 Johnsen, S.A. et al. (2009). Regulation of estrogen-dependent transcription by the LIM cofactors CLIM and RLIM in breast cancer. *Cancer Res.* 69: 128–136.

81 Liu, Z. et al. (2009). Human BRE1 is an E3 ubiquitin ligase for Ebp1 tumor suppressor. *Mol. Biol. Cell* 20: 757–768.

82 Zhu, B. et al. (2005). Monoubiquitination of human histone H2B: the factors involved and their roles in HOX gene regulation. *Mol. Cell* 20: 601–611.

83 Sheren, J.E. and Kassenbrock, C.K. (2013). RNF38 encodes a nuclear ubiquitin protein ligase that modifies p53. *Biochem. Biophys. Res. Commun.* 440: 473–478.

84 Haselbach, D. et al. (2018). Structure and conformational dynamics of the human spliceosomal B(act) complex. *Cell* 172: 454–464.e411.

85 Brickner, J.R. et al. (2017). A ubiquitin-dependent signalling axis specific for ALKBH-mediated DNA dealkylation repair. *Nature* 551: 389–393.

86 Lear, T. et al. (2017). RING finger protein 113A regulates C-X-C chemokine receptor type 4 stability and signaling. *Am. J. Physiol. Cell Physiol.* 313: C584–C592.

87 Kelly, C.E. et al. (2013). Rnf165/Ark2C enhances BMP-Smad signaling to mediate motor axon extension. *PLoS Biol.* 11: e1001538.

88 Doil, C. et al. (2009). RNF168 binds and amplifies ubiquitin conjugates on damaged chromosomes to allow accumulation of repair proteins. *Cell* 136: 435–446.

89 Pinato, S., Gatti, M., Scandiuzzi, C. et al. (2011). UMI, a novel RNF168 ubiquitin binding domain involved in the DNA damage signaling pathway. *Mol. Cell. Biol.* 31: 118–126.

90 Mattiroli, F. et al. (2012). RNF168 ubiquitinates K13-15 on H2A/H2AX to drive DNA damage signaling. *Cell* 150: 1182–1195.

91 Mallette, F.A. et al. (2012). RNF8- and RNF168-dependent degradation of KDM4A/JMJD2A triggers 53BP1 recruitment to DNA damage sites. *EMBO J.* 31: 1865–1878.

92 Chen, J., Feng, W., Jiang, J. et al. (2012). Ring finger protein RNF169 antagonizes the ubiquitin-dependent signaling cascade at sites of DNA damage. *J. Biol. Chem.* 287: 27715–27722.

93 Poulsen, M., Lukas, C., Lukas, J. et al. (2012). Human RNF169 is a negative regulator of the ubiquitin-dependent response to DNA double-strand breaks. *J. Cell Biol.* 197: 189–199.

94 Panier, S. et al. (2012). Tandem protein interaction modules organize the ubiquitin-dependent response to DNA double-strand breaks. *Mol. Cell* 47: 383–395.

95 Cai, Y. et al. (2010). Subunit composition and substrate specificity of a MOF-containing histone acetyltransferase distinct from the male-specific lethal (MSL) complex. *J. Biol. Chem.* 285: 4268–4272.

96 Ismail, I.H. et al. (2015). The RNF138 E3 ligase displaces Ku to promote DNA end resection and regulate DNA repair pathway choice. *Nat. Cell Biol.* 17: 1446–1457.

97 Schmidt, C.K. et al. (2015). Systematic E2 screening reveals a UBE2D-RNF138-CtIP axis promoting DNA repair. *Nat. Cell Biol.* 17: 1458–1470.

98 Yamada, M. et al. (2006). NARF, an nemo-like kinase (NLK)-associated ring finger protein regulates the ubiquitylation and degradation of T cell factor/lymphoid enhancer factor (TCF/LEF). *J. Biol. Chem.* 281: 20749–20760.

99 Coulombe, P. et al. (2019). The ORC ubiquitin ligase OBI1 promotes DNA replication origin firing. *Nat. Commun.* 10: 2426.

100 Gaudet, P., Livstone, M.S., Lewis, S.E., and Thomas, P.D. (2011). Phylogenetic-based propagation of functional annotations within the gene ontology consortium. *Brief. Bioinform.* 12: 449–462.

101 Tatham, M.H. et al. (2008). RNF4 is a poly-SUMO-specific E3 ubiquitin ligase required for arsenic-induced PML degradation. *Nat. Cell Biol.* 10: 538–546.

102 Guo, B. and Sharrocks, A.D. (2009). Extracellular signal-regulated kinase mitogen-activated protein kinase signaling initiates a dynamic interplay between sumoylation and ubiquitination to regulate the activity of the transcriptional activator PEA3. *Mol. Cell. Biol.* 29: 3204–3218.

103 van Hagen, M., Overmeer, R.M., Abolvardi, S.S., and Vertegaal, A.C. (2010). RNF4 and VHL regulate the proteasomal degradation of SUMO-conjugated hypoxia-inducible factor-2alpha. *Nucleic Acids Res.* 38: 1922–1931.

104 Mukhopadhyay, D., Arnaoutov, A., and Dasso, M. (2010). The SUMO protease SENP6 is essential for inner kinetochore assembly. *J. Cell Biol.* 188: 681–692.

105 Kaiser, F.J., Moroy, T., Chang, G.T. et al. (2003). The RING finger protein RNF4, a co-regulator of transcription, interacts with the TRPS1 transcription factor. *J. Biol. Chem.* 278: 38780–38785.

106 Tursun, B. et al. (2005). The ubiquitin ligase Rnf6 regulates local LIM kinase 1 levels in axonal growth cones. *Genes Dev.* 19: 2307–2319.

107 Xu, K. et al. (2009). Regulation of androgen receptor transcriptional activity and specificity by RNF6-induced ubiquitination. *Cancer Cell* 15: 270–282.

108 Zhang, S. et al. (2013). Identification of RNF8 as a ubiquitin ligase involved in targeting the p12 subunit of DNA polymerase delta for degradation in response to DNA damage. *J. Biol. Chem.* 288: 2941–2950.

109 Mailand, N. et al. (2007). RNF8 ubiquitylates histones at DNA double-strand breaks and promotes assembly of repair proteins. *Cell* 131: 887–900.

110 Zhang, S. et al. (2008). PCNA is ubiquitinated by RNF8. *Cell Cycle* 7: 3399–3404.

111 Hoshikawa, S., Ogata, T., Fujiwara, S. et al. (2008). A novel function of RING finger protein 10 in transcriptional regulation of the myelin-associated glycoprotein gene and myelin formation in Schwann cells. *PLoS One* 3: e3464.

112 Lin, J. et al. (2005). Characterization of mesenchyme Homeobox 2 (MEOX2) transcription factor binding to RING finger protein 10. *Mol. Cell. Biochem.* 275: 75–84.

113 Garzia, A., Meyer, C., and Tuschl, T. (2021). The E3 ubiquitin ligase RNF10 modifies 40S ribosomal subunits of ribosomes compromised in translation. *Cell Rep.* 36: 109468.

114 Pan, J. et al. (2005). RNF17, a component of the mammalian germ cell nuage, is essential for spermiogenesis. *Development* 132: 4029–4039.

115 Yin, X.Y., Gupta, K., Han, W.P. et al. (1999). Mmip-2, a novel RING finger protein that interacts with mad members of the Myc oncoprotein network. *Oncogene* 18: 6621–6634.

116 Ding, W. et al. (2008). EGF receptor-independent action of TGF-alpha protects Naked2 from AO7-mediated ubiquitylation and proteasomal degradation. *Proc. Natl. Acad. Sci. U.S.A.* 105: 13433–13438.

117 Liu, W. et al. (2006). Axin is a scaffold protein in TGF-beta signaling that promotes degradation of Smad7 by Arkadia. *EMBO J.* 25: 1646–1658.

118 Poulsen, S.L. et al. (2013). RNF111/Arkadia is a SUMO-targeted ubiquitin ligase that facilitates the DNA damage response. *J. Cell Biol.* 201: 797–807.

119 Koinuma, D. et al. (2003). Arkadia amplifies TGF-beta superfamily signalling through degradation of Smad7. *EMBO J.* 22: 6458–6470.

120 Han, J. et al. (2013). ZNF313 is a novel cell cycle activator with an E3 ligase activity inhibiting cellular senescence by destabilizing p21(WAF1.). *Cell Death Differ.* 20: 1055–1067.

121 Wang, S. et al. (2016). RNF123 has an E3 ligase-independent function in RIG-I-like receptor-mediated antiviral signaling. *EMBO Rep.* 17: 1155–1168.

122 Kamura, T. et al. (2004). Cytoplasmic ubiquitin ligase KPC regulates proteolysis of p27(Kip1) at G1 phase. *Nat. Cell Biol.* 6: 1229–1235.

123 Zhi, X. et al. (2013). E3 ubiquitin ligase RNF126 promotes cancer cell proliferation by targeting the tumor suppressor p21 for ubiquitin-mediated degradation. *Cancer Res.* 73: 385–394.

124 Callow, M.G. et al. (2011). Ubiquitin ligase RNF146 regulates tankyrase and Axin to promote Wnt signaling. *PLoS One* 6: e22595.

125 Kang, H.C. et al. (2011). Iduna is a poly(ADP-ribose) (PAR)-dependent E3 ubiquitin ligase that regulates DNA damage. *Proc. Natl. Acad. Sci. U.S.A.* 108: 14103–14108.

126 Nian, H. et al. (2007). RNF151, a testis-specific RING finger protein, interacts with dysbindin. *Arch. Biochem. Biophys.* 465: 157–163.

127 Davies, C.C. et al. (2010). Identification of a co-activator that links growth factor signalling to c-Jun/AP-1 activation. *Nat. Cell Biol.* 12: 963–972.

128 Pang, K. et al. (2019). RNF208, an estrogen-inducible E3 ligase, targets soluble vimentin to suppress metastasis in triple-negative breast cancers. *Nat. Commun.* 10: 5805.

129 McDonald, E.R. III and El-Deiry, W.S. (2004). Suppression of caspase-8- and −10-associated RING proteins results in sensitization to death ligands and inhibition of tumor cell growth. *Proc. Natl. Acad. Sci. U.S.A.* 101: 6170–6175.

130 Yang, W. et al. (2007). CARPs are ubiquitin ligases that promote MDM2-independent p53 and phospho-p53ser20 degradation. *J. Biol. Chem.* 282: 3273–3281.

131 Wei, P., Pan, D., Mao, C., and Wang, Y.X. (2012). RNF34 is a cold-regulated E3 ubiquitin ligase for PGC-1alpha and modulates brown fat cell metabolism. *Mol. Cell. Biol.* 32: 266–275.

132 Zhang, R. et al. (2014). The E3 ligase RNF34 is a novel negative regulator of the NOD1 pathway. *Cell. Physiol. Biochem.* 33: 1954–1962.

133 Connor, M.K., Azmi, P.B., Subramaniam, V. et al. (2005). Molecular characterization of ring finger protein 11. *Mol. Cancer Res.* 3: 453–461.

134 Scharaw, S. et al. (2016). The endosomal transcriptional regulator RNF11 integrates degradation and transport of EGFR. *J. Cell Biol.* 215: 543–558.

135 Koo, B.K. et al. (2012). Tumour suppressor RNF43 is a stem-cell E3 ligase that induces endocytosis of Wnt receptors. *Nature* 488: 665–669.

136 van Baren, M.J. et al. (2002). A double RING-H2 domain in RNF32, a gene expressed during sperm formation. *Biochem. Biophys. Res. Commun.* 292: 58–65.

137 Wang, W. et al. (2021). RNF39 mediates K48-linked ubiquitination of DDX3X and inhibits RLR-dependent antiviral immunity. *Sci. Adv.* 7.

138 Guais, A. et al. (2006). h-Goliath, paralog of GRAIL, is a new E3 ligase protein, expressed in human leukocytes. *Gene* 374: 112–120.

139 Matz, A. et al. (2015). Regulation of neuronal survival and morphology by the E3 ubiquitin ligase RNF157. *Cell Death Differ.* 22: 626–642.

140 Dogan, T. et al. (2017). Role of the E3 ubiquitin ligase RNF157 as a novel downstream effector linking PI3K and MAPK signaling pathways to the cell cycle. *J. Biol. Chem.* 292: 14311–14324.

141 Chen, H.W. et al. (2015). Ring finger protein 166 potentiates RNA virus-induced interferon-beta production via enhancing the ubiquitination of TRAF3 and TRAF6. *Sci. Rep.* 5: 14770.

142 Yamada, H.Y. and Gorbsky, G.J. (2006). Tumor suppressor candidate TSSC5 is regulated by UbcH6 and a novel ubiquitin ligase RING105. *Oncogene* 25: 1330–1339.

143 Brophy, T.M. et al. (2008). RN181, a novel ubiquitin E3 ligase that interacts with the KVGFFKR motif of platelet integrin alpha(IIb)beta3. *Biochem. Biophys. Res. Commun.* 369: 1088–1093.

144 Liu, Q.Y., Lei, J.X., Sikorska, M., and Liu, R. (2008). A novel brain-enriched E3 ubiquitin ligase RNF182 is up regulated in the brains of Alzheimer's patients and targets ATP6V0C for degradation. *Mol. Neurodegener* 3: 4.

145 Cao, Y., Sun, Y., Chang, H. et al. (2019). The E3 ubiquitin ligase RNF182 inhibits TLR-triggered cytokine production through promoting p65 ubiquitination and degradation. *FEBS Lett.* 593: 3210–3219.

146 Roder, K. et al. (2014). RING finger protein RNF207, a novel regulator of cardiac excitation. *J. Biol. Chem.* 289: 33730–33740.

147 Liu, W. et al. (2011). Identification of RNF213 as a susceptibility gene for moyamoya disease and its possible role in vascular development. *PLoS One* 6: e22542.

148 Otten, E.G. et al. (2021). Ubiquitylation of lipopolysaccharide by RNF213 during bacterial infection. *Nature* 594: 111–116.

149 Kong, Q. et al. (2010). RNF220, an E3 ubiquitin ligase that targets Sin3B for ubiquitination. *Biochem. Biophys. Res. Commun.* 393: 708–713.

150 Gao, D. et al. (2009). REUL is a novel E3 ubiquitin ligase and stimulator of retinoic-acid-inducible gene-I. *PLoS One* 4: e5760.

151 Oshiumi, H., Miyashita, M., Matsumoto, M., and Seya, T. (2013). A distinct role of Riplet-mediated K63-linked polyubiquitination of the RIG-I repressor domain in human antiviral innate immune responses. *PLoS Pathog.* 9: e1003533.

152 Oshiumi, H., Matsumoto, M., Hatakeyama, S., and Seya, T. (2009). Riplet/RNF135, a RING finger protein, ubiquitinates RIG-I to promote interferon-beta induction during the early phase of viral infection. *J. Biol. Chem.* 284: 807–817.

153 Qiu, X.B. and Goldberg, A.L. (2002). Nrdp1/FLRF is a ubiquitin ligase promoting ubiquitination and degradation of the epidermal growth factor receptor family member, ErbB3. *Proc. Natl. Acad. Sci. U.S.A.* 99: 14843–14848.

154 Qiu, X.B., Markant, S.L., Yuan, J., and Goldberg, A.L. (2004). Nrdp1-mediated degradation of the gigantic IAP, BRUCE, is a novel pathway for triggering apoptosis. *EMBO J.* 23: 800–810.

155 Meng, Z. et al. (2021). A20/Nrdp1 interaction alters the inflammatory signaling profile by mediating K48- and K63-linked polyubiquitination of effectors MyD88 and TBK1. *J. Biol. Chem.* 297: 100811.

156 Jing, X., Infante, J., Nachtman, R.G., and Jurecic, R. (2008). E3 ligase FLRF (Rnf41) regulates differentiation of hematopoietic progenitors by governing steady-state levels of cytokine and retinoic acid receptors. *Exp. Hematol.* 36: 1110–1120.

157 Arshad, M. et al. (2013). RNF13, a RING finger protein, mediates endoplasmic reticulum stress-induced apoptosis through the inositol-requiring enzyme (IRE1alpha)/c-Jun NH2-terminal kinase pathway. *J. Biol. Chem.* 288: 8726–8736.

158 Jin, X., Cheng, H., Chen, J., and Zhu, D. (2011). RNF13: an emerging RING finger ubiquitin ligase important in cell proliferation. *FEBS J.* 278: 78–84.

159 Maruyama, Y., Yamada, M., Takahashi, K., and Yamada, M. (2008). Ubiquitin ligase Kf-1 is involved in the endoplasmic reticulum-associated degradation pathway. *Biochem. Biophys. Res. Commun.* 374: 737–741.

160 Nian, H. et al. (2008). Mouse RING finger protein Rnf133 is a testis-specific endoplasmic reticulum-associated E3 ubiquitin ligase. *Cell Res.* 18: 800–802.

161 Gemmill, R.M. et al. (2002). The TRC8 hereditary kidney cancer gene suppresses growth and functions with VHL in a common pathway. *Oncogene* 21: 3507–3516.

162 Jo, Y., Lee, P.C., Sguigna, P.V., and DeBose-Boyd, R.A. (2011). Sterol-induced degradation of HMG CoA reductase depends on interplay of two Insigs and two ubiquitin ligases, gp78 and Trc8. *Proc. Natl. Acad. Sci. U.S.A.* 108: 20503–20508.

163 Jo, Y., Hartman, I.Z., and DeBose-Boyd, R.A. (2013). Ancient ubiquitous protein-1 mediates sterol-induced ubiquitination of 3-hydroxy-3-methylglutaryl CoA reductase in lipid droplet-associated endoplasmic reticulum membranes. *Mol. Biol. Cell* 24: 169–183.

164 Lee, J.P. et al. (2010). The TRC8 ubiquitin ligase is sterol regulated and interacts with lipid and protein biosynthetic pathways. *Mol. Cancer Res.* 8: 93–106.

165 Stagg, H.R. et al. (2009). The TRC8 E3 ligase ubiquitinates MHC class I molecules before dislocation from the ER. *J. Cell Biol.* 186: 685–692.

166 Zhang, L. et al. (2017). Inhibition of cholesterol biosynthesis through RNF145-dependent ubiquitination of SCAP. *Elife* 6.

167 Jiang, L.Y. et al. (2018). Ring finger protein 145 (RNF145) is a ubiquitin ligase for sterol-induced degradation of HMG-CoA reductase. *J. Biol. Chem.* 293: 4047–4055.

168 Fenech, E.J. et al. (2020). Interaction mapping of endoplasmic reticulum ubiquitin ligases identifies modulators of innate immune signalling. *Elife* 9.

169 Lu, J.P., Wang, Y., Sliter, D.A. et al. (2011). RNF170 protein, an endoplasmic reticulum membrane ubiquitin ligase, mediates inositol 1,4,5-trisphosphate receptor ubiquitination and degradation. *J. Biol. Chem.* 286: 24426–24433.

170 Song, X. et al. (2020). E3 ubiquitin ligase RNF170 inhibits innate immune responses by targeting and degrading TLR3 in murine cells. *Cell. Mol. Immunol.* 17: 865–874.

171 Wang, P., Wu, Y., Li, Y. et al. (2013). A novel RING finger E3 ligase RNF186 regulate ER stress-mediated apoptosis through interaction with BNip1. *Cell. Signal.* 25: 2320–2333.

172 Jongsma, M.L. et al. (2016). An ER-associated pathway defines endosomal architecture for controlled cargo transport. *Cell* 166: 152–166.

173 Qin, Y. et al. (2014). RNF26 temporally regulates virus-triggered type I interferon induction by two distinct mechanisms. *PLoS Pathog.* 10: e1004358.

174 Matsuda, N., Suzuki, T., Tanaka, K., and Nakano, A. (2001). Rma1, a novel type of RING finger protein conserved from Arabidopsis to human, is a membrane-bound ubiquitin ligase. *J. Cell Sci.* 114: 1949–1957.

175 Didier, C. et al. (2003). RNF5, a RING finger protein that regulates cell motility by targeting paxillin ubiquitination and altered localization. *Mol. Cell. Biol.* 23: 5331–5345.

176 Zhang, Y., Higashide, W., Dai, S. et al. (2005). Recognition and ubiquitination of *Salmonella* type III effector SopA by a ubiquitin E3 ligase, HsRMA1. *J. Biol. Chem.* 280: 38682–38688.

177 Tcherpakov, M. et al. (2009). Regulation of endoplasmic reticulum-associated degradation by RNF5-dependent ubiquitination of JNK-associated membrane protein (JAMP). *J. Biol. Chem.* 284: 12099–12109.

178 Zhong, B. et al. (2009). The ubiquitin ligase RNF5 regulates antiviral responses by mediating degradation of the adaptor protein MITA. *Immunity* 30: 397–407.

179 Tang, F. et al. (2011). RNF185, a novel mitochondrial ubiquitin E3 ligase, regulates autophagy through interaction with BNIP1. *PLoS One* 6: e24367.

180 El Khouri, E., Le Pavec, G., Toledano, M.B., and Delaunay-Moisan, A. (2013). RNF185 is a novel E3 ligase of endoplasmic reticulum-associated degradation (ERAD) that targets cystic fibrosis transmembrane conductance regulator (CFTR). *J. Biol. Chem.* 288: 31177–31191.

181 Wang, L. et al. (2006). Cloning, expression and subcellular localization of a novel human gene-RNF122. *Beijing Da Xue Xue Bao Yi Xue Ban* 38: 239–243.

182 Wu, Y. et al. (2018). Transmembrane E3 ligase RNF183 mediates ER stress-induced apoptosis by degrading Bcl-xL. *Proc. Natl. Acad. Sci. U.S.A.* 115: E2762–E2771.

183 Ichikawa, D., Mizuno, M., Yamamura, T., and Miyake, S. (2011). GRAIL (gene related to anergy in lymphocytes) regulates cytoskeletal reorganization through ubiquitination and degradation of Arp2/3 subunit 5 and coronin 1A. *J. Biol. Chem.* 286: 43465–43474.

184 Anandasabapathy, N. et al. (2003). GRAIL: an E3 ubiquitin ligase that inhibits cytokine gene transcription is expressed in anergic CD4+ T cells. *Immunity* 18: 535–547.

185 Lussier, M.P., Lepage, P.K., Bousquet, S.M., and Boulay, G. (2008). RNF24, a new TRPC interacting protein, causes the intracellular retention of TRPC. *Cell Calcium* 43: 432–443.

186 Arimoto, K. et al. (2007). Negative regulation of the RIG-I signaling by the ubiquitin ligase RNF125. *Proc. Natl. Acad. Sci. U.S.A.* 104: 7500–7505.

187 Giannini, A.L., Gao, Y., and Bijlmakers, M.J. (2008). T-cell regulator RNF125/TRAC-1 belongs to a novel family of ubiquitin ligases with zinc fingers and a ubiquitin-binding domain. *Biochem. J.* 410: 101–111.

188 Kim, H. et al. (2015). Downregulation of the ubiquitin ligase RNF125 underlies resistance of melanoma cells to BRAF inhibitors via JAK1 deregulation. *Cell Rep.* 11: 1458–1473.

189 Yang, L. et al. (2015). RNF125 is a ubiquitin-protein ligase that promotes p53 degradation. *Cell. Physiol. Biochem.* 35: 237–245.

190 Deng, L. et al. (2015). The ubiquitination of RagA GTPase by RNF152 negatively regulates mTORC1 activation. *Mol. Cell* 58: 804–818.

191 Zhang, S. et al. (2010). RNF152, a novel lysosome localized E3 ligase with pro-apoptotic activities. *Protein Cell* 1: 656–663.

192 Li, Y.Y. et al. (2017). Degradation of AMPK-alpha1 sensitizes BRAF inhibitor-resistant melanoma cells to arginine deprivation. *Mol. Oncol.* 11: 1806–1825.

193 Hong, S.W. et al. (2012). Ring finger protein 149 is an E3 ubiquitin ligase active on wild-type v-Raf murine sarcoma viral oncogene homolog B1 (BRAF). *J. Biol. Chem.* 287: 24017–24025.

194 Wu, Y. et al. (2021). Development of an individualized ubiquitin prognostic signature for clear cell renal cell carcinoma. *Front. Cell Dev. Biol.* 9: 684643.

195 Liu, D. et al. (2021). Identification of hub ubiquitin ligase genes affecting Alzheimer's disease by analyzing transcriptome data from multiple brain regions. *Sci. Prog.* 104, https://doi.org/10.1177/00368504211001146.

196 Choudhury, R. et al. (2016). APC/C and SCF(cyclin F) constitute a reciprocal feedback circuit controlling S-phase entry. *Cell Rep.* 16: 3359–3372.

197 Choudhury, R. et al. (2017). The E3 ubiquitin ligase SCF(cyclin F) transmits AKT signaling to the cell-cycle machinery. *Cell Rep.* 20: 3212–3222.

198 Mavrommati, I. et al. (2018). beta-TrCP- and casein kinase II-mediated degradation of cyclin F controls timely mitotic progression. *Cell Rep.* 24: 3404–3412.

199 Janjusevic, R., Abramovitch, R.B., Martin, G.B., and Stebbins, C.E. (2006). A bacterial inhibitor of host programmed cell death defenses is an E3 ubiquitin ligase. *Science* 311: 222–226.

200 Lin, D.Y., Diao, J., and Chen, J. (2012). Crystal structures of two bacterial HECT-like E3 ligases in complex with a human E2 reveal atomic details of pathogen-host interactions. *Proc. Natl. Acad. Sci. U.S.A.* 109: 1925–1930.

201 Huibregtse, J.M., Scheffner, M., Beaudenon, S., and Howley, P.M. (1995). A family of proteins structurally and functionally related to the E6-AP ubiquitin-protein ligase. *Proc. Natl. Acad. Sci. U.S.A.* 92: 2563–2567.

202 Scheffner, M. and Staub, O. (2007). HECT E3s and human disease. *BMC Biochem.* 8: S6.

203 Rotin, D. and Kumar, S. (2009). Physiological functions of the HECT family of ubiquitin ligases. *Nat. Rev. Mol. Cell Biol.* 10: 398–409.

204 Jäckl, M. et al. (2018). β-Sheet augmentation is a conserved mechanism of priming HECT E3 ligases for ubiquitin ligation. *J. Mol. Biol.* 430: 3218–3233.

205 Ingham, R.J., Gish, G., and Pawson, T. (2004). The Nedd4 family of E3 ubiquitin ligases: functional diversity within a common modular architecture. *Oncogene* 23: 1972–1984.

206 Hochrainer, K. et al. (2005). The human HERC family of ubiquitin ligases: novel members, genomic organization, expression profiling, and evolutionary aspects. *Genomics* 85: 153–164.

207 Hunkeler, M. et al. (2021). Solenoid architecture of HUWE1 contributes to ligase activity and substrate recognition. *Mol. Cell* 81: 3468–3480.e3467.

208 Grabarczyk, D.B. et al. (2021). HUWE1 employs a giant substrate-binding ring to feed and regulate its HECT E3 domain. *Nat. Chem. Biol.* 17: 1084–1092.

209 Rosa, J.L. and Barbacid, M. (1997). A giant protein that stimulates guanine nucleotide exchange on ARF1 and Rab proteins forms a cytosolic ternary complex with clathrin and Hsp70. *Oncogene* 15: 1–6.
210 Huang, L. et al. (1999). Structure of an E6AP-UbcH7 complex: insights into ubiquitination by the E2-E3 enzyme cascade. *Science* 286: 1321–1326.
211 Verdecia, M.A. et al. (2003). Conformational flexibility underlies ubiquitin ligation mediated by the WWP1 HECT domain E3 ligase. *Mol. Cell* 11: 249–259.
212 Kamadurai, H.B. et al. (2009). Insights into ubiquitin transfer cascades from a structure of a UbcH5B~ubiquitin-HECTNEDD4L complex. *Mol. Cell* 36: 1095–1102.
213 Kamadurai, H.B. et al. (2013). Mechanism of ubiquitin ligation and lysine prioritization by a HECT E3. *Elife* 2: e00828.
214 Maspero, E. et al. (2013). Structure of a ubiquitin-loaded HECT ligase reveals the molecular basis for catalytic priming. *Nat. Struct. Mol. Biol.* 20: 696–701.
215 Ogunjimi, A.A. et al. (2005). Regulation of Smurf2 ubiquitin ligase activity by anchoring the E2 to the HECT domain. *Mol. Cell* 19: 297–308.
216 Nair, R.M. et al. (2021). Reconstitution and structural analysis of a HECT ligase-ubiquitin complex via an activity-based probe. *ACS Chem. Biol.* 16: 1615–1621.
217 Kim, H.C., Steffen, A.M., Oldham, M.L. et al. (2011). Structure and function of a HECT domain ubiquitin-binding site. *EMBO Rep.* 12: 334.
218 Maspero, E. et al. (2011). Structure of the HECT:ubiquitin complex and its role in ubiquitin chain elongation. *EMBO Rep.* 12: 342.
219 Hochstrasser, M. (2006). Lingering mysteries of ubiquitin-chain assembly. *Cell* 124: 27–34.
220 Singh, S. and Sivaraman, J. (2020). Crystal structure of HECT domain of UBE3C E3 ligase and its ubiquitination activity. *Biochem. J.* 477: 905–923.
221 Singh, S., Ng, J., Nayak, D., and Sivaraman, J. (2019). Structural insights into a HECT-type E3 ligase AREL1 and its ubiquitination activities *in vitro*. *J. Biol. Chem.* 294: 19934–19949.
222 Salvat, C., Wang, G., Dastur, A. et al. (2004). The −4 phenylalanine is required for substrate ubiquitination catalyzed by HECT ubiquitin ligases*. *J. Biol. Chem.* 279: 18935–18943.
223 Kamadurai, H.B. et al. (2009). Insights into ubiquitin transfer cascades from a structure of a UbcH5B approximately ubiquitin-HECT(NEDD4L) complex. *Mol. Cell* 36: 1095–1102.
224 Riling, C. et al. (2015). Itch WW domains inhibit its E3 ubiquitin ligase activity by blocking E2-E3 ligase trans-thiolation*. *J. Biol. Chem.* 290: 23875–23887.
225 Ruetalo, N. et al. (2019). The WW1 domain enhances autoinhibition in Smurf ubiquitin ligases. *J. Mol. Biol.* 431: 4834–4847.
226 Wiesner, S. et al. (2007). Autoinhibition of the HECT-type ubiquitin ligase Smurf2 through its C2 domain. *Cell* 130: 651–662.
227 Wan, L. et al. (2011). Cdh1 regulates osteoblast function through an APC/C-independent modulation of Smurf1. *Mol. Cell* 44: 721–733.
228 Wang, J. et al. (2010). Calcium activates Nedd4 E3 ubiquitin ligases by releasing the C2 domain-mediated auto-inhibition *. *J. Biol. Chem.* 285: 12279–12288.

229 Escobedo, A. et al. (2014). Structural basis of the activation and degradation mechanisms of the E3 ubiquitin ligase Nedd4L. *Structure* 22: 1446–1457.

230 Sander, B., Xu, W., Eilers, M. et al. (2017). A conformational switch regulates the ubiquitin ligase HUWE1. *Elife* 6: e21036.

231 Ronchi, V.P., Klein, J.M., Edwards, D.J., and Haas, A.L. (2014). The active form of E6-associated protein (E6AP)/UBE3A ubiquitin ligase is an oligomer*. *J. Biol. Chem.* 289: 1033–1048.

232 Mund, T. and Pelham, H.R.B. (2009). Control of the activity of WW-HECT domain E3 ubiquitin ligases by NDFIP proteins. *EMBO Rep.* 10: 501–507.

233 Jiang, H., Thomas, S.N., Chen, Z. et al. (2019). Comparative analysis of the catalytic regulation of NEDD4-1 and WWP2 ubiquitin ligases. *J. Biol. Chem.* 294: 17421–17436.

234 Howitt, J. et al. (2012). Ndfip1 regulates nuclear Pten import *in vivo* to promote neuronal survival following cerebral ischemia. *J. Cell Biol.* 196: 29–36.

235 Trotman, L.C. et al. (2007). Ubiquitination regulates PTEN nuclear import and tumor suppression. *Cell* 128: 141–156.

236 Maddika, S. et al. (2011). WWP2 is an E3 ubiquitin ligase for PTEN. *Nat. Cell Biol.* 13: 728–733.

237 Shao, C., Li, Z., Ahmad, N., and Liu, X. (2017). Regulation of PTEN degradation and NEDD4-1 E3 ligase activity by Numb. *Cell Cycle (Georgetown, Tex.)* 16: 957–967.

238 Malakhova, O.A. and Zhang, D.-E. (2008). ISG15 inhibits Nedd4 ubiquitin E3 activity and enhances the innate antiviral response. *J. Biol. Chem.* 283: 8783.

239 Zhang, W. et al. (2016). System-wide modulation of HECT E3 ligases with selective ubiquitin variant probes. *Mol. Cell* 62: 121–136.

240 Nuber, U., Schwarz, S.E., and Scheffner, M. (1998). The ubiquitin-protein ligase E6-associated protein (E6-AP) serves as its own substrate. *Eur. J. Biochem.* 254: 643–649.

241 Bruce, M.C. et al. (2008). Regulation of Nedd4-2 self-ubiquitination and stability by a PY motif located within its HECT-domain. *Biochem. J.* 415: 155–163.

242 Liao, B. and Jin, Y. (2010). Wwp2 mediates Oct4 ubiquitination and its own auto-ubiquitination in a dosage-dependent manner. *Cell Res.* 20: 332–344.

243 Liu, X. et al. (2016). Trip12 is an E3 ubiquitin ligase for USP7/HAUSP involved in the DNA damage response. *FEBS Lett.* 590: 4213–4222.

244 Rutz, S. et al. (2015). Deubiquitinase DUBA is a post-translational brake on interleukin-17 production in T cells. *Nature* 518: 417–421.

245 MacDonald, C., Shields, S.B., Williams, C.A. et al. (2020). A cycle of ubiquitination regulates adaptor function of the Nedd4-family ubiquitin ligase Rsp5. *Curr. Biol.* 30: 465–479.e465.

246 Attali, I. et al. (2017). Ubiquitylation-dependent oligomerization regulates activity of Nedd4 ligases. *EMBO J.* 36: 425–440.

247 Persaud, A. et al. (2014). Tyrosine phosphorylation of NEDD4 activates its ubiquitin ligase activity. *Sci. Signal.* 7: ra95.

248 Lee, C.K., Yang, Y., Chen, C., and Liu, J. (2016). Syk-mediated tyrosine phosphorylation of Mule promotes TNF-induced JNK activation and cell death. *Oncogene* 35: 1988–1995.

249 Chandran, S. et al. (2011). Neural precursor cell-expressed developmentally down-regulated protein 4-2 (Nedd4-2) regulation by 14-3-3 protein binding at canonical serum and glucocorticoid kinase 1 (SGK1) phosphorylation sites*. *J. Biol. Chem.* 286: 37830–37840.

250 Chan, A.-L. et al. (2013). C-Abl phosphorylates E6AP and regulates its E3 ubiquitin ligase activity. *Biochemistry* 52: 3119–3129.

251 Huguenin-Dezot, N. et al. (2016). Synthesis of isomeric phosphoubiquitin chains reveals that phosphorylation controls deubiquitinase activity and specificity. *Cell Rep.* 16: 1180–1193.

252 Yang, Y. et al. (2010). E3 ubiquitin ligase Mule ubiquitinates Miz1 and is required for TNFα-induced JNK activation. *Proc. Natl. Acad. Sci. U.S.A.* 107: 13444–13449.

253 Coon, T.A. et al. (2015). The proinflammatory role of HECTD2 in innate immunity and experimental lung injury. *Sci. Transl. Med.* 7: 295ra109.

254 Shu, J. et al. (2016). Nedd8 targets ubiquitin ligase Smurf2 for neddylation and promote its degradation. *Biochem. Biophys. Res. Commun.* 474: 51–56.

255 Xie, P. et al. (2014). The covalent modifier Nedd8 is critical for the activation of Smurf1 ubiquitin ligase in tumorigenesis. *Nat. Commun.* 5: 3733.

256 He, S., Cao, Y., Xie, P. et al. (2017). The Nedd8 non-covalent binding region in the Smurf HECT domain is critical to its ubiquitn ligase function. *Sci. Rep.* 7: 41364.

257 Chandhoke, A.S. et al. (2016). The ubiquitin ligase Smurf2 suppresses TGFβ-induced epithelial–mesenchymal transition in a sumoylation-regulated manner. *Cell Death Differ.* 23: 876–888.

258 Schneider, T. et al. (2018). The E3 ubiquitin ligase HERC1 controls the ERK signaling pathway targeting C-RAF for degradation. *Oncotarget* 9: 31531–31548.

259 Pedrazza, L., Schneider, T., Bartrons, R. et al. (2020). The ubiquitin ligase HERC1 regulates cell migration via RAF-dependent regulation of MKK3/p38 signaling. *Sci. Rep.* 10: 824.

260 Bachiller, S. et al. (2018). HERC1 ubiquitin ligase is required for normal axonal myelination in the peripheral nervous system. *Mol. Neurobiol.* 55: 8856–8868.

261 Diouf, B. et al. (2011). Somatic deletions of genes regulating MSH2 protein stability cause DNA mismatch repair deficiency and drug resistance in human leukemia cells. *Nat. Med.* 17: 1298–1303.

262 Rosa, J.L., Casaroli-Marano, R.P., Buckler, A.J. et al. (1996). p619, a giant protein related to the chromosome condensation regulator RCC1, stimulates guanine nucleotide exchange on ARF1 and Rab proteins. *EMBO J.* 15: 4262–4273.

263 Garcia-Gonzalo, F.R., Bartrons, R., Ventura, F., and Rosa, J.L. (2005). Requirement of phosphatidylinositol-4,5-bisphosphate for HERC1-mediated guanine nucleotide release from ARF proteins. *FEBS Lett.* 579: 343–348.

264 Wu, W. et al. (2010). HERC2 is an E3 ligase that targets BRCA1 for degradation. *Cancer Res.* 70: 6384–6392.

265 Moroishi, T., Yamauchi, T., Nishiyama, M., and Nakayama, K.I. (2014). HERC2 targets the iron regulator FBXL5 for degradation and modulates iron metabolism. *J. Biol. Chem.* 289: 16430–16441.

266 Bekker-Jensen, S. et al. (2010). HERC2 coordinates ubiquitin-dependent assembly of DNA repair factors on damaged chromosomes. *Nat. Cell Biol.* 12: 80–86.

267 Cubillos-Rojas, M. et al. (2014). The E3 ubiquitin protein ligase HERC2 modulates the activity of tumor protein p53 by regulating its oligomerization. *J. Biol. Chem.* 289: 14782–14795.

268 García-Cano, J. et al. (2020). Regulation of the MDM2-p53 pathway by the ubiquitin ligase HERC2. *Mol. Oncol.* 14: 69–86.

269 Li, H. et al. (2019). HERC3-mediated SMAD7 ubiquitination degradation promotes autophagy-induced EMT and chemoresistance in glioblastoma. *Clin. Cancer Res.* 25: 3602–3616.

270 Shi, H.-X. et al. (2010). Positive regulation of interferon regulatory factor 3 activation by Herc5 via ISG15 modification. *Mol. Cell. Biol.* 30: 2424–2436.

271 Zhao, C., Hsiang, T.-Y., Kuo, R.-L., and Krug, R.M. (2010). ISG15 conjugation system targets the viral NS1 protein in influenza A virus–infected cells. *Proc. Natl. Acad. Sci. U.S.A.* 107: 2253–2258.

272 Wei, W., Li, M., Wang, J. et al. (2012). The E3 ubiquitin ligase ITCH negatively regulates canonical Wnt signaling by targeting dishevelled protein. *Mol. Cell. Biol.* 32: 3903–3912.

273 Goto, J. et al. (2020). HECT (homologous to the E6-AP carboxyl terminus)-type ubiquitin E3 ligase ITCH attenuates cardiac hypertrophy by suppressing the Wnt/β-catenin signaling pathway. *Hypertension* 76: 1868–1878.

274 Mössinger, J. et al. (2012). Phosphatidylinositol 4-kinase IIα function at endosomes is regulated by the ubiquitin ligase Itch. *EMBO Rep.* 13: 1087–1094.

275 Lee, Y.-R. et al. (2019). Reactivation of PTEN tumor suppressor for cancer treatment through inhibition of a MYC-WWP1 inhibitory pathway. *Science (New York, NY)* 364: eaau0159.

276 Lee, Y.-R. et al. (2020). WWP1 gain-of-function inactivation of PTEN in cancer predisposition. *N. Engl. J. Med.* 382: 2103–2116.

277 Wang, K. et al. (2020). WWP2 regulates proliferation of gastric cancer cells in a PTEN-dependent manner. *Biochem. Biophys. Res. Commun.* 521: 652–659.

278 Margolis, S.S. et al. (2010). EphB-mediated degradation of the RhoA GEF Ephexin5 relieves a developmental brake on excitatory synapse formation. *Cell* 143: 442–455.

279 Sell, G.L. et al. (2021). Deleting a UBE3A substrate rescues impaired hippocampal physiology and learning in Angelman syndrome mice. *Sci. Rep.* 11: 19414.

280 Olabarria, M. et al. (2019). Dysfunction of the ubiquitin ligase E3A Ube3A/E6-AP contributes to synaptic pathology in Alzheimer's disease. *Commun. Biol.* 2: 1–14.

281 Shirakura, M. et al. (2007). E6AP ubiquitin ligase mediates Ubiquitylation and degradation of hepatitis C virus Core protein. *J. Virol.* 81: 1174–1185.

282 Greer, P.L. et al. (2010). The Angelman Syndrome protein Ube3A regulates synapse development by ubiquitinating arc. *Cell* 140: 704–716.

283 Yamashita, M. et al. (2005). Ubiquitin ligase Smurf1 controls osteoblast activity and bone homeostasis by targeting MEKK2 for degradation. *Cell* 121: 101–113.

284 Kaneki, H. et al. (2006). Tumor necrosis factor promotes Runx2 degradation through up-regulation of Smurf1 and Smurf2 in osteoblasts. *J. Biol. Chem.* 281: 4326–4333.

285 Wei, J. et al. (2014). Bone-specific insulin resistance disrupts whole-body glucose homeostasis via decreased osteocalcin activation. *J. Clin. Invest.* 124: 1781–1793.

286 Shimazu, J., Wei, J., and Karsenty, G. (2016). Smurf1 inhibits osteoblast differentiation, bone formation and glucose homeostasis through Serine 148. *Cell Rep.* 15: 27–35.

287 Zhao, M., Qiao, M., Oyajobi, B.O. et al. (2003). E3 ubiquitin ligase Smurf1 mediates core-binding factor α1/Runx2 degradation and plays a specific role in osteoblast differentiation*. *J. Biol. Chem.* 278: 27939–27944.

288 Zhao, M. et al. (2004). Smurf1 inhibits osteoblast differentiation and bone formation *in vitro* and *in vivo*. *J. Biol. Chem.* 279: 12854–12859.

289 Zhang, J. et al. (2011). Mule determines the apoptotic response to HDAC inhibitors by targeted ubiquitination and destruction of HDAC2. *Genes Dev.* 25: 2610–2618.

290 Franco, L.H. et al. (2017). The ubiquitin ligase Smurf1 functions in selective autophagy of mycobacterium tuberculosis and anti-tuberculous host defense. *Cell Host Microbe* 21: 59–72.

291 Zhang, Y., Chang, C., Gehling, D.J. et al. (2001). Regulation of Smad degradation and activity by Smurf2, an E3 ubiquitin ligase. *Proc. Natl. Acad. Sci. U.S.A.* 98: 974–979.

292 Lin, X., Liang, M., and Feng, X.-H. (2000). Smurf2 is a ubiquitin E3 ligase mediating proteasome-dependent degradation of Smad2 in transforming growth factor-β signaling*210. *J. Biol. Chem.* 275: 36818–36822.

293 Fukuchi, M. et al. (2002). High-level expression of the Smad ubiquitin ligase Smurf2 correlates with poor prognosis in patients with esophageal squamous cell carcinoma1. *Cancer Res.* 62: 7162–7165.

294 Yang, Q. et al. (2009). Smurf2 participates in human trophoblast cell invasion by inhibiting TGF-β type I receptor. *J. Histochem. Cytochem.* 57: 605–612.

295 Yu, L. et al. (2020). Ubiquitination-mediated degradation of SIRT1 by SMURF2 suppresses CRC cell proliferation and tumorigenesis. *Oncogene* 39: 4450–4464.

296 Bonni, S. et al. (2001). TGF-β induces assembly of a Smad2–Smurf2 ubiquitin ligase complex that targets SnoN for degradation. *Nat. Cell Biol.* 3: 587–595.

297 Shukla, S. et al. (2014). KRAS protein stability is regulated through SMURF2: UBCH5 complex-mediated β-TrCP1 degradation. *Neoplasia* 16: 115–W115.

298 Moore, F.E. et al. (2010). The WW-HECT protein Smurf2 interacts with the Docking Protein NEDD9/HEF1 for Aurora A activation. *Cell Div.* 5: 22.

299 Zang, C.-x. et al. (2022). HACE1 negatively regulates neuroinflammation through ubiquitylating and degrading Rac1 in Parkinson's disease models. *Acta Pharmacol. Sin.* 43: 285–294.

300 Torrino, S. et al. (2011). The E3 ubiquitin-ligase HACE1 catalyzes the ubiquitylation of active Rac1. *Dev. Cell* 21: 959–965.

301 Zhang, L. et al. (2014). HACE1-dependent protein degradation provides cardiac protection in response to haemodynamic stress. *Nat. Commun.* 5: 3430.

302 Cho, J.J. et al. (2019). Hectd3 promotes pathogenic Th17 lineage through Stat3 activation and Malt1 signaling in neuroinflammation. *Nat. Commun.* 10: 701.

303 Li, F. et al. (2018). HECTD3 mediates TRAF3 polyubiquitination and type I interferon induction during bacterial infection. *J. Clin. Invest.* 128: 4148–4162.

304 King, B. et al. (2016). The ubiquitin ligase Huwe1 regulates the maintenance and lymphoid commitment of hematopoietic stem cells. *Nat. Immunol.* 17: 1312–1321.

305 Zhao, X. et al. (2009). The N-Myc-DLL3 cascade is suppressed by the ubiquitin ligase Huwe1 to inhibit proliferation and promote neurogenesis in the developing brain. *Dev. Cell* 17: 210–221.

306 Dominguez-Brauer, C. et al. (2017). E3 ubiquitin ligase mule targets β-catenin under conditions of hyperactive Wnt signaling. *Proc. Natl. Acad. Sci. U.S.A.* 114: E1148–E1157.

307 Cho, H.I. et al. (2020). BRPF3-HUWE1-mediated regulation of MYST2 is required for differentiation and cell-cycle progression in embryonic stem cells. *Cell Death Differ.* 27: 3273–3288.

308 He, Y., Zhou, J., and Wan, Q. (2021). The E3 ligase HUWE1 mediates TGFBR2 ubiquitination and promotes gastric cancer cell proliferation, migration, and invasion. *Invest. New Drugs* 39: 713–723.

309 Zhu, Q. et al. (2020). HUWE1 promotes EGFR ubiquitination and degradation to protect against renal tubulointerstitial fibrosis. *FASEB J.* 34: 4591–4601.

310 Zhong, Q., Gao, W., Du, F., and Wang, X. (2005). Mule/ARF-BP1, a BH3-only E3 ubiquitin ligase, catalyzes the polyubiquitination of Mcl-1 and regulates apoptosis. *Cell* 121: 1085–1095.

311 Friez, M.J. et al. (2016). HUWE1 mutations in Juberg-Marsidi and brooks syndromes: the results of an X-chromosome exome sequencing study. *BMJ Open* 6: e009537.

312 Chen, D. et al. (2005). ARF-BP1/Mule is a critical mediator of the ARF tumor suppressor. *Cell* 121: 1071–1083.

313 Hao, Z. et al. (2012). The E3 ubiquitin ligase Mule acts through the ATM–p53 axis to maintain B lymphocyte homeostasis. *J. Exp. Med.* 209: 173–186.

314 Yang, D. et al. (2018). HUWE1 controls the development of non-small cell lung cancer through down-regulation of p53. *Theranostics* 8: 3517–3529.

315 Liu, Z., Oughtred, R., and Wing, S.S. (2005). Characterization of E3Histone, a novel testis ubiquitin protein ligase which ubiquitinates histones. *Mol. Cell. Biol.* 25: 2819–2831.

316 Inoue, S. et al. (2013). Mule/Huwe1/Arf-BP1 suppresses Ras-driven tumorigenesis by preventing c-Myc/Miz1-mediated down-regulation of p21 and p15. *Genes Dev.* 27: 1101–1114.

317 Vaughan, L. et al. (2015). HUWE1 ubiquitylates and degrades the RAC activator TIAM1 promoting cell-cell adhesion disassembly, migration, and invasion. *Cell Rep.* 10: 88–102.

318 Cheng, Y.-F., Tong, M., and Edge, A.S.B. (2016). Destabilization of Atoh1 by E3 ubiquitin ligase Huwe1 and casein kinase 1 is essential for normal sensory hair cell development*. *J. Biol. Chem.* 291: 21096–21109.

319 Adhikary, S. et al. (2005). The ubiquitin ligase HectH9 regulates transcriptional activation by Myc and is essential for tumor cell proliferation. *Cell* 123: 409–421.

320 de Groot, R.E.A. et al. (2014). Huwe1-mediated ubiquitylation of dishevelled defines a negative feedback loop in the Wnt signaling pathway. *Sci. Signal.* 7: ra26.

321 Vandewalle, J. et al. (2013). Ubiquitin ligase HUWE1 regulates axon branching through the Wnt/β-catenin pathway in a *Drosophila* model for intellectual disability. *PLoS One* 8: e81791.

322 Wu, H.-T. et al. (2016). K63-polyubiquitinated HAUSP deubiquitinates HIF-1α and dictates H3K56 acetylation promoting hypoxia-induced tumour progression. *Nat. Commun.* 7: 13644.

323 Parsons, J.L. et al. (2009). Ubiquitin ligase ARF-BP1/Mule modulates base excision repair. *EMBO J.* 28: 3207.

324 Choe, K.N. et al. (2016). HUWE1 interacts with PCNA to alleviate replication stress. *EMBO Rep.* 17: 874–886.

325 Morett, E. and Bork, P. (1999). A novel transactivation domain in parkin. *Trends Biochem. Sci.* 24: 229–231.

326 van der Reijden, B.A., Erpelinck-Verschueren, C.A., Lowenberg, B., and Jansen, J.H. (1999). TRIADs: a new class of proteins with a novel cysteine-rich signature. *Protein Sci.* 8: 1557–1561.

327 Shimura, H. et al. (2000). Familial Parkinson disease gene product, parkin, is a ubiquitin-protein ligase. *Nat. Genet.* 25: 302–305.

328 Imai, Y., Soda, M., and Takahashi, R. (2000). Parkin suppresses unfolded protein stress-induced cell death through its E3 ubiquitin-protein ligase activity. *J. Biol. Chem.* 275: 35661–35664.

329 Wenzel, D.M., Lissounov, A., Brzovic, P.S., and Klevit, R.E. (2011). UBCH7 reactivity profile reveals parkin and HHARI to be RING/HECT hybrids. *Nature* 474: 105–108.

330 Spratt, D.E., Walden, H., and Shaw, G.S. (2014). RBR E3 ubiquitin ligases: new structures, new insights, new questions. *Biochem. J.* 458: 421–437.

331 Dove, K.K. and Klevit, R.E. (2017). RING-between-RING E3 ligases: emerging themes amid the variations. *J. Mol. Biol.* 429: 3363–3375.

332 Stieglitz, B. et al. (2013). Structural basis for ligase-specific conjugation of linear ubiquitin chains by HOIP. *Nature* 503: 422–426.

333 Kelsall, I.R., Zhang, J., Knebel, A. et al. (2019). The E3 ligase HOIL-1 catalyses ester bond formation between ubiquitin and components of the Myddosome in mammalian cells. *Proc. Natl. Acad. Sci. U.S.A.* 116: 13293–13298.

334 Li, C., Nelson, T.G., Vertegaal, A.C.O., and Thibault, P. (2021). Proteomic strategies for characterizing ubiquitin-like modifications. *Nat. Rev. Methods Primers* 1: 53.

335 Chen, Z. et al. (2022). Disease-associated KBTBD4 mutations in medulloblastoma elicit neomorphic ubiquitylation activity to promote CoREST degradation. *Cell Death Differ.* .

336 Mayor-Ruiz, C. et al. (2019). Plasticity of the Cullin-RING ligase repertoire shapes sensitivity to ligand-induced protein degradation. *Mol. Cell* 75: 849–858.e848.

337 Mayor-Ruiz, C. et al. (2020). Rational discovery of molecular glue degraders via scalable chemical profiling. *Nat. Chem. Biol.* 16: 1199–1207.

338 Shirasaki, R. et al. (2021). Functional genomics identify distinct and overlapping genes mediating resistance to different classes of heterobifunctional degraders of oncoproteins. *Cell Rep.* 34: 108532.

4

A Structural and Biophysical Perspective of Degrader Activity Through Ternary Complex Formation

Morgan S. Gadd and Marine C. Aublette

Lancaster University, Division of Biomedical and Life Sciences, Lancaster, UK

4.1 Introduction

Small-molecule-based targeted protein degraders seek to recruit together an E3 ubiquitin ligase protein (E3) with a target protein of interest to hijack the ubiquitin-proteasome system so as to result in the polyubiquitination and degradation of the target protein. To date, such molecules have generally come in two broad classes: proteolysis-targeting chimaeras (PROTACs) and molecular glues (MGs). PROTACs are bifunctional molecules containing moieties that act as ligands for both the E3 and the target and will generally function through the formation of random-order ternary complexes. MGs, on the other hand, will typically have affinity for only one binding partner or even only very weak affinity for either. Complex formation is a product of the MG altering the surface properties of one or both partner proteins to encourage the recruitment of the other. Thus, MGs function either via sequential order or simultaneous ternary complex formation, as at least one binding partner cannot be recruited independently by the MG. While in both instances a functional degrader must induce effective ternary complex formation, only MGs (by their very nature) must form de novo protein–protein interactions (neo-PPIs) that interface the two partner proteins. Because of their modularity, PROTACs form ternary complexes where the partners may or may not interface, with any such contacts, such as neo-PPIs, potentially being beneficial, neutral, or detrimental to the overall productivity of the complex, depending on the partners and the arrangements they can be recruited in. In this chapter, we hope to explore the current structural understanding of various ternary complexes of PROTAC- and MG-induced complexes and their physical bases through the emerging diversity of examples produced by the field.

Inducing Targeted Protein Degradation: From Chemical Biology to Drug Discovery and Clinical Applications, First Edition. Edited by Philipp Cromm.

4.1.1 Mechanism of Degraders Through Ternary Complexes

While PROTACs and MGs recruit their binding partners into ternary complexes by different ordered mechanisms, both share the same ultimate recruitment step and initial productive step of ternary complex formation. Having brought the E3 ligase into proximity with the target to allow ubiquitination of the latter, the degrader facilitates the monoubiquitination of at least one lysine residue on the target. Two key requirements here include the positioning of the target so that it can be reached by the E2 enzyme and ubiquitin and that the target has an accessible lysine in this location. To proceed, the ternary complex must also facilitate the subsequent Lys48-linked ubiquitination of successive ubiquitin molecules to grow the polyubiquitin chain. The final step is the dissociation of the polyubiquitinated target from the ternary complex so that it can be directed to 26S proteasome for degradation. Having successfully modified a target protein, the degrader is once again available and can be reused in another cycle, facilitating the catalytic mode of action of these molecules. Each step in this process will be influenced by the behavior of the ternary complex, and thus in turn each intermediate and transition state at each step may be correspondingly stabilized or destabilized by the nature of the ternary complex.

4.1.2 Ternary Complex Behavior

While ostensibly simply a process of bringing two molecules together via the activity of a third, there are a number of features of ternary complexes that influence not only their successful formation but in particular their productivity as degraders. These include, but are not limited to, binding pose, affinity, cooperativity, stoichiometry, residency, plasticity, and flexibility (Figure 4.1).

4.1.2.1 Binding Pose

The binding pose simply reflects in what arrangement the ternary complex comes together, in terms of positioning, orientation, and conformation of the partner proteins relative to one another. The binding pose will be a product of the manner in which the two partner proteins have been brought together (i.e. which binding sites are liganded), the properties of the linker, and the ways in which the two proteins can or cannot interface with one another. The binding pose is critical as, based on the structure of the E3 ligase and its recruitment of associated ubiquitination machinery and the overall structure of the target (and in particular location of surface lysines), this will determine if the target can potentially be successfully ubiquitinated at all.

4.1.2.2 Affinity and Cooperativity

Affinity and cooperativity go hand-in-hand as the latter is effectively a modifier of the former. Affinity drives the formation of ternary complexes by enabling the three partners to form a complex with each other. For PROTACs, each binding moiety will have its own affinity (K_d) for its respective partner protein, while for MGs, there will be (physiologically relevant) affinity either for only one partner,

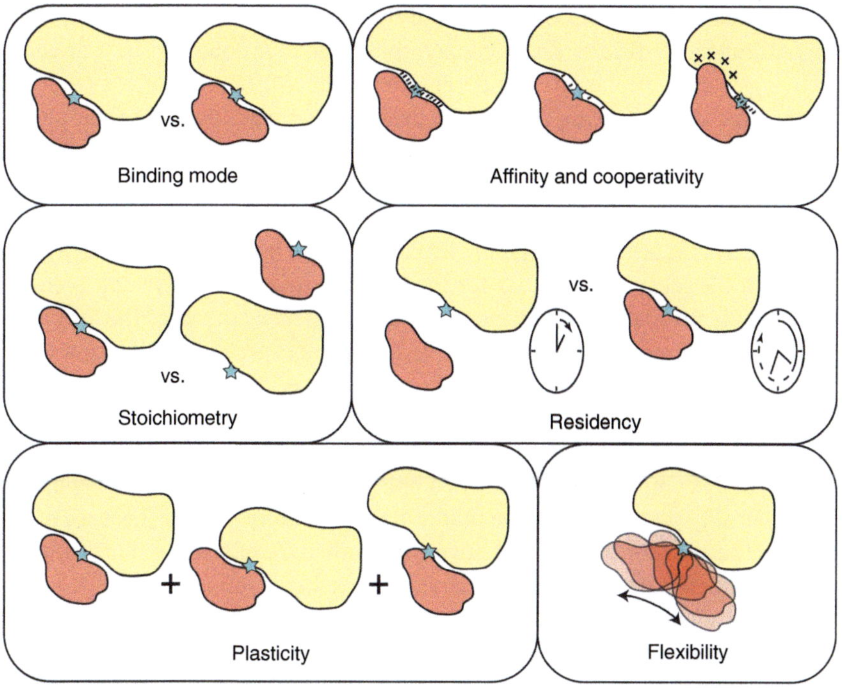

Figure 4.1 A non-exhaustive illustration of some behaviors of ternary complexes: binding mode, affinity, cooperativity, stoichiometry, residency, plasticity, and flexibility. The ternary complex bridging molecule is represented by a blue star. The partner proteins as yellow and red shapes. Behaviors are exhibited by the red molecule relative to yellow but can be displayed by both.

or neither, with ternary complex formation driven largely by cooperativity. Cooperativity is essentially a measure of how much additional or less affinity there is within a ternary (or greater) complex than the sum of the individual binary affinities. The cooperativity, often termed "α", is said to be positive when $\alpha = K_d(\text{binary})/K_d(\text{ternary}) > 1$ [1]. In this case, the ternary complex formation is favorable, and additional interactions are formed. It is negative when $\alpha < 1$, meaning that the formation of ternary complex is diminished because of steric clashes or entropic unfavorability. When $\alpha = 1$, the system is non-cooperative, indicating that the K_d remains unchanged for the two steps. Cooperativity is a balance of many binding energies against each other, both enthalpic and entropic. For PROTACs, cooperativity will be driven by the way in which the two partner proteins interact with one another in the induced complex, as well as any new interactions or conformational changes within the PROTAC, either further promoting ternary complex formation or opposing it. MGs on the other hand are entirely dependent on cooperativity for their activity, as the molecule itself has no affinity for at least one protein and thus effectively relies on highly positive cooperativity driven by favorable contacts between the partner proteins in order to facilitate ternary complex formation. As cooperative interactions are typically driven by weak interactions on surfaces of the proteins, adjacent to or even away from binding sites, differences in cooperativity are often found to be a driver of selectivity, as different targets and E3 ligases will have different surfaces that can be complementary, favoring specific E3 ligase–target pairs over others for some degraders [2–5].

4.1.2.3 Stoichiometry

Stoichiometry is another key factor for degraders, as the ternary complex must (typically) be in the format of 1 : 1 : 1 for the ligase:degrader:target system to enable productive ubiquitination. While increased affinity is a key driver of the formation of ternary complexes, it also acts in opposition. For most proteins, as the concentration of degrader increases beyond the K_d values for each binding partner, a self-inhibition process known as the "hook" effect will occur, where additional degrader molecules preferentially form binary complexes with either partner protein, disrupting ternary complexes [1]. Ternary complex formation at values below the K_d of the high-affinity partner and above that of the low-affinity partner (because of the hook effect) can be promoted by positive cooperativity by effectively increasing ternary complex affinities relative to binary complex formation. The opposite is true for negative cooperativity, although to a more limited extent, being dependent on binary K_d values and partner protein concentrations [1]. The hook effect in particular is a significant factor in tuning PROTAC activity, whereas it is a non-issue for MGs as they lack meaningful affinity for at least one of their binding partners.

4.1.2.4 Residency

The residency time of a ternary complex is also important. The complex must maintain sufficient proximity for a long-enough time for the ubiquitination events to occur. This will be typically reflected in the dissociation rate (k_{off}) of the ternary complex, which is a reflection of the mean time the ternary complex will stay together. Slow k_{off} values should give the ubiquitination machinery sufficient time (on the molecular scale) to successfully ubiquitinate the target, holding it within a limited space relative to the substrate receptor. Fast k_{off} rates, on the other hand, may lack sufficient residency time for ubiquitination to happen, although E3 ligase–target systems with sufficiently liberal ubiquitination requirements may be able to make do with fast association rates (k_{on}), largely keeping the target within the local environment of the ligase, if not engaged with it. On the flip side, slow k_{off} rates may contribute to "locking" the ternary complex in unproductive binding poses.

4.1.2.5 Plasticity

Plasticity in PPIs is the concept that a single surface can be plastic so as to accommodate mutation or host different binding partners through overlapping binding interfaces [6]. This is inherently true of MG-induced ternary complexes, which will often recruit many different target proteins to a well-defined interface, which in turn is often the site at which native substrates bind. For PROTACs, however, plasticity operates on a more fundamental level. As these typically induce neo-PPIs that are by themselves very weak, there will likely be a diverse population of different binding poses of equally weak neo-PPI interfaces that contribute toward ternary complex formation [7]. High plasticity may increase the degrader activity for certain E3 ligase–target pairs by increasing the number of binding poses explored or the potential for more dynamic flexibility, both of which may avoid the complex being trapped in an unproductive form. Alternatively, complexes with low plasticity would be more stable and "monomorphic," which may be critical for providing the stability for certain E3 ligases to successfully ubiquitinate their targets [8], akin to slow k_{off} rates leading to longer residency times.

4.1.2.6 Flexibility

PROTAC ternary complexes were originally thought to be largely flexible, as the aim of the molecules was simply to induce proximity between E3 ligase and target, not make them interact [9]. All ternary complexes will exhibit some degree of dynamism and flexibility, and while many potent degraders likely operate as a function of high levels of flexibility in their ternary complexes, others have revealed stable or plastic interfaces that would appear to restrict the partner proteins to a limited set of (or even potentially a single) binding poses [3, 7, 10, 11]. To date, there are no in-depth studies investigating the dynamic nature of a degrader-induced ternary complex (given flexibility is intrinsically hard to study); however, there will no doubt be certain parameters around it that will drive productive degrader activity, for example, movements in particular directions, within a set range, or potentially even the rate or randomness of movement exhibited.

4.1.3 Observing and Quantifying Ternary Complex Behavior

A large variety of approaches can be used for detecting/observing the formation of ternary complexes in one form or another. Perhaps, the most valuable are those that enable the identification and quantification of ternary complex formation in the cellular environment, such as coimmunoprecipitation or pull-downs [12–14] and Promega's NanoBRET [15, 16]. Pull-downs suffer from usually only capturing stronger interactors, while on the other hand, NanoBRET requires special labeling of the partner proteins, and doing this for endogenous proteins is labor intensive. Most importantly, however, these approaches allow validation and evaluation of ternary complex formation in physiologically relevant environments and samples.

4.1.3.1 Biophysics

Many different biophysical approaches enable the quantification of specific aspects of ternary complex behavior. Time-resolved Förster resonance energy transfer (TR-FRET) and PerkinElmer's AlphaLISA/AlphaScreen enable the quantification of ternary complexes as they form as direct measurements [3, 7, 17–22]. Competition experiments provide more insightful data, with the ability to calculate apparent affinities and cooperativities of ternary complexes using AlphaLISA, TR-FRET, fluorescence polarization (FP), microscale thermophoresis and ^{19}F nuclear magnetic resonance (NMR), and other approaches [15, 23–26].

Isothermal titration calorimetry (ITC) has been a staple of ternary complex measurement [3, 5, 15, 27] and provides highly accurate quantification of both affinity and cooperativity. As a calorimetric technique, it is also capable of providing quantitative data on enthalpic and entropic contributions to the K_d of ternary complex formation, which will reflect ternary complex features such as neo-PPI interfaces, plasticity, and linker folding. Its main drawbacks are that it has relatively low throughput and normally requires sample concentrations well above those that would be physiologically relevant. Surface plasmon resonance (SPR), on the other hand, relies on sample flow to measure binding affinities, and as such enables measurement of kinetic binding, in particular k_{on} and k_{off}, which yield the K_d for both binary and ternary complexes [28]. Biolayer interferometry (BLI) yields similar data to SPR, although without the use of sample flow that improves data quality, but has been successfully used to characterize degrader ternary complexes [29]. Both SPR and BLI can provide information on both cooperativity and residency of the ternary complexes measured.

4.1.3.2 Structural Biology

Structural approaches provide a means for actually observing the nature of ternary complexes and deriving a rational basis for the observed behaviors and biological degrader activities. Structures exhibiting polymorphism, such as flexibility, plasticity, or simply a diversity of populated species, are typically an anathema to most structural biology techniques, which may at best be able to capture single, potentially unrepresentative, snapshots of ternary complex behavior. ^{15}N-heteronuclear-single-quantum-coherence (HSQC) NMR is one example of an approach that can be used to explore flexibility; however, it relies on having a relatively small construct for at least one partner protein, such as was the case for the cIAP1 Bir3 domain (cIAP1^{Bir3}) [29].

Mass spectrometry (MS) also provides numerous avenues to study ternary complex formation. For recombinant constructs of partner proteins, native MS can not only provide information on the efficacy of degraders but also features such as complex assembly and cooperativity [30–32]. Hydrogen-deuterium exchange (HDX)-MS on the other hand yields critical information on which interfaces are shielded from solution, providing insights into both binding poses and stability of ternary complexes [33].

The main workhorses of structural biology, cryogenic electron microscopy (cryo-EM), NMR, and X-ray crystallography all have much to contribute to the structural resolution of ternary complexes, but each comes with drawbacks.

Cryo-EM has been successfully utilized in two studies of MG-induced complexes to elucidate the overall ternary complex assembly [34, 35]; however, these required X-ray crystallographic data for the finer details of MG engagement and the induced contacts. Cryo-EM has clear advantages in its capacity to elucidate the structural details for very large complexes (recently often to atomic resolution) and the fact that samples do not need to be crystallized. However, sample preparation is challenging, resolutions are not always high enough to visualize binding ligands and the details of interfacing residues, and data analysis can still be confounded by multiple conformations and dynamics. As an extremely nascent approach relative to its cousins, NMR and X-ray crystallography, innovations in the technology, and modeling capabilities may make these challenges non-issues within the next 5–10 years [36] to make it the central tool for elucidating ternary complex structures.

At first glance, NMR would seem to be the ultimate approach for structural resolution of ternary complexes, being conducted in solution, amenable to disordered species, and having a plethora of different spectroscopic approaches that could provide insights into various aspects of ternary complex behavior. Unfortunately, complexes larger than about 15 kDa do not typically yield high-quality spectra in the absence of isotopic labeling beyond the standard ^{13}C and ^{15}N. As most E3 ligases or their targets generally require relatively large recombinant constructs to engage with the degrader molecules and in the ternary complexes, there are no studies to date utilizing this structural approach.

X-ray crystallography is currently the best situated structural approach for the resolution of ternary complex structures [37]. As a relatively mature technique that has experienced major innovations in the past two decades, it has become accessible even for groups with limited expertise and resources. Structures that can be solved will typically be of sufficient resolution to see interfaces and ideally degrader molecules, and it is tolerant of very large complex sizes. The key challenge for X-ray crystallography is the need to generate diffraction-quality crystals, which can greatly limit the throughput.

The vast majority of ternary complex structures have been generated by X-ray crystallography, and these will be explored through the rest of this chapter.

4.2 X-ray Crystal Structures of Ternary Complexes

For macromolecules, the generation of crystals and the solution of their structures remains no easy feat, although advances in approaches, robotics, and general know-how have improved the rates at which structures can be solved. Two of the main parameters that influence the success of macromolecular crystallization are the monodispersity and monomorphism of the sample. As the terms suggest, samples prefer to crystallize when they are a single species that adopts a single shape, as this provides the best template for crystal growth. Unfortunately, beyond the standard challenges crystallographers face in overcoming these for their samples, degraders (in particular, PROTACs) introduce additional problems via stoichiometry, plasticity, and flexibility in their ternary complexes. As the induced interactions via the PROTAC molecule will not always be favorable, the interplay of affinities and cooperativity with stoichiometry need to be considered to yield the most monodisperse sample possible. On the other hand, ternary complexes are likely to exhibit some degree of flexibility, given the two proteins are being "made to meet," usually through otherwise very limited contacts. Particularly flexible or plastic ternary complexes are much less likely to yield crystals because of their polymorphism, and any samples that do crystallize will never represent the true population distribution of binding poses, as a single crystal will (typically) only crystallize with a single, closely related set of binding poses.

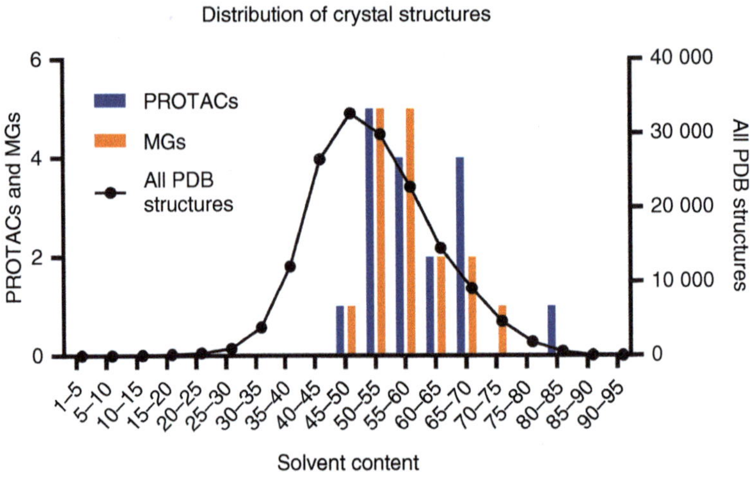

Figure 4.2 The distribution of the solvent contents for PROTAC (blue) and MG (orange) structures compared to all those in the PDB. *Source:* Data retrieved from rcsb.org on 21st November 2021.

Perhaps one interesting feature of ternary complex crystal structures solved to date is their crystal solvent contents. An oft-ignored property of the crystal, the solvent content is effectively a reflection of how much space is available in the crystallographic unit cell per molecule/complex. Most macromolecular crystal structures have solvent contents around 50% (the median structure is roughly 50.4%); however, the ternary complexes are decidedly biased toward higher solvent contents, with only two out of more than 30 structures solved to date being below 50% (Figure 4.2). While these numbers are still relatively small, and there are a number of different drivers of solvent content, this tendency may be an indication that ternary complex structures require a high degree of flexibility (and therefore space to occupy) at the crystal growing interface. Employment of approaches to stabilize crystal contacts, such as additives and surface functional group modifications, as well as the use of strategies such as crystal dehydration to reduce disorder, may make ternary complexes more amenable to crystallization and structural resolution.

This section will be divided into two parts, between ternary complex structures of PROTAC (bifunctional) degraders and those of MGs, relevant to targeted degradation of proteins in human cells.

4.2.1 PROTAC-Induced Ternary Complex Structures

4.2.1.1 PROTACs Recruiting von Hippel–Lindau Protein (VHL)

The majority of PROTAC-induced ternary structures have been solved for von Hippel–Lindau protein (VHL)-targeting degraders and cover a variety of target classes, including bromodomains and kinases. VHL is most amenable to structural investigation in the presence of its adaptor proteins, elongin-B and elongin-C, which are present in every described structure, but to date have not been observed to influence ternary complex formation and are thus not discussed.

4.2.1.1.1 VHL and BRD4

The structures of three PROTAC molecules inducing complexes between VHL and the BET protein BRD4 have been solved, two recruiting the second bromodomain ($BRD4^{BD2}$) and two recruiting the first ($BRD4^{BD1}$).

$BRD4^{BD2}$

The structure of MZ1 with both VHL and $BRD4^{BD2}$ (PDB code 5T35) represented the first crystal structure of a PROTAC degrader in complex with both binding partners [3]. MZ1 was discovered by linking the ester of JQ1 with the acetamide of VH032 via a diethylene glycol linker (Figure 4.3) [38]. MZ1 was found to be an effective degrader of all BET proteins but had particular selectivity toward the degradation of BRD4. Investigation by ITC, SPR, and AlphaLISA uncovered that these differences in selectivity were likely driven by the cooperativities of the ternary complexes formed with the different bromodomains [3, 28]. Correspondingly, the structure reveals highly cooperative complex formation between all three binding partners.

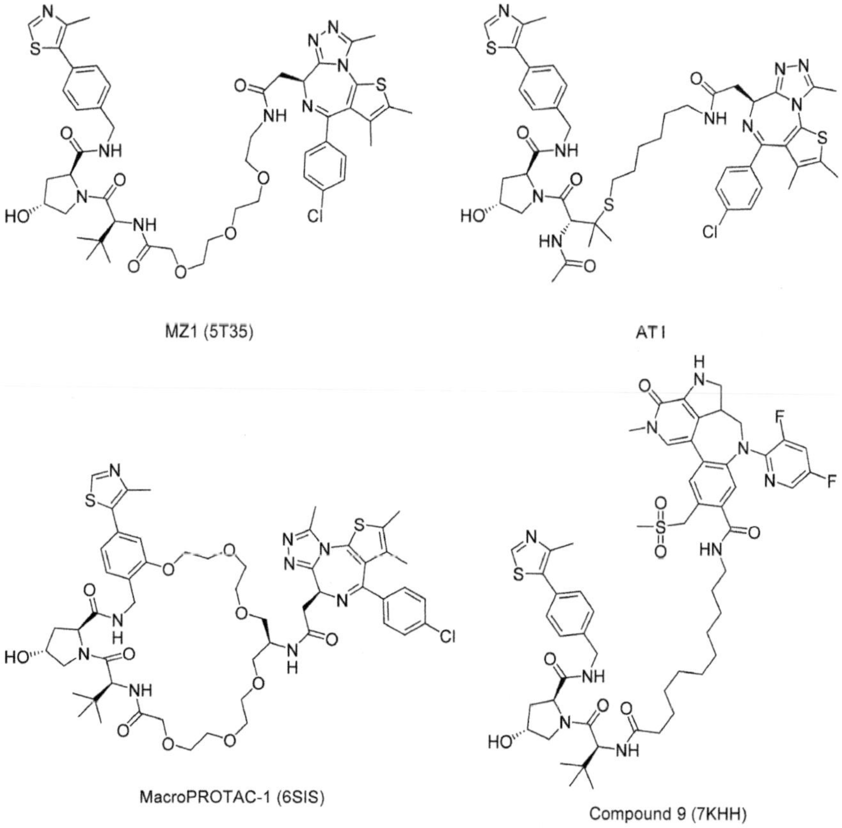

Figure 4.3 Structures of MZ1, AT1, and MacroPROTAC1 recruiting $BRD4^{BD2}$ and compound 9 recruiting $BRD4^{BD1}$.

A small, but not insignificant, complementary hydrophobic interface is formed between the two proteins. This interface is focused around sites adjacent to the ligand-binding sites, including the ZA-loop of BRD4 and the β1 and β4 strands and adjacent loops of the VHL substrate-binding domain (VHL_{SBD}), and is exemplified in an extension of $BRD4^{BD2}$'s WPF shelf into Pro71 of VHL. Hydrogen bonds are formed between Arg107 of VHL and Glu383 of BRD4 and His110 of VHL and Ala384 of BRD4. These are reinforced by salt bridges at the edges of the interface, forming between Arg108 of VHL and Asp381 and Glu383 of BRD4 as well as Arg69 of VHL and Glu438 of BRD4 (Figure 4.4a).

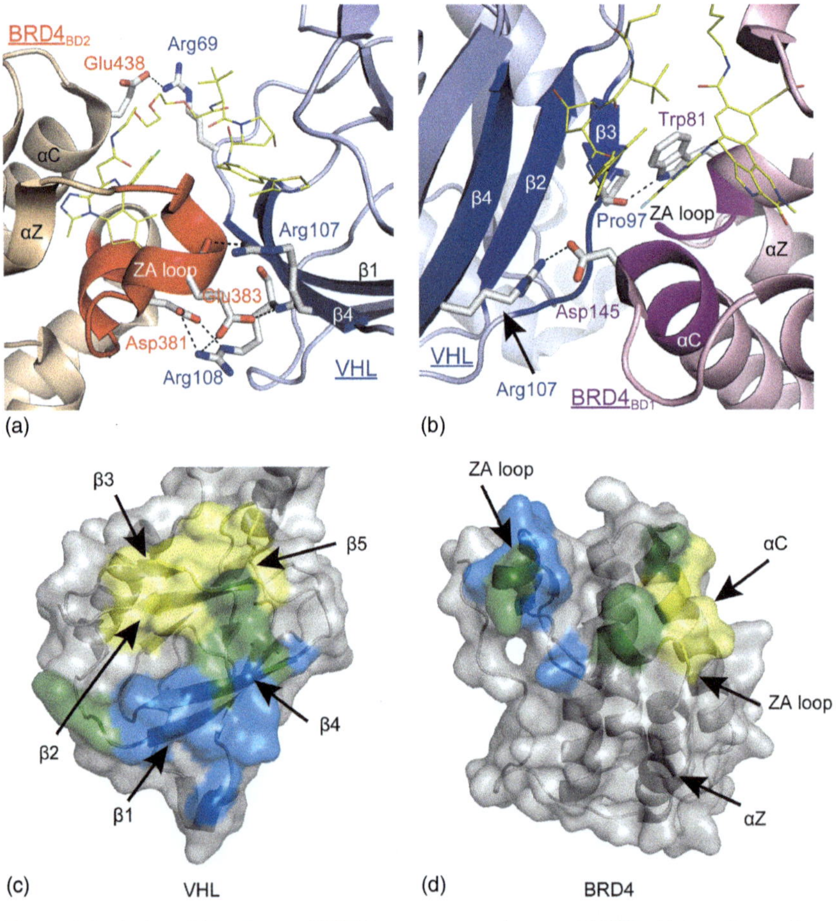

Figure 4.4 Induced interfaces of BRD4 ternary complexes with VHL. (a) Interfaces of $Brd4^{BD2}$ (red) and VHL (blue) induced to interact by MZ1 (yellow sticks) in PDB structure 5T35 and (b) $Brd4^{BD1}$ (magenta) and VHL (blue) induced to interact by compound 9 (yellow sticks) in PDB structure 7KHH. Key elements of secondary structure and interfacing residues are indicated in darker colors and stick representation, respectively. (c, d) Comparison of VHL (c) and BRD4 bromodomain (d) binding surfaces in the induced ternary complexes. Residues forming PPIs in the MZ1 complex (5T35) in blue, in the compound 9 complex (7KHH) in yellow, and in both complexes in green.

The interactions between BRD4 and VHL result in an interface area of 343 Å^2. A small number of noncognate van der Waals contacts are observed between the linker and BRD4, as well as the individual moieties and the opposite binding partners, that contribute to the induced interaction interface. Including the contacts of the ligands in their binding pockets, the interface areas for MZ1:VHL and MZ1:BRD4 are 489 and 506 Å^2, respectively, leading to a total interface area of 1338 Å^2 for the ternary complex. Additionally, intramolecular contacts are found within MZ1, although these largely serve to allow the PROTAC to "fold in" to a compact form that stabilizes the neo-PPIs of the induced VHL:BRD4$_{BD2}$ interface.

Two efforts were pursued to exploit these structural data to improve the activity of the BET-degrading PROTACs. Based on the complex that had been observed, AT1 was designed to exploit the proximity of the *tert*-butyl group of the VH032 to the location of the JQ1 ester (Figure 4.3), in the hopes that this would further restrict the recruitment of the BET bromodomains to this particular conformation, which was believed to be privileged for the recruitment of BRD4^{BD2}. AT1 was found to be significantly more selective for degradation of BRD4 but at the cost of cooperativity across all targets and also degradation potency toward BRD4 itself.

A second effort took MZ1 and added another diethyl glycol linker, this time tethered to the phenyl ring of VH032 to generate a PROTAC effectively linked by a macrocycle, dubbed MacroPROTAC-1 (Figure 4.3) [39]. A structure of this molecule in complex with VHL and BRD4^{BD2} (PDB code 6SIS) was found to yield the same interface between the two proteins. The second arm of the macrocyclic linker nestles within a groove of the ZA-loop of BRD4^{BD2}, and sequence alignments indicate that this binding mode is better accommodated by the second bromodomains of the BET proteins than the first. While MacroPROTAC-1 exhibited significantly worse binding affinity toward the bromodomains, its ternary complex had slightly higher affinity than MZ1 and had favorable changes in cooperativity that led to equal degradation potency (see Figure 4.10a).

BRD4^{BD1}

Compound 9 was discovered by taking a simultaneously described novel BET inhibitor and incorporating this into a PROTAC with VH032 (Figure 4.3) [40]. The design of this molecule is most different from that of MZ1 by having a linker that is alkyl-based and using a vector from the BET inhibitor that projects from the opposite site of the binding pocket, across the WPF shelf. Despite compound 9 having little difference in binding affinity for BD1 or BD2 of BRD4, the ternary complex formed with VHL and BRD4^{BD1} is roughly 100 times longer lived than that of BRD4^{BD2}, as determined by SPR. This is most striking in that compound 8, a PROTAC of the same structure but instead with a polyethylene glycol (PEG) linker of the same length, exhibits only a twofold higher stability of BRD4^{BD2} in the ternary complex compared to BRD4^{BD1}. This is ultimately reflected in their cellular activities, with compound 9 exhibiting a roughly 50-fold increase in both degradation and antiproliferation potency over compound 8.

The structure of VHL:compound 9:BRD4^{BD1} (PDB code 7KHH) reveals why this is the case. The hydrophobicity of the alkyl linker, the VHL ligand's *tert*-butyl group, and the BET ligand itself allow the compound to effectively collapse within the ternary complex, folding into a compact state that stabilizes the neo-PPI interface between VHL and $BRD4^{BD1}$. Compound 9 recruits the region at the end of $BRD4^{BD1}$'s αZ helix and the N-terminal portion of the αC helix to VHL's β2, β4, and particularly β3 strands (Figure 4.4b). This results in an interface that mediates a very different orientation and binding pose to the MZ1 complex (Figure 4.4c,d) and facilitates a hydrogen bond between Trp81 of BRD4 and Pro97 of VHL and a salt bridge between Asp145 of BRD4 and Arg107 of VHL. When taken together, the interactions between $BRD4^{BD1}$ and VHL result in an interface area of 353 $Å^2$. The interface areas for compound 9:VHL and compound 9:$BRD4^{BD1}$ are 384 and 499 $Å^2$, respectively, which lead to a total surface area of 1236 $Å^2$ for the ternary complex induced by compound 9.

One noteworthy aspect of compound 9's ternary structure is that the phenylmethylthiazole group on the right-hand side of the VHL pocket is displaced and filled by Arg107 and Ile109. This arrangement mimics the conformation of Arg107 in the unbound form of VHL [41] and enables the residue to form its salt bridge with Asp145 of BRD4. In this conformation, the phenylmethylthiazole appears only to form a π–π interaction with His110 of VHL. Given that this pocket is induced by the presence of phenylthiazoles or phenyloxazoles [42], this observation offers an insight into opportunities for design and modification around even the ligand moieties of PROTAC molecules, potentially vastly expanding the scope of PROTAC optimization beyond linkers and their vectors, to complete reimagining of ligand-binding sites in the context of ternary, rather than binary, complexes. This is underscored, with a caveat, by compound 12, which exhibits an oxypiperidine addition to the phenyl ring of the VHL ligand and has an even greater half-life, presumably because of further stabilization of the complex. This, however, comes in hand with a decrease in cellular potencies back to the level of the PEG-linked compound 8, suggesting either too much stabilization or some other disruption of productive ubiquitination and degradation has taken place.

4.2.1.1.2 VHL and SMARCA

Degraders for SMARCA2 and SMARCA4, two subunits of the SWI/SNF or BAF chromatin remodeling complex, were discovered by a joint team at Dundee and Boehringer Ingelheim (BI). While ostensibly tumor suppressors, several cancer cell lines have been found to be SMARCA2 or SMARCA4 dependent, particularly acute myeloid leukemia [43]. As such, degradation of SMARCA2 and SMARCA4 has been investigated for its therapeutic potential and led the Dundee-BI team to discover degraders PROTAC 1, PROTAC 2, and ACBI1 through an iterative approach using structure-guided design (Figure 4.5a).

Based on their own structural data, the team took a disclosed 2-(6-aminopyridazin-3-yl)phenol-based SMARCA bromodomain inhibitor [44] and chose a piperazine derivative as a good attachment point [26]. This was linked to a high-affinity VHL ligand, VH101, with a fluorocyclopropyl group [45], to design a small series of compounds that included PROTAC 1, containing a diethylene glycol linker attached

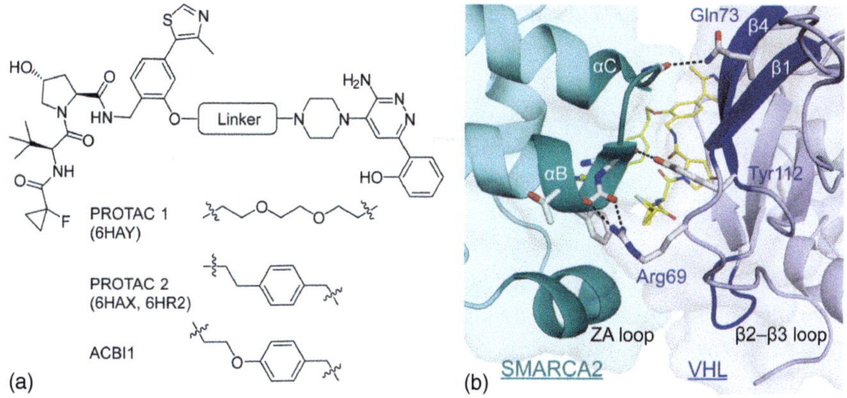

Figure 4.5 Degradation of SMARCA BDs by VHL-recruiting PROTACs. (a) Structures of SMARCA-targeting PROTAC 1, PROTAC 2, and ACBI1. (b) Interfaces of SMARCA2 (turquoise) and VHL (blue) induced to interact by PROTAC 2 (yellow sticks) in PDB structure 6HAX. Key elements of secondary structure and interfacing residues are indicated in darker colors and stick representation, respectively.

to VH101 through a phenol. Despite a roughly 20-fold loss in binding affinity to the bromodomains, PROTAC 1 successfully degraded SMARCA2, SMARCA4, and related protein PBRM1 and stabilized their ternary complexes. The activity was attributed to positive cooperativity for the bromodomains (α = 4.4–14) as measured by FP and TR-FRET. To understand the observations made about cooperativity and its potential for further design of SMARCA PROTACs, the crystal structure of VHL:PROTAC 1:SMARCA2^{BD} was solved (PDB code 6HAY).

Overall, the binding of PROTAC 1 is the same as each binder to their respective protein in a binary system, with only a small rearrangement in the BC loop of SMARCA2. SMARCA2 and VHL showed de novo interactions with VHL's N-terminal section, β1 and β4 strands, and β2–β3 loop binding to SMARCA2^{BD}'s BC loop and second short helix in the ZA loop. Several hydrogen bonds are captured, including from the side chains of VHL residues Gln73 and Tyr112 to the backbone carbonyls of Gly1467 and Asn1464, respectively. Additionally, two strong hydrogen bonds are mediated by Arg69 of VHL to the highly electronegative carbonyls of Thr1462 and Phe1463 at the C-terminal end of SMARCA2^{BD}'s αB helix – the importance of which was confirmed by mutagenesis (Figure 4.5b). The interactions between SMARCA2 and VHL result in an interface area of 329 Å^2. The interfaces for PROTAC 1:VHL and PROTAC 1:SMARCA2 are 476 and 365 Å^2, respectively, leading to a total surface area of 1171 Å^2.

The authors observed that a number of noncognate interactions were coming from the fluorocyclopropyl group of the VHL ligand to SMARCA2^{BD}, validating the choice of linker attachment point, but that the phenol-attached PEG linker packed in closely to the VHL residue Tyr98. Thus, the PEG linker was replaced with a 1,4-substituted phenyl with an additional three methylenes for the attachment, hoping to take advantage of the hydrophobicity and aromaticity of the environment of the linker, yielding PROTAC 2. This compound was cocrystallized with VHL and both SMARCA2^{BD} and SMARCA4^{BD} (PDB codes 6HAX and 6HR2, respectively).

The PROTAC 2 complex forms the same induced interactions with VHL and SMARCA2$_{BD}$ as can be seen for PROTAC 1, and this is recapitulated for SMARCA4$_{BD}$ as the interfacing residues are identical (Figure 4.5b). The new phenyl ring in the linker mediates a T-shaped π-stacking interaction to Tyr98 of VHL. The phenyl ring reproduces a similar conformation for the PROTAC as the flexible PEG linker. PROTAC 2 generates cooperativity α values of between 13 and 21 for the various bromodomains, suggesting greater favorability of stabilizing the complexes. This was reflected in improved degradation and potency of PROTAC 2 relative to PROTAC 1. The structural insights led to the incorporation of a phenolic ether oxygen within the linker to generate a new PROTAC, ACBI1, with even greater cooperativity values, presumably in part because of some additional slack in the linker allowing the adoption of a more favorable conformation and contacts (see Figure 4.10b). ACBI1 was found to be a significantly more potent PROTAC, with DC_{50} values of 6 nM for SMARCA2 and 11 nM for SMARCA4. Ultimately, this study illustrates how identifying a stable induced ternary complex can help rationalize optimization for some target and E3 ligase pairs. The combination of biophysical assays and crystallography was instrumental for the structure-guided design that led to a highly efficacious PROTAC.

4.2.1.1.3 VHL and Bcl-xL

A team at GlaxoSmithKline (GSK) discovered PROTAC 6 using the inhibitor A-1155463 [10], which had been found to be selective for B-cell lymphoma extra large (Bcl-xL) over Bcl-2 [46]. This PROTAC was designed by replacing a terminal and solvent-exposed tertiary amine with a pentaethylene glycol linker, which was coupled directly to the acetamide of VH032. PROTAC 6 was found to be a potent degrader, with a DC_{50} value of about 5 nM and exhibited marginal negative cooperativity ($\alpha = 0.72$), as determined by SPR.

The structure of VHL:PROTAC 6:Bcl-xL (PDB code 6ZHC) revealed that, despite the negative cooperativity, PROTAC 6 induces a significant number of neo-PPIs (Figure 4.6a). The VHL β2 and β3 strands and their linking β-hairpin make extensive contacts with the α2–α3 loop of Bcl-xL, while the N-terminal tail of the VHL$_{SBD}$ contacts the α4–α5 loop on the other side of the Bax/Bak-binding site of Bcl-xL. A hydrogen-bonding network is formed between Asn90, Phe91, and Gln96 of VHL with Arg103 and Ala104 of Bcl-xL, and a strong salt bridge is formed between Arg60 of VHL and Asp133 of Bcl-xL. Several van der Waals contacts are made too, in particular Phe91 of VHL sits within a shallow hydrophobic groove between Ala104 and Phe105 of Bcl-xL, and a π-stacking interaction with the latter.

Quite important noncognate interactions are also observed: the *tert*-butyl of VH032 interfaces with the α2–α3 loop of Bcl-xL and sandwiches Tyr101 between itself, the A-1155463-like moiety, and the linker. The carboxylic acid of A-1155463 is also a focal point – normally coordinated by Asn136 and Arg139 of Bcl-xL, both Asn67 and Arg69 of VHL also contact the acid, with the latter forming a salt bridge. Several bridging water molecules make further neo-PPI and noncognate hydrogen

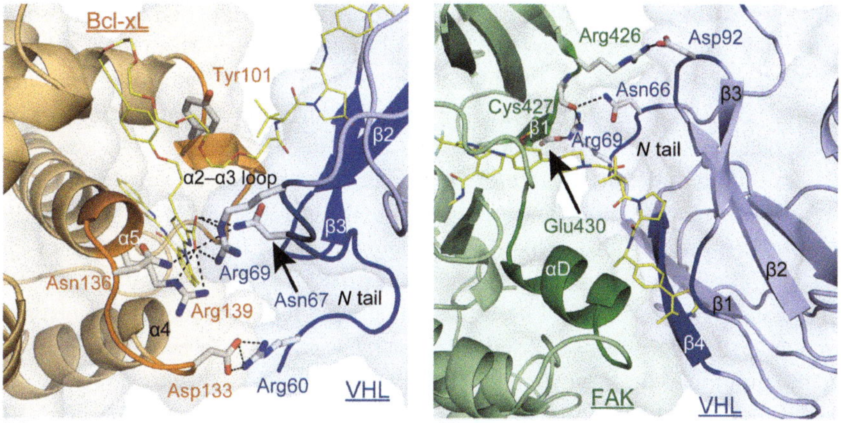

(a) (b)

Figure 4.6 Induced interfaces of Bcl-xL and FAK ternary complexes with VHL. (a) Interfaces of Bcl-xL (orange) and VHL (blue) induced to interact by PROTAC 6 (yellow sticks) in PDB structure 6ZHC and (b) FAK (green) and VHL (blue) induced to interact by GSK215 (yellow sticks) in PDB structure 7PI4. Key elements of secondary structure and interfacing residues are indicated in darker colors and stick representation, respectively.

bonds. The interactions between Bcl-xL and VHL produce an interface of 308 Å^2. The interface area for PROTAC 6:VHL and PROTAC 6:Bcl-xL is 469 and 785 Å^2, respectively, giving a total surface area of 1561 Å^2.

The most curious feature of this ternary complex is the fact that, in spite of a relatively large number of induced contacts, PROTAC 6 exhibits a very slight negative cooperativity. This is most likely attributable to the conformation of the PEG linker, which is forced to fold back on the phenol ether portion of the A-1155463 analog. As described by the authors, this will pose a significant entropic penalty to formation of this ternary complex posed by PROTAC 6 [10], outweighing the enthalpic gains and resulting in the observed negative cooperativity. Most clearly, as the authors point out, this ternary complex structure illustrates the potential for non-optimal PROTACs to yield structural information that leads to design insights that may not be accessible by empiricism or SAR. Both the linker and the ligand moieties themselves could be altered to leverage these structural data into a PROTAC better suited to recruit this ternary complex pose (see Figure 4.10c). Indeed, more broadly, there may be a plethora of inactive, entropically inhibited PROTAC molecules that do in fact allow the formation of productive ternary complex poses with recombinant proteins that could generate structural insights to design PROTACs more capable of taking advantage of favorable ternary complex contacts.

4.2.1.1.4 VHL and FAK

Focal adhesion kinase (FAK) has been the target of several targeted protein degradation studies from a variety of groups in recent years [47–49]. GSK215 (also discovered by GSK scientists) was generated by replacing the morpholine of VS-4718 with a 4-piperazineacetic acid to couple with the free amine of VHL-021 (equivalent of

VH032 with a benzylic methyl), producing a compound of the two moieties effectively attached directly together [11]. TR-FRET and SPR found GSK215 to exhibit an $\alpha = 104$ for its ternary complex formation with VHL and FAK, indicating very high levels of positive cooperativity, which in turn was found to strongly correlate with the degradation as evaluated by DC_{50} levels.

The structure of VHL:GSK215:FAK (PDB code 7PI4) reveals a tightly bound complex of the three – naturally, given that any true linker is essentially absent from the PROTAC molecule (Figure 4.6b). The N-terminal coil and the β2–β3 hairpin of the VHL_{SBD} contact the β1 strand of FAK's N-terminal lobe. Separately, VHL's β1, β3–β4 loop and β4 contact αD in FAK's C-terminal lobe. The side chains of Asn66 and Arg69 in VHL form hydrogen bonds with FAK's Cys427, while two borderline salt bridges are formed between Arg69 and Asp92 in VHL with Glu430 and Arg426 in FAK, respectively, all concentrated on FAK's N-terminal lobe. Ultimately, the FAK:VHL interface comprises a surface area of 365.9 $Å^2$ and forms a virtual cage around GSK215. This leads to αD of FAK having a large degree of van der Waals contact with the normally open phenylmethylthiazole and methyl groups of the VHL-021 ligand, leading to a total FAK:GSK215 interface area of 590.3 $Å^2$. Additionally, the VHL:GSK215 interface has an area of 401.8 $Å^2$, producing a total ternary complex interface area of 1358 $Å^2$.

One key finding of this study was that compound 2, akin to GSK215 but with an additional eight methylenes in the linker, had an even higher cooperativity value ($\alpha = 130$) than GSK215, but roughly fivefold lower degradation potency. Given the tightly packed nature of the GSK215 structure and the fact that this complex did not seem to be amenable to crystallization, it was speculated that the compound 2 complex is more flexible, leading to less-efficient degradation. Further structural investigation would be required to definitively say whether compound 2 results in a flexible and dynamic ternary complex or somehow traps it into an unproductive conformational arrangement.

4.2.1.1.5 VHL and WDR5

Degraders targeting WD40 repeat domain protein 5 (WDR5), a key histone methyltransferase complex component, were discovered by a mix of empirical exploration and structure-guided design [27]. In the first round of discovery, the WDR5 inhibitor was coupled by converting its morpholine group into a piperazine, allowing amide coupling of a variety of PEG and alkyl linkers to both VH032- and pomalidomide-based ligands as E3 ligase recruiters. MS33, containing a nine-carbon linker to VH032 (Figure 4.7), was found to yield the best degradation of WDR5, and its complex with VHL and WDR5 was determined by ITC to have very slightly positive cooperativity ($\alpha = 1.66$) and was successfully resolved to 1.7 Å in a crystal structure (PDB code 7JTO). The structure reveals a very small neo-PPI interface (129 $Å^2$) between the VHL N-terminal tail and the β2–β3 hairpin and the loops between blades 4/5 and 5/6 on the bottom face of WDR5. This is stabilized only by salt bridges between Arg69 and Asp92 of VHL with Asp172 and Lys259 of WDR, respectively, as well as a few hydrogen bonds. Very limited van der Waals contacts are observed, and the interacting loops are generally quite disordered.

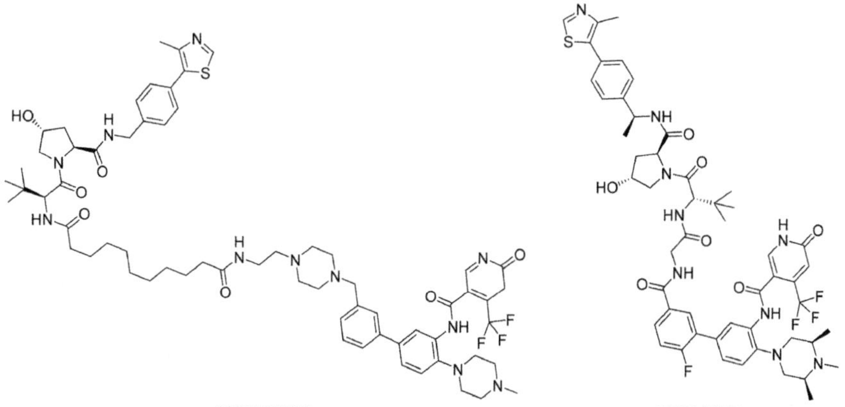

MS33 (7JTO) MS67 (7JTP)

Figure 4.7 Structures of MS33 and MS67.

With the insights of their crystal structure, the authors resolved to generate PROTACs with shorter linkages between the binding sites of the VHL and WDR5 ligands as the longer linker clearly did not facilitate contacts between the two proteins (see Figure 4.10d). Several optimizations to the ligands were made, including using the VHL-021 ligand and removing the methylpiperazine from the WDR5 ligand. These efforts yielded MS67, containing two amides to join the ligands linked by a methylene (Figure 4.7), which was found to exhibit higher levels of degradation and great potency than MS33. ITC revealed an increase in affinity of all interactions, in particular ternary complex formation, which had a K_d improvement of 10-fold and a slightly raised overall cooperativity to $\alpha = 2.74$. A more significant interface is mediated by MS67 (401 Å^2; PDB code 7JTP) than was seen for MS33, with the N-terminal tail, β1 and β4 strands of VHL forming interactions with the loops of blades 3, 4, and 5, again on the bottom face of WDR5. Far more van der Waals contacts are observed, supported by a π–π interaction between His110 and Tyr191, a salt bridge from Glu70 to Lys259, and hydrogen bonding from Arg109 and Arg108 to Ser171 and Asp192, when considering VHL and WDR5, respectively. There are also several van der Waals contacts mediated between the VHL-021 moiety and WDR5, as well as a hydrogen bond from the benzamide of the WDR5-binding moiety to Tyr112 of VHL. Combined with the interfaces of MS67 with VHL (470 Å^2) and WDR5 (566 Å^2), the total surface area of the ternary complex interface is 1437 Å^2.

4.2.1.2 PROTACs Recruiting Other E3 Ligases

4.2.1.2.1 Cereblon (CRBN) and BRD4

To date, the only structures of PROTACs recruiting cereblon (CRBN) as the E3 ligase are those deriving from the dBET series, targeting the BET bromodomain proteins [50, 51]. The team at the Dana–Farber Cancer Institute sought a structural and

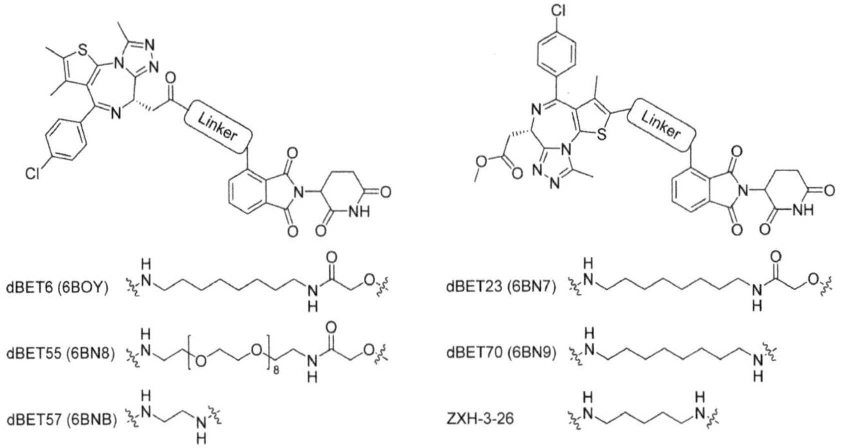

Figure 4.8 Structures of dBET6, dBET55, dBET57, dBET23, dBET70, and ZXH-3-26.

biophysical understanding of the ternary complexes formed by their degraders in the hopes of identifying pathways to improved potency and selectivity [7]. These PROTACs were generally found to have negative or close-to-neutral cooperativity ($\alpha = 0.1–0.8$) by TR-FRET, but typically with greater cooperativity for engaging with $BRD4^{BD1}$ compared to $BRD4^{BD2}$, which correlated with degradation activity. Mutagenesis of both CRBN and $BRD4^{BD1}$ revealed that each dBET molecule generally has distinct requirements for ternary complex formation, suggesting that while they may generally engage common interfaces, these are relatively plastic, and each degrader may induce interactions with them differently.

Induced CRBN:$BRD4^{BD1}$ structures were solved for dBET6 (PDB code 6BOY) and dBET55 (6BN8), which use the ester of JQ1 for amide coupling as a linkage, and dBET23 (6BN7) and dBET70 (6BN9), which is attached by replacing a methyl in the thiophene group (Figure 4.8). Each is linked to thalidomide via functionalization of the heteroatom at the C4 group. The structures of the induced complex were all found to adopt the same binding pose. A major interaction surface is formed between the $CRBN^{NTD}$ and $BRD4^{BD1}$'s ZA loop and αC helix, largely composed of van der Waals interactions, but additionally hydrogen bonds between Gln78 of BRD4 and Gln100 of CRBN as well as Asp145 of BRD4 and His103 of CRBN are created. Intriguingly, despite being tethered to the $CRBN^{TBD}$, $BRD4^{BD1}$ only marginally interacts here by engaging β10–β11 loop residues in CRBN via ZA loop residues that are already engaged with the $CRBN^{NTD}$. These induced interactions lead to an interface surface area of 520–570 $Å^2$, depending on the degrader. The isoindoline of the thalidomide moiety of the PROTAC molecules form a π-stacking interaction with Trp40 of $BRD4^{BD1}$ as an additional noncognate-induced interaction that promotes the ternary complex.

Because of the lack of suitable electron density of the PROTAC molecules in some structures, the conformations and degree to which each of the dBET degraders interface with each partner protein is unclear. The orientation of the isoindoline ring of the thalidomide moiety flips to accommodate the different linkage vectors of the BET binders – dBET23 links through the traditional C4 group orientation seen for CRBN molecular glue structures (see Section 4.2.2.1), whereas dBET6 is flipped 180° and projects in the opposite direction. The linker of dBET23 has a degree of van der Waals contacts with the first short helix of BRD4^{BD1}'s ZA loop, while dBET6's acetamide carbonyl hydrogen bonds with the Asn351 side chain of CRBN. dBET6 makes noncognate van der Waals interactions from the aryl chloride of JQ1 with a small projection formed between His353 and Tyr355 of CRBN; however, they appear to adopt this arrangement because of the disturbance by the acetamide linkage, as they exhibit different conformers for dBET23 and the chlorobenzene only interfaces with His353. These residues are observed to change conformation upon target recruitment following the binding of IMiDs, suggesting that either set of conformations may contribute positively to recruiting BRD4^{BD1} via the different degraders, depending on the needs of the linkers. For those structures with visible ligands, total ternary complex interface surface areas of 1290–1330 $Å^2$ are observed.

A final CRBN:BRD4^{BD1} structure induced by dBET57 (PDB code 6BNB), which uses the JQ1-ester linkage point and possesses a very short linker of only two methylenes (Figure 4.8), was solved and revealed a unique binding pose compared to others [7]. It was observed that neo-PPIs created between BRD4 and CRBN were in this case focused on the CRBN^{TBD}, in particular β12 interfaces with Trp81 of the ZA loop and the beginning of αC, while the β10–β11 and β13–β14 loops interface with residues 90–96 of the ZA loop and the end of αB. The absence of the PROTAC molecule from the electron density again makes estimating the total interface area difficult, but the neo-PPIs have a surface of 479 $Å^2$.

Molecular modeling established that there are a large number of weak, less-populated binding poses for CRBN:BRD4^{BD1} complexes in the absence of a ligand. The authors speculated that the main observed binding pose may be an artifact of the crystal contacts, and this would seem to be reinforced by the differing mutagenesis patterns for each degrader [7]. HDX MS studies of dBET6 further suggested that the observed binding pose is not a genuine population of the complex [33]. However, this approach would fail to observe interface shielding in the case of the plastic complexes that may explore multiple interfaces, emphasized by the study identifying shielding only for their degrader, CFT-1297, which was found to be much more stable and cooperative ($\alpha = 21$) than dBET6 using AlphaLISA [33]. Ultimately, the main requirement for the major binding pose observed for the dBET compounds appears to be having a linker of sufficient length, and the overall neo-PPI interface areas of both binding poses discovered within the study are larger than any mediated by a PROTAC-induced ternary complex involving VHL and roughly equivalent to those generated by IMiDs for CRBN, both of which have been observed to generate highly stable cooperative complexes. Thus, these plastic binding poses may easily be important populations of the complexes induced by these degraders that are entropically disfavored, but further biophysical and structural studies are needed to dissect this. A key finding of the work was that the negatively cooperative dBET degraders could still induce profound degradation of the target protein and that selectivity was governed by which target exhibited the least negative cooperativity, reinforcing findings with VHL-based PROTACs targeting BET proteins via an iBET726 moiety [5].

4.2.1.2.2 Cellular Inhibitor of Apoptosis Protein 1 (cIAP1) and BTK

Bifunctional molecules recruiting cellular inhibitor of apoptosis protein 1 (cIAP1) are typically called specific and non-genetic IAP-dependent protein erasers (SNIPERs) but are otherwise functionally analogs to PROTACs [52]. Two structures of cIAP1 in induced ternary complexes with Bruton's tyrosine kinase (BTK) have been solved by a team at Pfizer in an effort to understand the structural basis of the degrader activity mediated by cIAP1 recruitment [29]. BTK has been a popular target for PROTAC development in recent years, with early efforts focusing on CRBN-, VHL-, and MDM2-based degraders [17, 53, 54]. For cIAP1-based PROTACs (i.e. SNIPERS), BC5P was chosen as the starting point for characterizing BTK degradation. BC5P is composed of a pentaethylene glycol linker to couple the BTK recruiter, PF-06250112 (based on previous work with CRBN-linked PROTACs) [17], to a derivative of a cIAP1 antagonist that acts through the Bir3 domain (Figure 4.9a) [55].

The BC5P-induced complex of BTK and cIAP1^{Bir3} was cocrystallized (PDB code 6W8I) and revealed a high degree of flexibility [29]. The conformation of the linker in the crystal structure appeared to be unclear, and different poses of the ternary complex were observed in each copy of the complex in the asymmetric unit. Combined with a ^{15}N-HSQC and molecular modeling, this suggested that the structures represented only a small fraction of a broad distribution of ternary complexes with a flexible assembly, indicating a certain plasticity and dynamism in the induced interaction. Each complex in the asymmetric unit reveals a different interface (Figure 4.9b), with the contacts on cIAP1^{Bir3} focused around either its central β-sheet or more so with the C-terminal three-helix bundle, while for BTK, the interactions happen variously with the β1–β3 strands of the N-terminal lobe, hinge region, and N-terminal activation loop. This leads to induced PPI interfaces of between 95 and 367 Å^2 across the three complexes, highlighting the variation between them.

Using this structural information, a new degrader BCPyr was designed, containing a 2,5-pyrazine linker to accommodate the length and vector of the linker that was

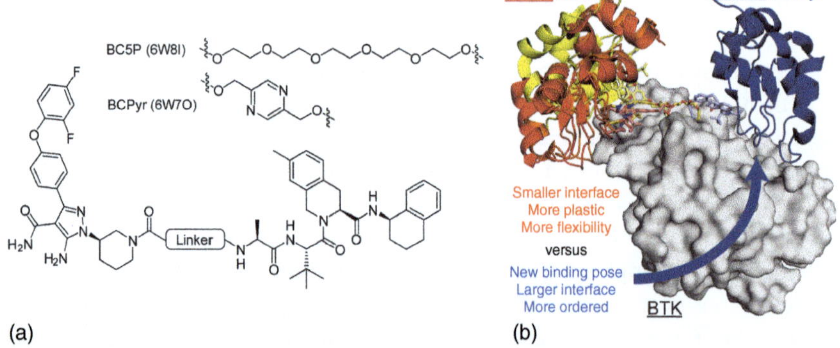

Figure 4.9 Degradation of BTK by cIAP1-recruiting PROTACs. (a) Structures of BC5P and BCPyr. (b) Alignment of the BC5P- and BCPyr-induced ternary complexes through BTK (gray surface). cIAP1 is shown in ribbon form (red, orange, yellow for BC5P, blue for BCPyr). PROTACs are shown as complementary colored sticks.

observed for one of the conformations with BC5P (~12 Å), with less capacity to rotate (Figure 4.9a). BCPyr in complex with cIAP1 and BTK was solved (PDB code 6W7O) and revealed a completely new pose to the structure compared with BC5P that was largely consistent between the two complexes in the asymmetric unit (Figure 4.9b). From BTK, the β1 strand in the N-terminal lobe and αD, αF, and the αF–αG loop in the C-terminal lobe interact with the loops beneath the peptide-binding site across the full αβ fold of $cIAP1^{Bir3}$. An extensive hydrogen bonding network is formed among these residues and a single salt bridge between Asp303 of $cIAP1^{Bir3}$ and Arg487 of BTK. The BCPyr complex results in an interface between cIAP1 and BTK of 512.9 $Å^2$. Additional interactions are observed between the carbonyl and the pyrazine of the linker with Cys481 and Asn484 of BTK, respectively, contributing to an interface area of 532 $Å^2$ for BCPyr:BTK. With the BCPyr:$cIAP1^{Bir3}$ interface of 390 $Å^2$, the total surface area of the induced ternary complex is 1435 $Å^2$. The complex is further stabilized by intramolecular interactions within the ligand, with the pyrazine of the linker making van der Waals contacts with the *tert*-butyl of the cIAP1-binding moiety.

The key finding for BCPyr was that, in spite of showing an extensive interface and an increase in positive cooperativity, as measured by BLI for multiple cIAP1 constructs, there was a greater than fourfold decrease in degradation potency (see Figure 4.10f). The resulting orderedness of the more cooperative complex was confirmed by ^{15}N-HSQC NMR and further molecular modeling, suggesting that it may be "trapped" in a less productive form for degradation activity. Overall, the two crystal structures showed that an increase in cooperativity does not necessarily lead to better degradation for cIAP1-recruiting degraders and that either more flexibility or plasticity to access particular binding poses may be necessary for optimal degrader activity.

4.2.1.3 Assessment of Structure-Guided Design of PROTAC Degraders

The majority of the studies reported above took the opportunity to utilize their ternary complex structures for structure-guided design of new PROTAC degraders (Figure 4.10). Structural changes included optimizing the binding ligands or linker for contacts within the ternary complex environment, shortening linkers to encourage tighter or specific interfaces, and new linkage arrangements to promote a desired binding pose. For those studies where design efforts focused on improvements of the observed binding pose, increases in selectivity and potency were observed, depending on the objective of the linkage (Figure 4.10a,b) [3, 26]. On the other hand, those that attempted to capture new binding poses had mixed luck with some finding increases in selectivity or degradation potency (Figure 4.10d,e) [7, 27], while another seemingly fell into an energy minimum that did not facilitate degradation activity (Figure 4.10f) [29]. For the dBET series degrader ZXH-3-26, careful analysis of trends within a large population of molecular modeling poses and tuning of linker length was key to generating a highly selective BRD4 degrader (Figure 4.10e) [7]. While these studies are still only a small number of efforts to draw significant conclusions from, they attest to structure-guided design of PROTACs as being a key tool in the armory for more rational and directed degrader discovery and development.

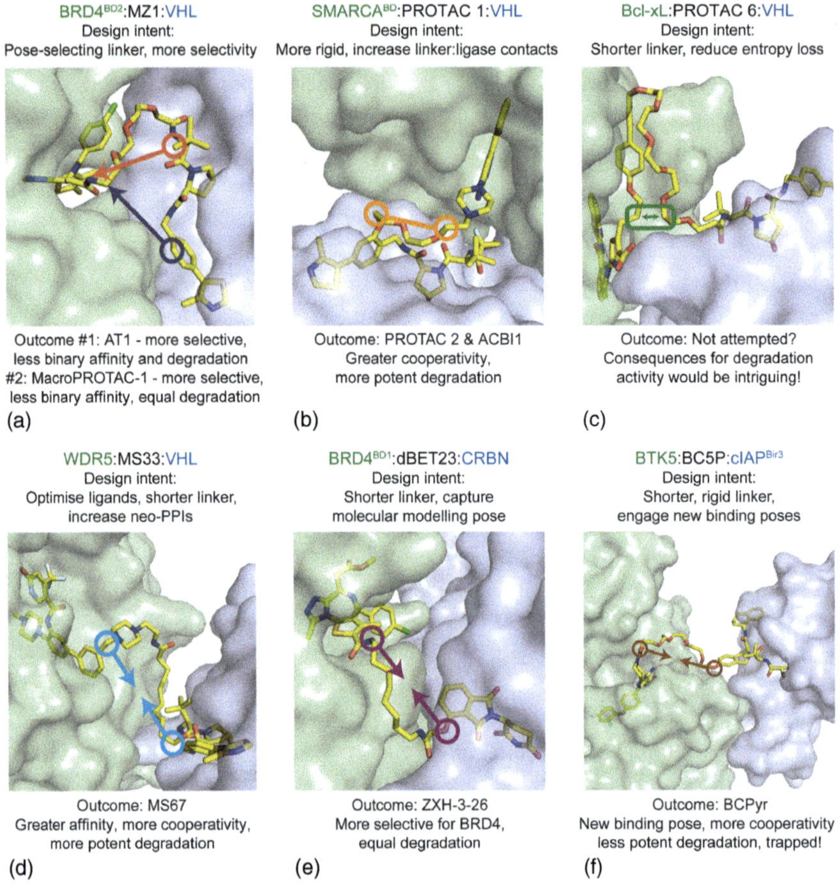

Figure 4.10 Overview of the structure-guided design efforts for PROTACs. Target proteins as green surface, PROTACs as yellow sticks, and E3 ligases as blue surfaces. (a) BRD4^{BD2}:MZ1:VHL (5T35) showing attachment points and vector for AT1 linkage (red) and MacroPROTAC-1 cyclizing linker (dark blue). (b) SMARCA2^{BD}:PROTAC 1:VHL (6HAY) showing atoms between which more rigid, aromatic linkers were substituted (orange) to give PROTAC 2 and ACBI1. (c) Bcl-xL:PROTAC 6:VHL (6ZHC) showing a potential linkage vector (dark green) that may yield very different degrader properties. (d) WDR5:MS33:VHL (7JTO) showing new attachment points (light blue) for MS67 linkage with a very short linker. (e) BRD^{BD1}:dBET23:CRBN (6BN7) showing atoms between which a shorter linker was used (purple) to yield ZXH-3-26 to capture a new binding pose. (f) BTK:BC5P:cIAP1^{Bir3} (6W8I) showing the atoms between which a much shorter, rigid linker was implemented (brown) to obtain BCPyr.

4.2.2 Molecular-Glue-Induced Ternary Complex Structures

To date, the vast majority of discovered or identified MGs that can function as degraders in human cells hijack the activity of the DDB1-CUL4B (CRL4) E3 ligase complex. As with other CRL E3 ligases, CRL4 mediates its activity through a variety of substrate receptors, dubbed DDB1-CUL4B-associated factors (DCAFs), which in turn recruit targets for ubiquitination. The MG degraders generally modify the

surface of the DCAF in order to recruit a novel substrate target protein (neosubstrate) to the substrate-binding interface. Several DCAF:MG:neosubstrate complex structures have now been solved. The induced PPI interfaces are larger than those generated by the MG, underlining how MGs modify the substrate-recruiting surface rather than recruit substrates themselves.

4.2.2.1 Molecular Glues Recruiting Cereblon (CRBN)

While the adverse effects of thalidomide and its analogs (e.g. lenalidomide and pomalidomide; Figure 4.11a), often termed immunomodulatory imide drugs (IMiDs), have been well known from the late 1950s, these were only tied to the E3 ligase activity of CRBN and MG behavior of the IMiDs in the previous decade [56–58]. The general binding mode for IMiDs is for the glutarimide to bind into a "tritryptophan pocket" of CRBN's thalidomide binding domain (TBD) lined by Trp380, Trp386, Trp400, and Phe402 and the backbone of the β12–β13 loop, forming a complementary hydrogen bond network with the backbone amide of Trp380 and carbonyl and imidazole of His378. The isoindoline aligns adjacent to the β10–β11 loop, buffeted by the Asn351, Pro352, and His353 side chains, and an isoindoline carbonyl hydrogen bonds with the side chain amide of Asn351. IMiDs with a C4 amino group are additionally found to form a hydrogen bond with Glu377. Thalidomide analogs generally bind to a surface area of 230–240 $Å^2$ of CRBN.

To recruit neosubstrates, CRBN forms a pocket with the IMiD using its β10–β11 loop and β12, β13, and β14 strands that perfectly accommodates a class 3 β-hairpin where the fourth residue in the turn is a glycine. To accommodate the hairpin, CRBN residues His353 and Tyr355 reorient to line the pocket, and the side chains of CRBN residues Asn351, His357, and Trp400 align to the hydrogen bond with the backbone carbonyls of the first, second, and third residues of the hairpin, respectively. The glycine at position 4 is critical, as the side chain projects into the isoindoline ring of the IMiD and Trp386 of CRBN, forming some key CH–π interactions to stabilize the hairpin of the neosubstrate. Conversely, any other amino acid identity here would abrogate binding because of steric clashes. Ultimately, this structure acts as the degron of IMiD substrates (Figure 4.11b).

A wide range of neosubstrates recruited to CRBN by the binding of IMiD MGs have since been identified, with individual MGs having their own preferences for neosubstrate engagement. The structures of solved complexes with neosubstrates are described briefly below.

4.2.2.1.1 CRBN and CK1α

The first structure of a neosubstrate-bound MG complex with CRBN was that of lenalidomide and casein kinase 1α (CK1α; PDB code 5FQD [22]), which was solved shortly after its identification as a target [59]. The observation that thalidomide, pomalidomide, and CC-122 had little-to-no effect on CK1α levels indicated that the absence of a carbonyl in lenalidomide's phthalimide ring made a significant contribution to its capacity to recruit CK1α as a neosubstrate. The structure suggested that in order to facilitate CK1α recruitment, lenalidomide must pinch in closer to the β12–β13 loop of CRBN. To accommodate this binding mode, the carbonyls of the other

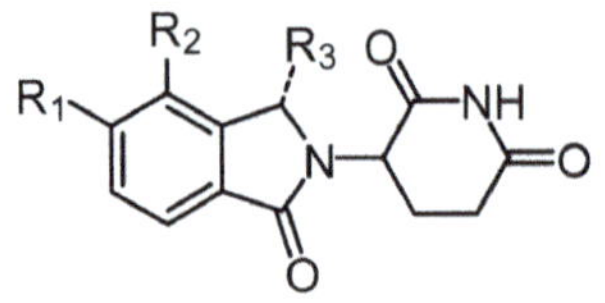

IMiD	R1	R2	R3	PDB codes
Thalidomide	—H	—H	=O	7BQU
5-hydroxythalidomide	—OH	—H	=O	7BQV
Lenalidomide	—H	—NH_2	—H	5QFD
Pomalidomide	—H	—NH_2	=O	6H0F, 6H0G, 6UML

(a)

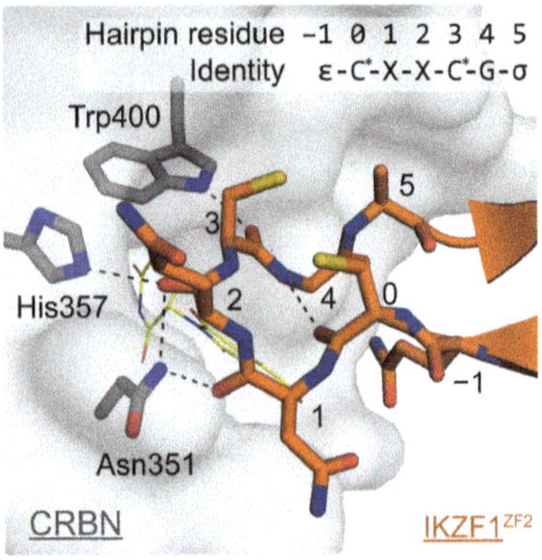

(b)

Figure 4.11 (a) Structure of thalidomide and its close analogs. (b) Representation of the IMiD degron using the induced IZKF1^{ZF2}:CRBN complex from PDB structure 6HOF. IKZF1^{ZF2} in ribbon and stick representation (orange) showing residues at the **β**-hairpin degron. **ε** represents the residue position that typically drives selectivity because of different isoindoline substituents. **σ** represents the residue position that is typically best accommodated by small side chains. Gray sticks highlight the surface of CRBN that coordinates residues 1–3 of the neosubstrate **β**-hairpin. Pomalidomide is shown in the pocket as thin yellow sticks. *Cysteines are only a requirement for the degron motif of zinc finger neosubstrates.

IMiDs would sterically clash with the backbone carbonyl of Glu377 in CRBN, thus explaining why only lenalidomide could induce CK1α degradation (see Figure 4.14a).

The interaction of CK1α is largely mediated by the β2–β3 loop of the kinase N-terminal lobe acting as the degron and binding into the β-hairpin-binding pocket of CRBN. Additionally, the N-terminal activation loop from the C-terminal lobe of the kinase packs into β12 of CRBN. The N-terminal loop and ends of the β4 and β5 strands, all adjacent to the CK1α β2–β3 loop, all make small additional contributions by interacting with CRBN residues surrounding the β-hairpin-binding pocket. The interface induced between CRBN and CK1α is 586 Å^2, while lenalidomide forms interfaces of 235 and 102 Å^2 with each protein, respectively, to yield a total interface area of 922 Å^2.

4.2.2.1.2 CRBN and GSPT1

Scientists at Celgene discovered thalidomide analog CC-885 as an IMiD capable of CRBN-mediated degradation of G1 to S phase transition protein 1 (GSPT1), a translation termination factor and a neosubstrate that is not affected by previously known IMiDs [60]. CC-885 is similar to lenalidomide; however, it lacks the C4 amino group and instead includes a C5-linked methylurea and a chloromethylphenyl ring attached to that (Figure 4.12). Subsequent efforts led to the discovery of CC-90009, which replaces the urea and phenyl with 4-chlorophenyldifluoroacetamide and is more selective for GSPT1, being incapable of degrading other neosubstrates such as IKZF1 or CK1α [61].

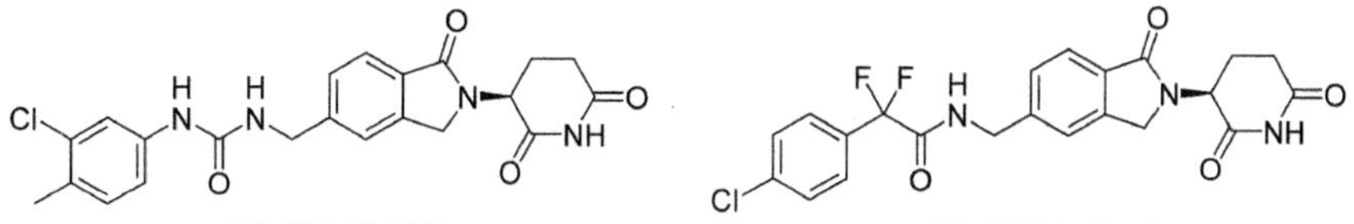

Figure 4.12 Structures of CC-885 and CC-90009.

The structural basis of IMiD-induced degradation of GSPT1 via CRBN has been elucidated via crystal structures of both CC-885 (PDB code 5HXB) and CC-90009 (6XK9) mediating complexes between the β-barrel of GSPT1's third domain ($GSPT1^{D3}$) and CRBN. Both structures reveal the same binding mode and architecture of the $CRBN^{TBD}$ and the CRBN/IMiD-binding β-hairpin of GSPT1, comprising residues 572–575 in the β3–β4 loop of the β-barrel. Compared to the structure with CK1α, there is conservation of the binding site in the $CRBN_{TBD}$; however, a 0.9 Å shift is observed in the β-hairpin of GSPT1 away from the IMiD, indicating that this motif needs to be positioned slightly differently to recruit GSPT1 to the complex and reflecting the movements of the isoindoline groups of the IMiDs in the binding pocket. For GSPT1, this is a shift from the uncomplexed form of the β-hairpin (PDB code 3E1Y) [62], having had to twist and come in toward the IMiD in order to bind CRBN. The combination of these two differences suggests that GSPT1 must compromise on the conformation of the β-hairpin in order to bind to CRBN and the IMiD.

CC-885 and CC-90009 mediate specific interactions with $GSPT1^{D3}$ via the C5 extension from the isoindoline group. GSPT1 accommodates the C5 functional group by having Val570 as the identity of the second-to-last residue before the β-hairpin. The carbonyls of the urea and amide of CC-885 and CC-90009, respectively, mediate hydrogen bonds with CRBN residue His353, however only the urea additionally hydrogen bonds with Glu377. Overall, this orients the urea/amide to point the phenyl ring of each molecule toward the β4–β5 loop of the $CRBN_{NTD}$. In both structures, the phenyl rings bind within a groove of $GSPT1^{D3}$ formed by Gln534 and Val536 of the β1 strand and Ile626 and Lys628 of the β6 strand. The only differences between the two structures here are slight rotations in Val536 and Ile626 that seem to accommodate CC-90009 projecting further and more closely to the β-barrel, albeit with a 60° rotation away from GSPT1. However, it is difficult to judge the significance of these at the resolution of the structures (~3.6 Å). Given that the two structures reveal very similar interface areas between the IMiDs and $GSPT1^{D3}$ (247 $Å^2$ for CC-885 and 236 $Å^2$ for CC-90009), it seems unlikely that stronger interactions mediate CC-90009's selectivity for $GSPT1^{D3}$. Instead, the improved selectivity of CC-90009 is likely attributable to the substitution of the urea with the difluoroacetamide, resulting in a sp^3 carbon in the place of the sp^2 nitrogen, or perhaps the disengagement of Glu377 of CRBN from the ligand. Both changes would likely restrict CC-90009's capacity to adopt a binding mode that accommodates the side chains for CK1α or IKZF1 at the Val570 position of GSPT1, but dissecting this awaits further investigation.

4.2.2.1.3 CRBN and C_2H_2 Zinc Fingers

The major class of target recruited to IMiD-modulated CRBN is classical C_2H_2 zinc fingers, but this is restricted to those with only two inter-cysteine residues and containing a glycine following the second zinc-ligating cysteine, generating the requisite β-hairpin structure and completing the degron for CRBN-mediated degradation. As such, several complexes of these neosubstrates bound to CRBN because of various IMiD molecules have now been solved. These zinc fingers generally bind into the IMiD-modified CRBN pocket using their β-hairpins, while the β2 strand and the helix interface with the β12–β14 sequence of strands and loops in CRBN.

Ikaros (IKZF1)

Ikaros (IKZF1) and Aiolos (IKZF3) are closely related B-cell transcription factors that share nearly identical second C_2H_2 zinc fingers, differing only between a serine and threonine, respectively, at the end of the helix. Both proteins are known to be sensitive to degradation in the presence of lenalidomide [63, 64] and pomalidomide, however are not degraded in cells as a result of thalidomide treatment [21].

The pomalidomide-induced structure of CRBN bound to $IKZF1^{ZF2}$ (PDB code 6HOF) defines the standard binding mode for IMiD-induced binding of C_2H_2 zinc fingers [21], with Gly151 (Gly152 in IKZF3) the key residue in the β-hairpin (Figure 4.11b). The C4 amino group of pomalidomide makes two key hydrogen bonds; one with Glu377 of CRBN to contribute to binding the E3 ligase and another to stabilize a bridging water molecule between Glu377 and Gln146 of $IKZF1^{ZF2}$. For IKZF3, the identity of Gln147 (equivalent of Gln146 from IKZF1) was found to be critical for its lenalidomide- or pomalidomide-induced degradation, with most other amino acid substitutions abrogating binding, suggesting that the mode of action for these IMiDs against IKZF1 and IKZF3 may be mediated through these interactions (see Figure 4.14b). Overall, the interface between CRBN and $IKZF1^{ZF2}$ was found to be 521 Å^2, pomalidomide and CRBN 237 Å^2, and 101 Å^2 between pomalidomide and $IKZF1^{ZF2}$, yielding a total interface area of 858 Å^2.

Zinc Finger Protein 692 (ZNF692)

Like Ikaros and Aiolos, ZNF692 is a transcription factor that was found to be degraded by CRBN following lenalidomide or pomalidomide treatment but is insensitive to thalidomide [21]. ZNF692 was found to exhibit the IMiD degron in its fourth zinc finger and a structure of the complex with pomalidomide and CRBN was solved (PDB code 6HOG). Overall, the structure reveals a highly conserved binding mode when compared with that of $IKZF1^{ZF2}$ and mediates largely the same contacts. While the bridging water is absent because of the resolution of the data, Glu377 of CRBN and Gln418 adopt the same conformers to capture the water with the C4 amino group of pomalidomide, suggesting conservation of these contacts that may drive selectivity. On the whole, the interface areas for $ZNF692^{ZF4}$ are similar to those of $IKZF1^{ZF2}$, the neo-PPI interface being 531.5 Å^2, the interfaces of CRBN and ZNF692 with pomalidomide 245 and 95 Å^2, respectively, resulting in a total ternary complex interface of 872 Å^2.

The key difference between the ZNF692^{ZF4} and IKZF1^{ZF2} structures is the small shift and the rotation between the two C_2H_2 zinc finger folds. ZNF692^{ZF4} is pushed away from CRBN's β12–β14 sequence of strands and loops, resulting in a slight displacement of the β-hairpin from the binding position of IKZF1^{ZF2}. This is most likely driven by Phe424, which substitutes for the equivalent Ala152 in IKZF1, being restricted and otherwise forming a steric clash with the β12–β14 sheet of CRBN. Ultimately, this difference highlights how the CRBN–IMiD pocket exhibits a degree of plasticity or "give" to recruit degrons in slightly different orientations.

Helios (IKZF2)

While the second zinc fingers of IKZF1 and IKZF3 each bear a glutamine as the residue before the first zinc-ligating residue of the β-hairpin degron, both Helios (IKZF2) and Eos (IKZF4) have a histidine in this position, precluding their degradation by lenalidomide or pomalidomide. Driven by the observation that the Q146H mutation of IKZF1 could facilitate an interaction with CRBN in the presence of the GSPT1-degrading IMiD CC-885, Wang et al. discovered ALV1 and ALV2 as IKZF2/4-degrading IMiDs (Figure 4.13a) [20]. ALV2 in particular was found to selectively degrade IKZF2/4, while ALV1 maintained activity toward IKZF1/3 as well. Both ALV1 and ALV2 contain an anilinomaleimide in the place of the isoindoline group of the traditional IMiDs and a 3-chloro-4-methylphenyl ring linked by either two sp^3 carbons and an amide or one sp^3 carbon and a urea, respectively.

The structure of ALV1 in complex with CRBN and IKZF2^{ZF2} (PDB code 7LPS) helped provide some insights into how this change in selectivity was mediated.

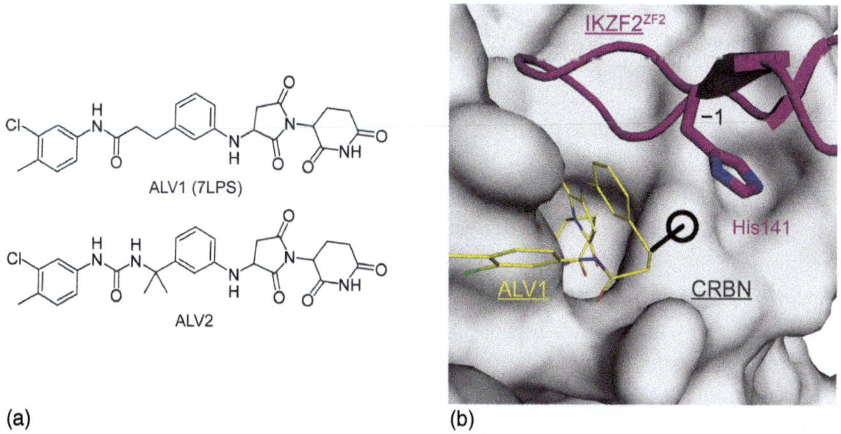

Figure 4.13 Engaging IKZF2 through IMiD alterations. (a) Structures of ALV1 and ALV2. (b) Structure of the ALV1-induced ternary complexes of CRBN (gray surface) and IKZF2^{ZF2} (purple ribbon). ALV1 is shown as yellow-colored sticks and the likely projection of a methyl group from ALV2 is marked with black lines, illustrating the limited space for certain amino acid identities at the −1 position of the **β**-hairpin (His141 in IKZF2).

Because of the profile of the IMiD-binding pocket, particularly when a neosubstrate is bound, the aniline ring is incapable of significant rotation, restricting it to the same plane as the isoindoline group would adopt. This significantly restricts the identity of the residue before the first cysteine (His141 in IKZF2), as anything other than a methyl or methylene in the Cβ will face significant clashes with the aniline ring. ALV2 could further restrict amino acid identity because of its methyl groups filling the space that larger side chains likely occupy for ALV1 binding but could be vacated by residues such as histidine (for IKZF2^{ZF2}), alanine, and asparagine (Figure 4.13b). To further stabilize the ALV1-induced complex, the 3-chloro-4-methylphenyl ring wraps around the β11–β12 loop of CRBN and the two phenyl rings contribute to a T-shaped π stack with His353; however, this interaction is unlikely to be preserved for ALV2 because of the presence of the urea restricting the bend of the molecule. An interface of 489 Å^2 is induced between CRBN and IKZF2^{ZF2}, 383 Å^2 between CRBN and ALV1, and 127 Å^2 between IKZF2^{ZF2} and ALV, giving a total interface area of 999 Å^2 for the ternary complex.

Spalt-Like Transcription Factor 4 (SALL4)

Spalt-like transcription factor 4 (SALL4) was discovered in 2018 to be one of the main targets of IMiD compounds that lead to the teratogenic effects associated with thalidomide and other IMiDs [56–58]. SALL4 is a C_2H_2 zinc finger transcription factor that drives a number of programs in embryonic development and its mutations have been associated with Duane-radial ray and associated syndromes, which share several similarities with thalidomide embryopathy [65]. Two teams generated structures of SALL4^{ZF2} with different IMiDs [18, 66], one using pomalidomide (PDB code 6UML) and another using thalidomide (7BQU) and 5-hydroxythalidomide (7BQV).

Overall, the three structures reveal extremely close alignment of CRBN^{TBD}, the IMiDs and the β-hairpin of SALL4^{ZF2}. The β-hairpin of SALL4^{ZF2} acts as the degron to bind to the IMiD-modulated CRBN^{TBD} and is captured in the structures of these complexes. In the pomalidomide complex, Tyr355 of CRBN adopts the conformer of the IMiD-only structures, whereas for the thalidomide complexes, Tyr355 matches the conformers of the other published neosubstrate-bound structures. The latter authors attribute this to an artifact of their construct design [18]; however, it is possible that the different IMiDs place different constraints on the exact binding position of the β-hairpin, resulting in the need for Tyr355 to adopt different conformations, as there would be a clash with the carbonyl of SALL4^{ZF2}'s Ser413 in the pomalidomide-bound structure if it adopted the same conformer as the thalidomide-bound structures.

The β2 strand and the helix of SALL4^{ZF2} pack against the β12–β14 sheet of CRBN, making some opportunistic hydrogen bonds from the side chains of Arg418 and Arg431 to the backbone carbonyls of Pro374 and Cys394 in CRBN, respectively. Val411 is the residue before the first cysteine of SALL4^{ZF2}, and its small size would appear to accommodate a variety of modifications at the C5 of IMiDs bearing isoindoline groups. Across the three structures, an interface of 350–480 Å^2 between the two proteins is observed (differences largely because of the movement of Tyr355 of CRBN), 220–240 Å^2 for the IMiD:CRBN interface, and 85–95 Å^2 for the IMiD:SALL4^{ZF2} interface, resulting in a total interface area of 680–800 Å^2.

The pomalidomide-induced complex reveals a 15° rotation in the binding mode of SALL4^{ZF2} compared to IKZF1$_{ZF2}$, and although the thalidomide-induced complexes exhibit a more intermediate degree of rotation, all four structures are likely confounded by crystal contacts impinging on the helices of the C_2H_2 fingers. However, Matyskiela et al. make excellent use of mutagenesis to illustrate that these differences are indeed significant and that the residue following the hairpin glycine (His417 in SALL4^{ZF2}) has a major influence on the ability of the IMiDs to degrade SALL4 because of clashes with CRBN Ile371. Ultimately, these structures further illustrate the subtly different poses that the β-hairpins may adopt in the binding pocket of CRBN, even for the same protein species, underlining how the plasticity of IMiD-based target engagement can accommodate a wide variety of amino acid substitutions within the hairpins to degrade a multitude of targets.

4.2.2.1.4 Question of Selectivity

With a series of molecular and structural studies of C_2H_2 zinc finger proteins degraded by IMiDs because of induced interactions with CRBN, a degron has begun to emerge. A motif of εCXXCG around the cysteine zinc-ligating residues is the key element recognized by the CRBN^{TBD}, where ε represents the residue most engaged with the IMiD molecule, such as Gln146 in IKZF1 [20, 21]. A similar degron likely exists for non-C_2H_2 neosubstrates, albeit slightly less restricted given the dispensability of the cysteines in positions 2 and 5. The degron could possibly be expanded to a seventh residue, with large residues following the glycine observed to induce a rotational shift in the binding mode of the β-hairpin. For SALL4 in particular, mutagenesis at His417 and CRBN's Ile371 revealed a clash that could be resolved by reducing the length of either side chain and improved the IMiD-induced CRBN binding of SALL4 [66]. Thus, potential neosubstrates with small side chains in this seventh position are most likely to be favored if they meet the other requirements of the degron.

The structural basis for selectivity of particular IMiDs is investigated in several cases, although is not so easily dissected. The structure of CRBN:lenalidomide:CK1α suggests that the susceptibility of CK1α to lenalidomide over other IMiDs is because of the absence of a carbonyl group which, because of lenalidomide's binding mode to recruit CK1α, would otherwise clash with the backbone carbonyl of Glu377 of CRBN [22]. However, the structure of IKZF1^{ZF2} bound in the presence of pomalidomide [21] reveals that the latter adopts a binding mode that very closely matches that of lenalidomide in the presence of CK1α (roughly 0.1 Å further away from Glu377; Figure 4.14a). As some binding of CK1α in the presence of thalidomide and pomalidomide is observed, this would suggest that this binding mode is right on the limit of tolerability for its recruitment with these IMiDs.

The preference for zinc fingers such as IKZF1, IKZF3, and ZNF692 to be recruited to CRBN by lenalidomide and pomalidomide, over thalidomide, was attributed to the ability of the C4 amino groups to stabilize a water-mediated hydrogen bond between Glu377 and the glutamine residue sitting in the first residue of the C_2H_2 degron [21]. Subsequent work on SALL4^{ZF2} using AlphaScreen revealed that, while thalidomide can induce a complex with SALL4 bearing a V411Q mutation at this

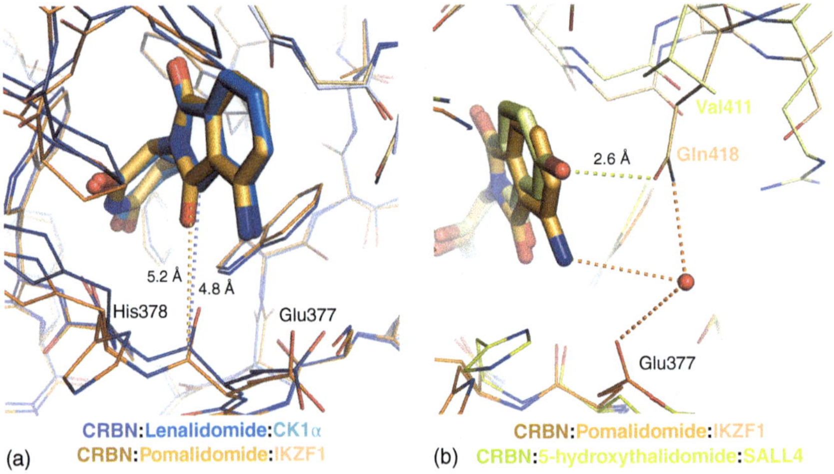

Figure 4.14 Insights into the selectivity of IMiDs. (a) Lenalidomide-induced CK1a structure (5FQD, blues) aligned with pomalidomide-induced IKZF1^{ZF2} structure (6H0F, oranges), shown as CRBN (dark lines), IMiD (medium sticks), and CK1a/IKZF1 (light lines). Measurements taken from C3 of the IMiD to the carbonyl carbon of Glu377 in CRBN are shown as dashed lines in respective colors. (b) Pomalidomide-induced IKZF1^{ZF2} structure (6H0F, oranges) aligned with 5-hydroxythalidomide-induced SALL4^{ZF2} structure (7BQV, yellows), shown as CRBN (dark lines), IMiD (medium sticks), and SALL4/IKZF1 (light lines). A bridging water coordinated in the CRBN:pomalidomide:IKZF1 structure is shown with hydrogen bonds as orange dashed lines, while the clash distance (2.6 Å) that prevents Gln418 from engaging with the water in the presence of 5-hydroxy substitutions on the IMiD ring is shown as a yellow dashed line.

position, 5-hydroxythalidomide, a common oxidative metabolite, cannot [18]. While this remains to be fully explained, it is possible that the C5 hydroxyl group disrupts Gln418 of IKZF1 to diminish the contribution of the water-mediated hydrogen bond (Figure 4.14b) and that its propensity to alter the target selectivity profiles of each IMiD may be a result of differential rates of metabolism for each.

The final case of interest is the selectivity of ALV-2 toward IKZF2 and its lack of degradation of the more widely appreciated IMiD neosubstrates, especially when compared to the precursor, ALV-1 [20]. As speculated above, the positioning of the aniline ring and the dimethyls close to the first residue of the degron appears to preclude the degradation of proteins bearing side chains that are either extended or have a tertiary Cβ. ALV-2 did not exhibit degradation of IKZF1 (glutamine in this position), CK1α (isoleucine), or GSPT1 (valine), whereas ALV-1 did. As such, ALV-2 may be restricted to residues such as alanine, asparagine, aspartate, and histidine in this position and degrade only a very limited set of targets. It would be interesting to know if ALV-2 is incapable of degrading SALL4 (valine in the position), as this may significantly reduce its teratogenicity relative to other IMiDs. Sadly, this protein was not captured in the proteomic analysis of the cell lines tested.

4.2.2.2 Molecular Glues Recruiting Other E3 Ligases

4.2.2.2.1 DDB1- and CUL4-Associated Factor 15 (DCAF15) and RBM39

Aryl sulfonamides were discovered to be involved in the recruitment of proteins to DCAF15 to allow polyubiquitination and further degradation [67, 68]. Termed splicing inhibitor sulfonamides (SPLAMs), these MGs promote the binding of DCAF15 to targets such as the RNA-recognition motif (RRM) of RNA-binding motif protein 39 (RBM39) and are molecules that appear to have the same mode of action as IMiDs. However, there was a need to study and understand the general binding mode of these molecules in order to make rational improvements. Three groups published their studies in late 2019 exploring the SPLAM-induced complexes and interactions of DCAF15 with RBM39 using biophysical assays, crystallization, and cryo-EM [34, 35, 69]. Using ITC and TR-FRET, the groups confirmed that the SPLAMs had only weak affinity for DCAF15 and none for RBM39 but could induce a strong ternary complex between the two. They solved several different structures induced by SPLAMS: E7820 (PDB codes 6PAI and 6Q0R, EMDB codes EMD-20553 and EMD-20554), tasisulam (6Q0V), indisulam (6Q0W, 6SJ7 and 6UD7, and EMD-10213), and 4-(aminomethyl)-*N*-(3-cyano-4-methyl-1*H*-indol-7-yl)benzenesulfonamide (6UE5) (Figure 4.15a).

DCAF15 is composed of five β sheets and five α helixes. It recruits the SPLAM on its surface through a pocket formed by α4 (Thr230, Gln232, and Phe235), α6 (Arg552, Val556, Val559, and Met560), and β16 (Val477 and Ile478) in the fifth sheet. A T-shaped π-stacking interaction is formed between the phenylsulfonamide and Phe235 of DCAF15. The oxygens of the sulfonamide form strong hydrogen bonds with DCAF15 backbone amides of Ala234 and Phe235 that lie at the N-terminal end of α4 (Figure 4.15a,b). The indole nitrogen of the SPLAMs (which tasisulam lacks) forms a hydrogen bond with Phe231. On the other hand, E7820 and 4-(aminomethyl)-*N*-(3-cyano-4-methyl-1*H*-indol-7-yl)benzenesulfonamide possess a methyl on C4 of the indole that projects into a hydrophobic pocket lined by Val477, Cys555, and

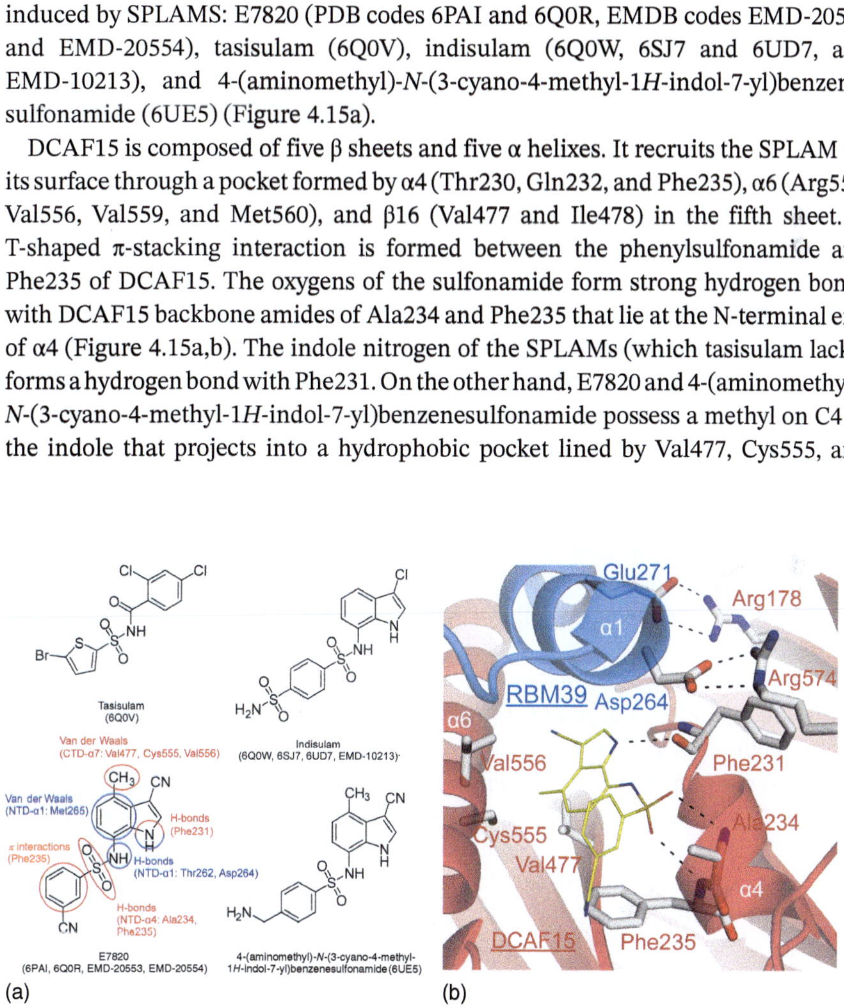

Figure 4.15 (a) Structures of DCAF15:RBM39 MGs: E7820, Indisulam, Tasisulam and 4-(aminomethyl)-*N*-(3-cyano-4-methyl-1*H*-indol-7-yl)benzenesulfonamide. Important interactions of E7820 with DCAF15 (in red) and RBM39 (in blue). (b) RBM39 (blue) and DCAF15 (red) induced to interact by E7820 (yellow sticks) in PDB structure 6PAI. Key neo-protein–protein and neo-protein–ligand interactions are indicated.

Val556, providing them with additional affinity for DCAF15. Across the structures, the DCAF15:SPLAM interface typically measures between 290 and 320 Å^2.

The SPLAM and its binding site create a large, shallow groove in between α6 and the nearby loops of the third β-sheet, from the C- and N-terminal portions of DCAF15, respectively. The second RRM of RBM39 (RBM39^{RRM2}) binds into this groove, with the key interface being the α1 helix of RBM39 interacting with the SPLAM and its binding pocket, particularly α6 of DCAF15. The β2 strand sits against the adjacent loops of the third β sheet, while the β2–β3 loop reaches the first β sheet and the N-terminal tail. Further, α2 of RBM39^{RRM2} interacts with α6 of DCAF, with the former effectively sitting above the ridge of the groove created by the latter. Some key interactions with the neosubstrate include the formation of a salt bridges between Arg178 and Arg574 of DCAF15 and Glu271 and Asp264 of RBM39^{RRM2}, respectively (Figure 4.15b). There are also significant van der Waals interactions between the indole of E7820 and the N-terminal end of α1, in particular Met265. Between the structures, the only significant difference is that 6PAI has the nitrile on its phenylsulfonamide pointing into DCAF15, whereas 6Q0V has it pointing into RBM39. The induced PPI interface between DCAF15 and RBM39 is between 930 and 1210 Å^2, depending on the structure (NB: these differences seem to relate to slight differences between the model fits to electron density), and the SPLAM:RBM39 interface is 125–162 Å^2. This leads to total ternary complex interface areas of 1390–1670 Å^2.

A key difference between IMiDs and SPLAMs is that the IMiDs bind to CRBN in a conserved and well-defined pocket, whereas SPLAMs bind in a less-conserved pocket that is not functional without the presence of the molecular glue. This is promising for the future as other interesting E3 ligases could possibly be targeted by MGs, even if they do not possess effective ligand-binding pockets, as the role of a MG is simply to modify a surface-exposed region. Discovery efforts to identify such MGs will likely be driven by the directed screening approaches such as those discussed below for inducing a DDB1:CDK12 interaction.

4.2.2.2.2 DNA Damage-Binding Protein 1 (DDB1) and CDK12

Of all the examples of degraders presented here, the molecule CR8 is perhaps the most unique. CR8 and a series of compounds with analogous activity, dCeMM2, 3, and 4, were discovered by screening against cell lines in which loss of the compounds' *in vitro* activity was linked with disruption of various elements of CRL activity [70, 71]. Each of these compounds were found to induce degradation of cyclin K; however, they act by binding to the active site of cyclin-dependent kinase 12 (CDK12, a partner kinase of cyclin K) and modifying its surface as a MG so that it can be recruited by DDB1. Another compound known as HQ461 was also found to exhibit the same MG activity following a separate effort seeking to understand the mechanistic basis of its Nrf2-suppressing activity [72].

The structure of DDB1:CR8:CDK12-cyclin K (PDB code 6TD3) reveals how this complex forms [70]. From the active site of CDK12, the phenylpyridyl group of CR8 is exposed and in the complex binds into a small groove lined by Asn907, Asn908,

Ile909, Arg928, Arg947, and Phe949 in β-propeller C (BPC) of DDB1. Intriguingly, this groove is largely unexplored as an interaction interface by native DCAFs, save for DCAF1, whose Glu1388 forms a salt bridge with DDB1's Arg947 [73]. β1 and β2 of the N-terminal lobe, plus the hinge region between the lobes, both form contacts with $DDB1_{BPC}$, while αD is held against the BPC by Arg1080 of the C-terminal domain acting almost as a finger. Interactions with B-propeller A (BPA) of DDB1 are mediated by the C-terminal lobe, particularly around the αF, αG, and αH loops and helices. Finally, CDK12's extended and typically disordered C-terminal tail, which has been observed to pack in next to the active site in the ATP-bound state [74], instead adopts a partially helical structure and binds within the large cleft between BPA and BPC. This mimics the way in which DCAFs form helix-loop-helix motifs to engage DDB1 in this region, although this binding by CDK12 was observed to be quite disordered, in line with the low propensity of the tail to form secondary structure.

Overall, this complex exhibits one of the largest interfaces, with the neo-PPI interface having a total surface area of 2086 $Å^2$, the CDK12:CR8 interaction a surface area of 423 $Å^2$, DDB1:CR8 149 $Å^2$, reaching a total of 2658 $Å^2$. This compares with interfaces of 2300–2400 $Å^2$ for CRBN and DCAF15 with DDB1. The result is a binding position and orientation of CDK12 that is very similar to that of DCAFs, essentially making it a neosubstrate receptor and pseudo-DCAF protein that, by virtue of its native complex, positions cyclin K for ubiquitination and degradation via the CRL activity [70]. Critically, this structure helps emphasize the potential of a largely underdeveloped approach for PPI inducers such as MGs or bifunctional molecules, in that novel targets can be recruited to cellular machinery (such as E3 ligases) in numerous ways without necessarily inducing the interaction directly at the interface of the native substrate receptor.

4.3 Future Perspective on the Importance of Ternary Complexes in PROTAC Discovery and Development

As the key role of both PROTAC and MG degraders is to induce proximity between and E3 ligase and target through ternary complex formation, its study is vital to deliver productive degrader molecules. As described in the introduction, there are a multitude of behaviors that ternary complexes can exhibit and the nature of these properties for each will impact on the activity of the degrader that induces them.

4.3.1 Ternary Complexes – Is Seeing Believing?

The first question that should be asked when observing and quantifying the behavior of degrader-induced ternary complexes is – "is this actually what the ternary complex is doing?" No technology currently in existence can tell us what all ternary complexes in a solution are doing at any moment in time, let alone in a cellular environment. At best we can capture snapshots of what some defined population complexes may be doing in a particular state or point in time, or derive the value of individual parameters, such as affinity or residency, without the context of others. Any binding pose or dynamic observed should not be seen as "the ternary complex," just a significant one within a wider population. For systems with highly stable or cooperative ternary complexes or large neo-PPI interfaces (see Tables 4.1 and 4.2 for a summary of interface areas for the described structures), it is likely that this is the majority state of the complex. However, even here alternative states need to be assumed to exist and be meaningful.

The prediction of ternary complex formation using computational methods has enabled questions to focus on what binding poses do form and how meaningful are they. Initial molecular modeling methods focused on simply explaining the behaviors of MZ1 and the dBET PROTACs, which were queried using CHARMM and Rosetta, respectively [3, 7]. Several methods have now been developed, including Model 4B, based on the Molecular Operating Environment [75], PRosettaC and PROTAC_ternary, based on Rosetta [76, 77], and PROTAC-Model, based on both FRODDOCK and Rosetta [78]. These methods have been predictive of known binding poses and reasonably expected ones, on top of the correct predictions relating to ternary complex cooperativity and degrader activity. These methods will be most powerful in their predicative modeling of degrader and ternary complex behavior in advance of molecule synthesis, allowing degrader candidates to be triaged and prioritized. Such approaches are only likely to become more powerful as computational, modeling, and artificial intelligence capabilities expand in the coming years, with the development of methods such as AlphaFold-Multimer possessing much promise for this area of the degrader field [79].

Donovan et al. demonstrated how, for a subset of CRBN-based kinase PROTACs, the existence of many ternary complexes is either so weak or fleeting that they cannot be observed in a pull-down experiment but only deduced from the induced ubiquitination and degradation of the target [12], akin to fundamental particles being discovered in the Large Hadron Collider by observing the aftermath of their formation and destruction. Several exciting (and potentially overlapping) possibilities arise from this: (i) that some ternary complexes may form robustly and productively through only very weak interactions; (ii) that some complexes may be very transient, associating and dissociating from each other on time scales that enable them to be separated; (iii) that some ternary complexes may not actually form as a three-body entity, instead simply drawing the partner proteins together with sufficient proximity and time for ubiquitination to happen.

Possibilities such as these go well with the framework developed by Rodriguez-Rivera and Levi for how ternary complex formation can influence the degradation activity [80]. They postulate that for many degraders, short-lived, low-population ternary complexes will provide the best degradation outcomes. This can be considered in terms of the kinetics and thermodynamics of the energy landscape between the degrader recruiting its partners and successful ubiquitination of the target, where stabilizing ternary complexes that promote a transition state, or destabilizing those of intermediate states, are most likely to be productive. Of course, while each of these ternary complexes will fundamentally remain the same through

Table 4.1 Summary of solvent contents (RCSB PDB website) and interface surface areas (PDBePISA) between the proteins and the PROTACs.

PROTAC ternary structure PDB code	Proteins (target E3 ligase)	Neo-PPI interface area (Å^2)	PROTAC:target interface area (Å^2)	PROTAC:E3 interface area (Å^2)	Total interface area (Å^2)	Solvent content (%)
6ZHC	**Bcl-XL VHL**	308	778	458	1543	58.4
7PI4	**FAK1 VHL**	366	590	402	1358	57.1
5T35	**BRD4^{BD2} VHL**	343	506	489	1338	68.1
6SIS		326	551	484	1361	67.2
7KHH	**BRD4^{BD1} VHL**	353	499	384	1236	56.6
7JTO	**WDR5 VHL**	129	615	446	1190	52.4
7JTP		399	566	469	1435	53.8
6HR2	**SMARCA4 VHL**	324	350	461	1135	53.7
6HAX	**SMARCA2 VHL**	320	348	456	1125	51.3
6HAY		329	365	476	1171	52.8
6BN9	**BRD4^{BD1} CRBN**	567	N/A	N/A	N/A	64.8
6BN8		536	N/A	N/A	N/A	64.6
6BN7		519	503	306	1328	66.9
6BNB		479	N/A	N/A	N/A	80.3
6BOY		550	424	321	1294	67.6
6W8I[a]	**BTK cIAP1**	95	598	396	1089	55.2
		206	701	387	1294	
		367	636	387	1390	
6W7O		513	532	390	1435	46.3

N/A – no PROTAC in the crystal structure.
[a] 6W8I is split into the three observed complexes in the asymmetric unit because of their conformational differences.

Table 4.2 Summary of solvent contents (RCSB PDB website) and interface surface areas (PDBePISA) for the proteins and MGs.

MG ternary structure PDB code	Proteins (target E3 ligase)	Neo-PPI interface area (Å^2)	MG:target interface area (Å^2)	MG:E3 interface area (Å^2)	Total interface area (Å^2)	Solvent content (%)
5FQD	CRBN CK1α	586	102	235	922	55
6XK9	CRBN GSPT1	638	236	328	1202	69.0
5HXB		632	247	312	1190	68.4
6H0G	CRBN ZNF692^{ZF4}	532	95	245	872	60.6
6H0F	CRBN IKZF1^{ZF2}	521	101	237	858	60.2
6UML	CRBN SALL4^{ZF2}	352	90	239	681	57.6
7BQV		479	93	230	802	56.8
7BQU		394	87	223	704	49.0
7LPS	CRBN IKZF2^{ZF2}	489	127	383	999	50.4
6PAI	DCAF15 RBM39	933	132	320	1386	54.2
6Q0R		1020	155	292	1467	53.6
6Q0V		1116	125	318	1559	54.9
6Q0W		1124	148	305	1577	54.7
6UD7		1210	162	298	1670	55.8
6UE5		1197	156	305	1658	56.8
6TD3	DDB1 CDK12	2086	423	149	2658	70.0

ubiquitination, the requirements for the behavior of the ternary complex to enable productive ubiquitination may differ. The idea that some ternary complexes may be "trapped" in unproductive forms has been demonstrated by the number of ternary complexes Donovan et al. could identify, but not observe degradation for, as well as in the discovery of BCPyr [12, 29].

4.3.2 Each (Ternary Complex) to Its Own

Of course, this discussion leaves out that many degraders do induce highly stable, long-lived ternary complexes that also lead to profound degradation of their targets, including all MGs and many PROTAC systems [8, 11, 26, 40]. In fact, while there are more limited studies of other E3 ligases, biophysical and structural investigations of PROTAC-mediated ternary complexes hijacking VHL have almost always found that increased affinity, cooperativity, and stability drive improved target degradation profiles, as for IMiDs with CRBN. A more limited pull-down study with VHL-based PROTAC promiscuous for kinases uncovered strong ternary complex formation for the majority of targets degraded [14]. All-in-all, this suggests that different degrader classes may be privileged for different mechanisms, relying on different degrees of all behaviors (as described in Section 4.1.2) to yield optimal degradation activity; VHL-based PROTACs generally relying on stable, cooperative complexes, CRBN-based PROTACs perhaps leveraging more transient and plastic interactions, and IMiDs and SPLAMs requiring high cooperativity and substrate complementarity.

The same principle is likely true for different targets, with preferences to be ubiquitinated by ternary complexes with different behaviors. Additionally, as each behavior is likely to differ from one degrader to another, even for the same E3 ligase–target pair, the requirements of each other behavior for productive degradation is likely to differ as a result. For example, a degrader that positions the substrate more effectively for ubiquitination by the E2–E3 complex may suddenly have fewer constraints on behaviors such as residency or flexibility, as there would be a larger window and larger population of ternary complexes amenable to degradation.

This then leads to the concept that each E3 ligase–degrader–target system is ultimately its own unique entity. When changing from one target or E3 ligase to another, or even simply altering the degrader, a perturbation in one behavior could completely alter the degradation activity as a result of changed demands on the others. While trends can be derived from related complexes and rational design considered, ultimately nothing about ternary complex formation or behavior can be taken for granted, as any step could be a step too far. To establish the rules for degrader design (particularly bifunctional degraders such as PROTACs) and thus what works and what does not, further exploration and empiricism is required, generating high-quality data and examples, for both productive and dead-end degraders, preferably for a diversity of compounds and targets [12]. Longer term advances in modeling, theories, and technologies to assess ternary complex behavior will drive the depth of understanding required to lead to true rational design of degraders, particularly for insights into currently hard-to-measure behaviors such as plasticity and flexibility.

References

1 Douglass, E.F. Jr., Miller, C.J., Sparer, G. et al. (2013). A comprehensive mathematical model for three-body binding equilibria. *J. Am. Chem. Soc.* 135 (16): 6092–6099.

2 Huang, H.-T., Dobrovolsky, D., Paulk, J. et al. (2018). A chemoproteomic approach to query the degradable kinome using a multi-kinase degrader. *Cell Chem. Biol.* 25 (1): 88–99.e6.

3 Gadd, M.S., Testa, A., Lucas, X. et al. (2017). Structural basis of PROTAC cooperative recognition for selective protein degradation. *Nat. Chem. Biol.* 13 (5): 514–521. https://doi.org/10.1038/nchembio.2329.

4 Burslem, G.M., Smith, B.E., Lai, A.C. et al. (2018). The advantages of targeted protein degradation over inhibition: an RTK case study. *Cell Chem. Biol.* 25 (1): 67–77.e3.

5 Chan, K.-H., Zengerle, M., Testa, A., and Ciulli, A. (2018). Impact of target warhead and linkage vector on inducing protein degradation: comparison of bromodomain and extra-terminal (BET) degraders derived from triazolodiazepine (JQ1) and tetrahydroquinoline (I-BET726) BET inhibitor scaffolds. *J. Med. Chem.* 61 (2): 504–513.

6 Sundberg, E.J. and Mariuzza, R.A. (2000). Luxury accomodation: the expanding role of structural plasticity in protein-protein interaction. *Structure* 8 (7): 137–142.

7 Nowak, R.P., Deangelo, S.L., Buckley, D. et al. (2018). Plasticity in binding confers selectivity in ligand-induced protein degradation article. *Nat. Chem. Biol.* 14 (7): 706–714. https://doi.org/10.1038/s41589-018-0055-y.

8 Imaide, S., Riching, K.M., Makukhin, N. et al. (2021). Trivalent PROTACs enhance protein degradation via combined avidity and cooperativity. *Nat. Chem. Biol.* 17 (11): 1157–1167.

9 Sakamoto, K.M. (2005). Chimeric molecules to target proteins for ubiquitination and degradation. In: *Ubiquitin and Protein Degradation, Part B*, 833–847. Academic Press. Available from: https://www.sciencedirect.com/science/article/pii/S007668790599054X.

10 Chung, C., Dai, H., Fernandez, E. et al. (2020). Structural insights into PROTAC-mediated degradation of Bcl-xL. *ACS Chem. Biol.* 15 (9): 2316–2323.

11 Law, R.P., Nunes, J., Chung, C. et al. (2021). Discovery and characterisation of highly cooperative FAK-degrading PROTACs. *Angew. Chem. Int. Ed.* 60 (43): 23327–23334. https://doi.org/10.1002/anie.202109237.

12 Donovan, K.A., Ferguson, F.M., Bushman, J.W. et al. (2020). Mapping the degradable kinome provides a resource for expedited degrader development. *Cell* 183 (6): 1741–1731. https://doi.org/10.1016/j.cell.2020.10.038.

13 Bondeson, D.P., Mares, A., Smith, I.E.D. et al. (2015). Catalytic *in vivo* protein knockdown by small-molecule PROTACs. *Nat. Chem. Biol.* 11 (8): 611–617.

14 Bondeson, D.P., Smith, B.E., Burslem, G.M. et al. (2018). Lessons in PROTAC design from selective degradation with a promiscuous warhead. *Cell Chem. Biol.* 25 (1): 78–87.e5. https://doi.org/10.1016/j.chembiol.2017.09.010.

15 Zoppi, V., Hughes, S.J., Maniaci, C. et al. (2019). Iterative design and optimization of initially inactive proteolysis targeting chimeras (PROTACs) identify VZ185 as a potent, fast, and selective von Hippel-Lindau (VHL) based dual degrader probe of BRD9 and BRD7. *J. Med. Chem.* 62 (2): 699–726. https://doi.org/10.1021/acs.jmedchem.8b01413.

16 Mahan, S.D., Riching, K.M., Urh, M., and Daniels, D.L. (2021). Kinetic detection of E3:PROTAC:Target ternary complexes using NanoBRETNanoBRET technology in live cells. In: *BT - Targeted Protein Degradation: Methods and Protocols* (ed. A.M. Cacace, C.M. Hickey and M. Békés), 151–171. New York: Springer US. https://doi.org/10.1007/978-1-0716-1665-9_8.

17 Zorba, A., Nguyen, C., Xu, Y. et al. (2018). Delineating the role of cooperativity in the design of potent PROTACs for BTK. *Proc. Natl. Acad. Sci. U.S.A.* 115 (31): E7285–E7292. https://doi.org/10.1073/pnas.1803662115.

18 Furihata, H., Yamanaka, S., Honda, T. et al. (2020). Structural bases of IMiD selectivity that emerges by 5-hydroxythalidomide. *Nat. Commun.* 11 (1): 4578. https://doi.org/10.1038/s41467-020-18488-4.

19 Khan, S., Zhang, X., Lv, D. et al. (2019). A selective BCL-XL PROTAC degrader achieves safe and potent antitumor activity. *Nat. Med.* 25 (12): 1938–1947. https://doi.org/10.1038/s41591-019-0668-z.

20 Wang, E.S., Verano, A.L., Nowak, R.P. et al. (2021). Acute pharmacological degradation of Helios destabilizes regulatory T cells. *Nat. Chem. Biol.* 17 (6): 711–717. https://doi.org/10.1038/s41589-021-00802-w.

21 Sievers, Q.L., Petzold, G., Bunker, R.D. et al. (2018). Defining the human C_2H_2 zinc finger degrome targeted by thalidomide analogs through CRBN. *Science* 362 (6414): eaat0572.

22 Petzold, G., Fischer, E.S., and Thomä, N.H. (2016). Structural basis of lenalidomide-induced CK1α degradation by the CRL4CRBN ubiquitin ligase. *Nature* 532 (7597): 127–130. https://doi.org/10.1038/nature16979.

23 Boutard, N., Białas, A., Sabiniarz, A. et al. (2019). Synthesis of amide and sulfonamide substituted N-aryl 6-aminoquinoxalines as PFKFB3 inhibitors with improved physicochemical properties. *Bioorg. Med. Chem. Lett.* 29 (4): 646–653.

24 de Castro, G.V. and Ciulli, A. (2021). Estimating the cooperativity of PROTAC-induced ternary complexes using 19F NMR displacement assay. *RSC Med. Chem.* 12 (10): 1765–1770. https://doi.org/10.1039/D1MD00215E.

25 Bartoschik, T., Zoephel, A., Rumpel, K. et al. (2021). MSTMicroScale thermophoresis (MST)and TRICTemperature related intensity change (TRIC) technology to reliably study PROTACProteolysis-targeting chimeras (PROTACs) binary and ternary binding in drug development. In: *Targeted Protein Degradation: Methods and Protocols* (ed. A.M. Cacace, C.M. Hickey and M. Békés), 115–133. New York: Springer US. https://doi.org/10.1007/978-1-0716-1665-9_6.

26 Farnaby, W., Koegl, M., Roy, M.J. et al. (2019). BAF complex vulnerabilities in cancer demonstrated via structure-based PROTAC design. *Nat. Chem. Biol.* 15 (7): 672–680. https://doi.org/10.1038/s41589-019-0294-6.

27 Xufen, Y., Dongxu, L., Jithesh, K. et al. (2021). A selective WDR5 degrader inhibits acute myeloid leukemia in patient-derived mouse models. *Sci. Transl. Med.* 13 (613): eabj1578. https://doi.org/10.1126/scitranslmed.abj1578.

28 Roy, M.J., Winkler, S., Hughes, S.J. et al. (2019). SPR-measured dissociation kinetics of PROTAC ternary complexes influence target degradation rate. *ACS Chem. Biol.* 14 (3): 361–368.

29 Schiemer, J., Horst, R., Meng, Y. et al. (2021). Snapshots and ensembles of BTK and cIAP1 protein degrader ternary complexes. *Nat. Chem. Biol.* 17 (2): 152–160. https://doi.org/10.1038/s41589-020-00686-2.

30 Song, J.H., Wagner, N.D., Yan, J. et al. (2021). Native mass spectrometry and gas-phase fragmentation provide rapid and in-depth topological characterization of a PROTAC ternary complex. *Cell Chem. Biol.* 28 (10): 1528–1538.e4.

31 Beveridge, R., Kessler, D., Rumpel, K. et al. (2020). Native mass spectrometry can effectively predict PROTAC efficacy. *ACS Cent. Sci.* 6 (7): 1223–1230. https://doi.org/10.1021/acscentsci.0c00049.

32 Sternicki, L.M., Nonomiya, J., Liu, M. et al. (2021). Native mass spectrometry for the study of PROTAC GNE-987-containing ternary complexes. *ChemMedChem* 16 (14): 2206–2210. https://doi.org/10.1002/cmdc.202100113.

33 Eron, S.J., Huang, H., Agafonov, R.V. et al. (2021). Structural characterization of degrader-induced ternary complexes using hydrogen–deuterium exchange mass spectrometry and computational modeling: implications for structure-based design. *ACS Chem. Biol.* 16 (11): 2228–2243. https://doi.org/10.1021/acschembio.1c00376.

34 Bussiere, D.E., Xie, L., Srinivas, H. et al. (2019). The structural basis of Indisulam-mediated recruitment of RBM39 to the DCAF15-DDB1-DDA1 E3 ligase complex. *bioRxiv* 737510.

35 Faust, T.B., Yoon, H., Nowak, R.P. et al. (2020). Structural complementarity facilitates E7820-mediated degradation of RBM39 by DCAF15. *Nat. Chem. Biol.* 16 (1): 7–14. https://doi.org/10.1038/s41589-019-0378-3.

36 Murata, K. and Wolf, M. (2018). Cryo-electron microscopy for structural analysis of dynamic biological macromolecules. *Biochim. Biophys. Acta, Gen. Subj.* 1862 (2): 324–334.

37 Leissing, T.M., Luh, L.M., and Cromm, P.M. (2020). Structure driven compound optimization in targeted protein degradation. *Drug Discov. Today Technol.* 37: 73–82.

38 Zengerle, M., Chan, K.H., and Ciulli, A. (2015). Selective small molecule induced degradation of the BET bromodomain protein BRD4. *ACS Chem. Biol.* 10 (8): 1770–1777. https://doi.org/10.1021/acschembio.5b00216.

39 Testa, A., Hughes, S.J., Lucas, X. et al. (2020). Structure-based design of a macrocyclic PROTAC. *Angew. Chem. Int. Ed.* 59 (4): 1727–1734. https://doi.org/10.1002/anie.201914396.

40 Dragovich, P.S., Pillow, T.H., Blake, R.A. et al. (2021). Antibody-mediated delivery of chimeric BRD4 degraders. Part 2: Improvement of *in vitro* antiproliferation activity and *in vivo* antitumor efficacy. *J. Med. Chem.* 64 (5): 2576–2607. https://doi.org/10.1021/acs.jmedchem.0c01846.

41 Stebbins, C.E., Kaelin, W.G. Jr., and Pavletich, N.P. (1999). Structure of the VHL-ElonginC-ElonginB complex: implications for VHL tumor suppressor function. *Science* 284 (5413): 455–461. https://doi.org/10.1126/science.284.5413.455.

42 Buckley, D.L., Van Molle, I., Gareiss, P.C. et al. (2012). Targeting the von Hippel-Lindau E3 ubiquitin ligase using small molecules to disrupt the VHL/HIF-1α interaction. *J. Am. Chem. Soc.* 134 (10): 4465–4468. https://doi.org/10.1021/ja209924v.

43 Shi, J., Whyte, W.A., Zepeda-Mendoza, C.J. et al. (2013). Role of SWI/SNF in acute leukemia maintenance and enhancer-mediated Myc regulation. *Genes Dev.* 27 (24): 2648–2662.

44 Albrecht, B.K., Cote, A., Crawford, T. et al. (2016). *Therapeutic pyridazine compounds and uses thereof.* WO2016138114 WIPO Patent.

45 Soares, P., Gadd, M.S., Frost, J. et al. (2018). Group-based optimization of potent and cell-active inhibitors of the von Hippel–Lindau (VHL) E3 ubiquitin ligase: structure–activity relationships leading to the chemical probe (2S,4R)-1-((S)-2-(1-cyanocyclopropanecarboxamido)-3,3-dimethylbutanoyl)-4-hydr. *J. Med. Chem.* 61 (2): 599–618. https://doi.org/10.1021/acs.jmedchem.7b00675.

46 Tao, Z.-F., Hasvold, L., Wang, L. et al. (2014). Discovery of a potent and selective BCL-XL inhibitor with *in vivo* activity. *ACS Med. Chem. Lett.* 5 (10): 1088–1093. https://doi.org/10.1021/ml5001867.

47 Popow, J., Arnhof, H., Bader, G. et al. (2019). Highly selective PTK2 proteolysis targeting chimeras to probe focal adhesion kinase scaffolding functions. *J. Med. Chem.* 62 (5): 2508–2520.

48 Cromm, P.M., Samarasinghe, K.T.G., Hines, J., and Crews, C.M. (2018). Addressing kinase-independent functions of Fak via PROTAC-mediated degradation. *J. Am. Chem. Soc.* 140 (49): 17019–17026.

49 Gao, H., Wu, Y., Sun, Y. et al. (2020). Design, synthesis, and evaluation of highly potent FAK-targeting PROTACs. *ACS Med. Chem. Lett.* 11 (10): 1855–1862.

50 Winter, G.E., Buckley, D.L., Paulk, J. et al. (2015). Phthalimide conjugation as a strategy for *in vivo* target protein degradation. *Science* 348 (6241): 1376–1381. https://doi.org/10.1126/science.aab1433.

51 Winter, G.E., Mayer, A., Buckley, D.L. et al. (2017). BET bromodomain proteins function as master transcription elongation factors independent of CDK9 recruitment. *Mol. Cell* 67 (1): 5–18.e19.

52 Okuhira, K., Demizu, Y., Hattori, T. et al. (2013). Development of hybrid small molecules that induce degradation of estrogen receptor-alpha and necrotic cell death in breast cancer cells. *Cancer Sci.* 104 (11): 1492–1498.

53 Buhimschi, A.D., Armstrong, H.A., Toure, M. et al. (2018). Targeting the C481S ibrutinib-resistance mutation in Bruton's tyrosine kinase using PROTAC-mediated degradation. *Biochemistry* 57 (26): 3564–3575. https://doi.org/10.1021/acs.biochem.8b00391.

54 Sun, Y., Zhao, X., Ding, N. et al. (2018). PROTAC-induced BTK degradation as a novel therapy for mutated BTK C481S induced ibrutinib-resistant B-cell malignancies. *Cell Res.* 28 (7): 779–781. https://doi.org/10.1038/s41422-018-0055-1.

55 Perez, H.L., Chaudhry, C., Emanuel, S.L. et al. (2015). Discovery of potent heterodimeric antagonists of inhibitor of apoptosis proteins (IAPs) with sustained antitumor activity. *J. Med. Chem.* 58 (3): 1556–1562. https://doi.org/10.1021/jm501482t.

56 Ito, T., Ando, H., Suzuki, T. et al. (2010). Identification of a primary target of thalidomide teratogenicity. *Science.* 327 (5971): 1345–1350. https://doi.org/10.1126/science.1177319.

57 Matyskiela, M.E., Couto, S., Zheng, X. et al. (2018). SALL4 mediates teratogenicity as a thalidomide-dependent cereblon substrate. *Nat. Chem. Biol.* 14 (10): 981–987.

58 Donovan, K.A., An, J., Nowak, R.P. et al. (2018). Thalidomide promotes degradation of SALL4, a transcription factor implicated in Duane Radial Ray syndrome. *Elife* 7: e38430.

59 Krönke, J., Fink, E.C., Hollenbach, P.W. et al. (2015). Lenalidomide induces ubiquitination and degradation of CK1α in del(5q) MDS. *Nature* 523 (7559): 183–188. https://doi.org/10.1038/nature14610.

60 Matyskiela, M.E., Lu, G., Ito, T. et al. (2016). A novel cereblon modulator recruits GSPT1 to the CRL4CRBN ubiquitin ligase. *Nature* 535 (7611): 252–257.

61 Surka, C., Jin, L., Mbong, N. et al. (2021). CC-90009, A novel cereblon E3 ligase modulator, targets acute myeloid leukemia blasts and leukemia stem cells. *Blood* 137 (5): 661–677. https://doi.org/10.1182/blood.2020008676.

62 Cheng, Z., Saito, K., Pisarev, A.V. et al. (2009). Structural insights into eRF3 and stop codon recognition by eRF1. *Genes Dev.* 23 (9): 1106–1118.

63 Lu, G., Middleton, R.E., Sun, H. et al. (2014). The myeloma drug lenalidomide promotes the cereblon-dependent destruction of ikaros proteins. *Science* 343 (6168): 305.

64 Krönke, J., Udeshi, N.D., Narla, A. et al. (2014). Lenalidomide causes selective degradation of IKZF1 and IKZF3 in multiple myeloma cells. *Science* 343 (6168): 301–305.

65 Kohlhase, J., Schubert, L., Liebers, M. et al. (2003). Mutations at the SALL4 locus on chromosome 20 result in a range of clinically overlapping phenotypes, including Okihiro syndrome, Holt-Oram syndrome, acro-renal-ocular syndrome, and patients previously reported to represent thalidomide embryopathy. *J. Med. Genet.* 40 (7): 473–478.

66 Matyskiela, M.E., Clayton, T., Zheng, X. et al. (2020). Crystal structure of the SALL4–pomalidomide–cereblon–DDB1 complex. *Nat. Struct. Mol. Biol.* 27 (4): 319–322. https://doi.org/10.1038/s41594-020-0405-9.

67 Uehara, T., Minoshima, Y., Sagane, K. et al. (2017). Selective degradation of splicing factor CAPERα by anticancer sulfonamides. *Nat. Chem. Biol.* 13 (6): 675–680.

68 Han, T., Goralski, M., Gaskill, N. et al. (2017). Anticancer sulfonamides target splicing by inducing RBM39 degradation via recruitment to DCAF15. *Science* 356 (6336): eaal3755.

69 Du, X., Volkov, O.A., Czerwinski, R.M. et al. (2019). Structural basis and kinetic pathway of RBM39 recruitment to DCAF15 by a sulfonamide molecular glue E7820. *Structure* 27 (11): 1625–1633.e3.

70 Słabicki, M., Kozicka, Z., Petzold, G. et al. (2020). The CDK inhibitor CR8 acts as a molecular glue degrader that depletes cyclin K. *Nature* 585 (7824): 293–297.

71 Mayor-Ruiz, C., Bauer, S., Brand, M. et al. (2020). Rational discovery of molecular glue degraders via scalable chemical profiling. *Nat. Chem. Biol.* 16 (11): 1199–1207. https://doi.org/10.1038/s41589-020-0594-x.

72 Lv, L., Chen, P., Cao, L. et al. (2020). Discovery of a molecular glue promoting cdk12-ddb1 interaction to trigger cyclin k degradation. *eLife* 9: 1–34.

73 Wu, Y., Zhou, X., Barnes, C.O. et al. (2016). The DDB1–DCAF1–Vpr–UNG2 crystal structure reveals how HIV-1 Vpr steers human UNG2 toward destruction. *Nat. Struct. Mol. Biol.* 23 (10): 933–940. https://doi.org/10.1038/nsmb.3284.

74 Dixon-Clarke, S.E., Elkins, J.M., Cheng, S.-W.G. et al. (2015). Structures of the CDK12/CycK complex with AMP-PNP reveal a flexible C-terminal kinase extension important for ATP binding. *Sci. Rep.* 5 (1): 17122. https://doi.org/10.1038/srep17122.

75 Drummond, M.L., Henry, A., Li, H., and Williams, C.I. (2020). Improved accuracy for modeling PROTAC-mediated ternary complex formation and targeted protein degradation via new *in silico* methodologies. *bioRxiv* 197186. http://biorxiv.org/content/early/2020/07/10/2020.07.10.197186.abstract.

76 Bai, N., Miller, S.A., Andrianov, G.V. et al. (2021). Rationalizing PROTAC-mediated ternary complex formation using Rosetta. *J. Chem. Inf. Model.* 61 (3): 1368–1382. https://doi.org/10.1021/acs.jcim.0c01451.

77 Zaidman, D., Prilusky, J., and London, N. (2020). PRosettaC: Rosetta based modeling of PROTAC mediated ternary complexes. *J. Chem. Inf. Model.* 60 (10): 4894–4903.

78 Weng, G., Li, D., Kang, Y., and Hou, T. (2021). Integrative modeling of PROTAC-mediated ternary complexes. *J. Med. Chem.* 64 (21): 16271–16281. https://doi.org/10.1021/acs.jmedchem.1c01576.

79 Evans, R., O'Neill, M., Pritzel, A. et al. (2021). Protein complex prediction with AlphaFold-multimer. *bioRxiv* 463034.

80 Rodriguez-Rivera, F.P. and Levi, S.M. (2021). Unifying catalysis framework to dissect proteasomal degradation paradigms. *ACS Cent. Sci.* 7 (7): 1117–1125. https://doi.org/10.1021/acscentsci.1c00389.

5

Computational Modeling of PROTAC Ternary Complexes and Linker Design

Sven A. Miller[1], Grigorii V. Andrianov[1,2], Victoria Mischley[1,3], Khadija A. Wharton[1], Jesse J. Chen[4] and John Karanicolas[1,5]

[1] *Molecular Therapeutics Program, Fox Chase Cancer Center, 333 Cottman Avenue, Philadelphia, PA, 19111, USA*
[2] *Kazan Federal University, Institute of Fundamental Medicine and Biology, 18 Kremlyovskaya str, Kazan, 420008, Russia*
[3] *Drexel University College of Medicine, Philadelphia, PA, 19102, USA*
[4] *Triana Biomedicines, Inc., 400 Totten Pond Rd. #120, Waltham, MA, 02451, USA*
[5] *Temple University School of Pharmacy, Moulder Center for Drug Discovery Research, Philadelphia, PA, 19140, USA*

5.1 Introduction

The ubiquitination pathway is used by eukaryotic cells to post-translationally modify selected proteins by covalently attaching one or more copies of the small protein ubiquitin. Ubiquitin is first bound as a thioester conjugate to a ubiquitin activating enzyme (E1), which then passes the ubiquitin to a ubiquitin conjugating enzyme (E2). The E2 then binds to a ubiquitin ligase (E3), and they together engage the ultimate ubiquitin acceptor (the substrate protein). Addition of ubiquitin can serve as a signal for a wide variety of processes affecting the substrate protein, including altered subcellular localization or protein interactions. Most notably, however, polyubiquitin can serve as a signal to induce proteasomal degradation of the substrate protein [1].

Proteolysis targeting chimeras (PROTACs) are designed molecules that hijack the final step of the E1–E2–E3 cascade by redirecting the E3 substrate specificity, thus inducing targeted degradation of a "neosubstrate" protein of interest (Figure 5.1a). To do so, PROTACs are built from three parts: a moiety that binds to the E3 ubiquitin ligase, a warhead that recruits the target protein, and a chemical linker that connects the two. In many cases, PROTACs are built by repurposing an existing inhibitor (or binder) of the target protein and linking to it an E3-recruiting moiety to obtain a degrader. This approach is especially appealing in scenarios for which the target protein has multiple functional roles: whereas an inhibitor may disrupt only one of these, destruction of the protein ablates all of its functions [2–4] (Figure 5.1b). Further, relative to the inhibitors on which they have been built, certain PROTACs

Inducing Targeted Protein Degradation: From Chemical Biology to Drug Discovery and Clinical Applications, First Edition. Edited by Philipp Cromm.

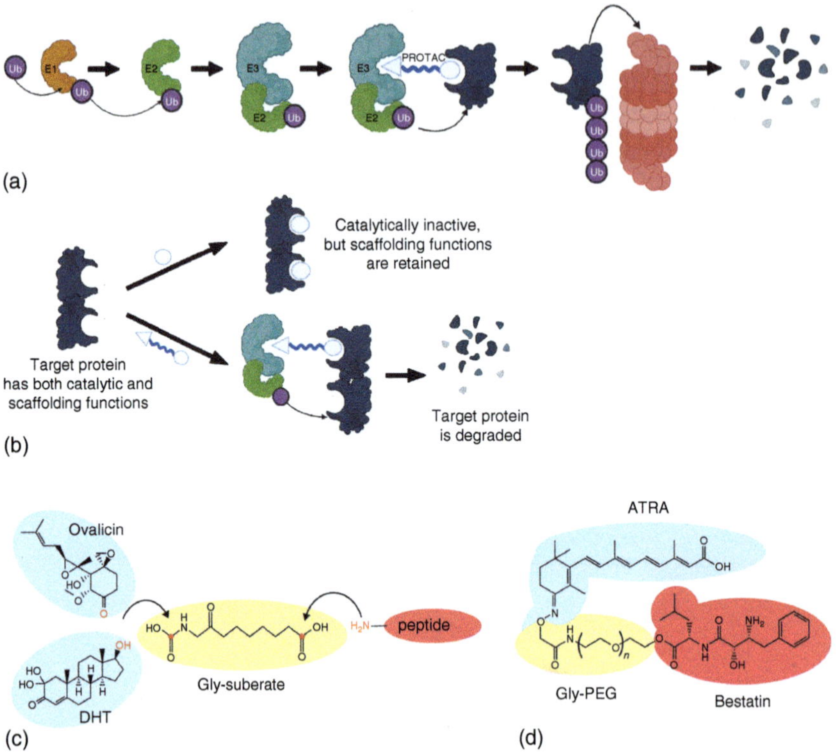

Figure 5.1 PROTAC activity and early examples. (a) The ubiquitination pathway entails activation of ubiquitin by an E1, followed by transfer to an E2. An E3 ubiquitin ligase binds to the E2. For HECT or RCR-type E3's, ubiquitin is transferred to the E3; for RING or U-box E3 ligases, ubiquitin remains conjugated to the E2. Rather than relying on binding by an endogenous substrate, PROTACs recruit a "neosubstrate" target protein to the E2–E3 complex. This proximity can be sufficient to induce ubiquitination and subsequent proteasome-mediated degradation of the target protein. (b) A key advantage of PROTACs relative to inhibitors is that protein destruction eliminates all functional roles of a target protein; by contrast, traditional competitive inhibitors only abrogate activities at the inhibitor's binding site. (c) Early PROTACs were built by using glycine-suberate linkers to affix E3-recruiting peptides onto natural products (e.g. ovalicin and DHT). (d) Subsequent developments moved toward non-peptidic E3-recruiting moieties (e.g. bestatin), shown here joined to all-*trans* retinoic acid (ATRA) via a polyethylene glycol (PEG) linker.

have been found to yield improved potency and/or more sustained biological effects [4–6]. Although PROTACs fall outside the "rule-of-five" and thus may suffer from poor cell penetrance [7], recent advances in tuning their properties have led to compounds that can be orally administered [8] or improve cellular accumulation [9]. Further promoting their efficacy, PROTACs' underlying mechanism of action can allow them to be catalytically active *in vivo* [10]: that is to say, substoichiometric amounts of the PROTAC can induce multiple ubiquitylation events. Consequently, PROTACs can provide a means for dramatically extending the utility of the already-available small molecules that address the desired protein target.

The earliest proof-of-concept PROTACs were built from the chemical tools that were most readily available at the time: peptides known to bind specific E3 ligases, connected using flexible amino acid or alkyl-carbon linkers to natural products that target the desired neosubstrate [11, 12] (Figure 5.1c). While such constructs provided important validation for the approach, these peptide-based PROTACs exhibited poor pharmacokinetics, which limited further development. Subsequent PROTACs began moving away from peptides as their E3-recruiting motifs, such as an early example that affixed methyl bestatin (to recruit cIAP1) to all-*trans* retinoic acid (a ligand of CRABPs) using a polyethylene glycol (PEG) linker [13, 14] (Figure 5.1d). This work, coupled with studies demonstrating that effective PROTACs could be readily adapted to degrade multiple diverse substrates [5], led to rapid and intense interest in this burgeoning field. In the few years since, PROTACs have been reported for degrading targets that include hormone receptors [15–17], BET family proteins [5, 18–20], kinases [3, 4, 21–36], anti-apoptotic proteins [37], E3 ligases [38, 39], tyrosinases [40], histone methyl transferases [41], cytochrome P450s [42, 43], IDO1 [44], and many more [45]. To manage this new wealth of information, two separate searchable databases of PROTACs have been assembled for community use [46] (PROTACpedia https://protacpedia.weizmann.ac.il and PROTAC-DB http://cadd.zju.edu.cn/protacdb/).

5.2 PROTAC Ternary Complexes

The crystal structures of ternary complexes (comprising the E3 ligase, the PROTAC, and the neosubstrate) have revealed the basis by which the components come together in a productive manner. In particular, such structures have shown that the typical schematic representations of ternary complexes – such as those in Figures 5.1a,b are misleading in an important way.

The traditional framing of PROTAC activity focuses on their heterobifunctional design, whereby one side of the PROTAC recruits the E3 ligase and the other side binds to the target protein; other additional potential interactions among the components are often not discussed. For example, the prototypical BRD4-degrading PROTAC MZ1 was designed by tethering the bromodomain inhibitor JQ1 to a VHL-recruiting moiety [20]. Surprisingly, however, the crystal structure of the BRD4–MZ1–VHL complex included numerous unexpected stabilizing interactions [47] (Figure 5.2a). Despite the fact that BRD4 is a neosubstrate for VHL, and thus there has been no evolutionary selection for their association, the MZ1 ternary complex includes a highly coordinated network of hydrophobic and electrostatic interactions between the two proteins. Moreover, the PEG linker that connects the PROTAC's two functional groups also makes favorable hydrogen bonding interactions with the protein components and therefore occludes solvent from otherwise-exposed regions of the warhead and E3-recruiting components of the PROTAC. Finally, this ternary complex even includes close contacts between BRD4 and the PROTAC's VHL-recruiting moiety. In this case, then, the PROTAC's ability to drive formation of the ternary complex cannot be neatly deconstructed into two distinct protein-recruiting moieties separated by an inert linker: the components of this PROTAC contribute to stabilizing the ternary complex in ways beyond those expected from this simple "heterobifunctional" paradigm, and protein–protein interactions also play a key role.

As a growing list of ternary complex structures have been solved and/or biophysically characterized [48–55], the importance of cooperativity in assembling the ternary complex has been hotly debated as a driver of efficient target degradation. Although important counterexamples have been reported [26, 48], many efficient PROTACs have been found to exhibit a cooperative assembly [47, 51, 54, 56–58]: that is to say, the components of the ternary complex come together more potently than expected from the binding affinities of the PROTAC with either protein alone. Collectively, this may suggest that the adventitious (non-evolved) protein–protein interactions observed in many crystal structures may indeed play a key role in facilitating ternary complex formation and in the ensuing neosubstrate ubiquitination.

Given that nearly every crystal structure of a PROTAC ternary complex includes extensive (adventitious) protein–protein interactions, it is remarkable to reflect on the fact that the protein pairs typically have no detectable binding to one another [59–61] (or at best extremely weak binding [62]) in the absence of the PROTAC. In light of ternary complexes having such complementary protein surfaces [26, 47, 63], it is also instructive to consider the breadth of potential neosubstrates that might be degraded by a given E3 ligase. In the case of VHL, for example, the crystal structures of the ternary complex that include vastly diverse neosubstrates confirm that the same surface of the VHL protein is involved in binding; however, the surface features of the partner proteins vary dramatically (Figure 5.2b). Thus, despite the apparent requirement for a complementary surface topology,

Figure 5.2 Adventitious interactions can stabilize PROTAC ternary complexes. (a) The crystal structure of the BRD4–MZ1–VHL ternary complex (PDB ID: 5T35) reveals both hydrophobic and hydrogen bonding interactions between the protein components of the ternary complex. Distinct hydrophobic regions on opposite ends of the binding interface, residues Leu385 and Trp374 of the "WPF" shelf on BRD4 (*orange*), form complementary interactions with VHL (*magenta*); these are further reinforced by hydrogen bonding between Glu438 and Arg69. The PEG linker of MZ1 PROTAC also engages Brd4's His437 through hydrogen bonding interactions. Finally, MZ1's VHL-recruiting moiety also engages BRD4 directly in this binding mode through contacts to the backbone of Ala384 and Leu385. (b) Crystal structures of ternary complexes from three different VHL-recruiting PROTACs that each targets a different neosubstrate (PDB IDs: 6HR2, 6SIS, and 7JTP). In each case, the protein–protein interface is shown in *red*. All the three examples include extensive complementarity between the protein components. Although the same binding surface of VHL is used in all the three examples, the surface patches used by the neosubstrates are very different from one another. (c) Plasticity of CRBN-BRD4 engagement is demonstrated through similar PROTACs with different linker lengths (PDB IDs: 6BNB and 6BN7). The crystal structure of the ternary complex containing dBET23 (8-carbon linker) shows one set of interactions between BRD4 (*magenta*) and CRBN (*blue*). When this linker is shortened to yield dBET57 (2-carbon linker), the resulting crystal structure shows a rotation of BRD4 (*yellow*) relative to CRBN. The PROTAC was not built into the latter complex because it could not be clearly resolved at the resolution of this crystal structure. Nonetheless, the altered binding mode highlights the fact that PROTAC-stabilized complexes of BRD4 and CRBN can engage the same protein surfaces using very different arrangements.

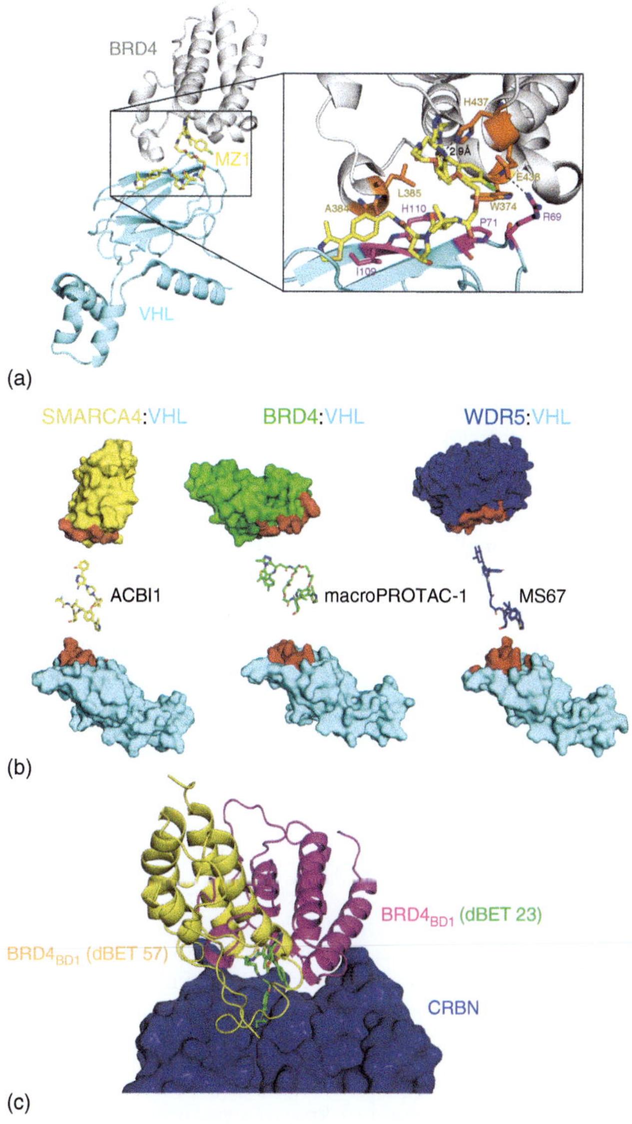

there do not appear to be any other surface features that are common to proteins amenable to degradation by VHL-based PROTACs.

That an E3 ligase can be repurposed to build degraders of diverse neosubstrates highlights the ability of at least some E3 ligases (such as CRBN and VHL) to form PROTAC-stabilized complementary interactions with many different protein partners. Remarkably, however, an E3 ligase can even recognize a *single target* with multiple different binding modes: structural characterization of CRBN–dBET–BRD4 complexes showed that simply varying the linker length (dBET23 versus dBET57) was sufficient to produce an alternate arrangement in the ternary complex [48]

(Figure 5.2c). The crystal structures do not report on the conformational diversity that might be present in solution; thus, it may be possible that a longer PROTAC linker allows for multiple binding modes, and a shorter linker is compatible with only a subset of these. To test the prospective consequences of selecting for a single binding mode, the authors then designed a short linker expected to bind to a distinct conformation and found that this construct yielded superior BRD4 selectivity (relative to other bromodomains) compared to its precursor PROTACs [48].

Further evidence for the importance of adventitious interactions in the ternary complex (typically protein–protein contacts) derives from the fact that the selectivity with which PROTACs degrade their targets are not necessarily retained directly from the warheads on which they are built. Beyond the BRD4-selective degraders described above, the phenomenon of "emergent" selectivity has been observed most often in PROTACs that repurpose the existing kinase inhibitors with a well-established selectivity [22–24, 30, 64, 65]. In these cases, it is often found that only a subset of the warhead's targets are actually degraded; this subset further depends on the details of the chosen E3 ligase and linker that are used. This paradigm has been emphasized most dramatically in studies that intentionally begin with low-affinity kinase inhibitors of broad specificity and then use large-scale proteomics to identify PROTAC derivatives (from a collection with varied linker lengths/compositions/attachment points) that can exhibit astonishing selectivity [66]. An additional conclusion reached by this work, however, was that formation of a stable ternary complex is not always sufficient to induce degradation of the target kinase [66]: thus, additional factors – such as the availability of surface lysine residues relative to the complete ubiquitination complex [67] – may be required to fully explain PROTAC target preferences.

5.3 Computational Modeling of PROTAC Ternary Complexes

Structure-based modeling of PROTAC ternary complexes represents an interesting and somewhat different challenge than those typically encountered in computer-aided drug discovery. There exist many well-validated approaches for modeling protein/small-molecule complexes, but these are intended for ligand/receptor systems in which the receptor is a single protein of known structure: application of such methods is complicated by the fact that the relative orientation of the two proteins in the ternary complex is not known *a priori*. There also exist many well-validated approaches for docking pairs of proteins to one another, but these are not intended for scenarios in which a flexible ligand occupies the center of their interface. In short, building up a model of a PROTAC ternary complex is challenging from a sampling perspective because all the three components must be correctly placed relative to one another, and the active conformation of the PROTAC is not known in advance (i.e. its internal degrees of freedom must be sampled as well).

From the standpoint that PROTACs are heterobifunctional constructs, however, the bound pose of each functional moiety relative to its cognate protein is known ahead of time: crystal structures are available for most of the commonly used

E3-recruiting groups bound to their respective E3 ligases, and PROTACs are usually built by repurposing an inhibitor that has been structurally characterized in complex with its target protein. From a sampling standpoint, then, one can envision tackling the problem either from a "ligand-centric" approach or from a "protein-centric" approach (Figure 5.3). From a ligand-centric standpoint, one would focus on sampling the potential conformations of the PROTAC itself. Given the coordinates of the two functional groups, the corresponding proteins can then be added, leading to a model of the ternary complex. Alternatively, from a protein-centric standpoint, one would focus on sampling the potential arrangements of the two protein components. Given the coordinates of the proteins, one could then build in the locations of their ligands; these might then be connected using the necessary linker to construct a model of the ternary complex.

The first published implementation of a general pipeline for modeling PROTAC ternary complexes was described by Drummond and Williams [68] using the

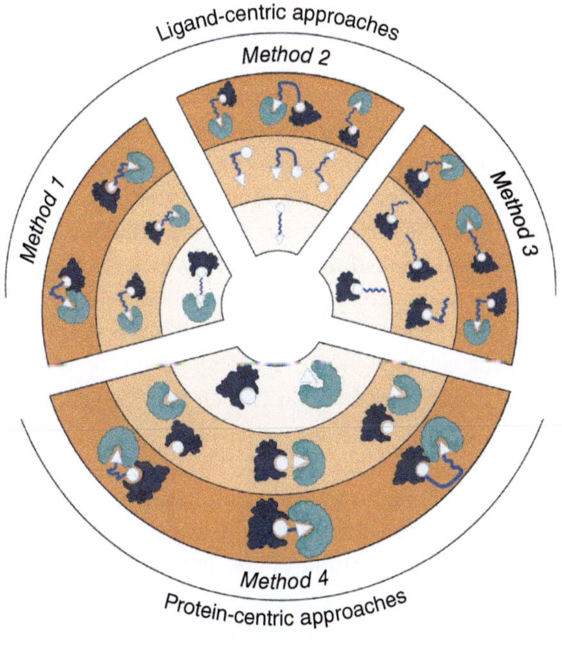

Figure 5.3 Ligand-centric and protein-centric approaches for modeling PROTAC ternary complexes. *Ligand-centric: Method 1* starts with the PROTAC linker in an extended conformation and then samples around each rotatable bond; the bound proteins follow along as the ends of the PROTAC are moved. *Method 2* identifies low-energy conformations of the free PROTAC and then builds on the protein components. *Method 3* starts with the PROTAC warhead and linker bound to the target protein (neosubstrate) and then varies the linker conformation; the E3-recruiting moiety and the E3 ligase are then added. *Protein-centric: Method 4* docks the protein components together to identify complementarity protein–protein interactions without considering the effect of the linker. These docked poses are then filtered to determine which ones are compatible with the linker of interest. Variations of *Method 4* have emerged as the *de facto* standard for currently used protocols to model PROTAC ternary complexes.

molecular operating environment (MOE)'s native scientific vector language (SVL) [69]. Their study described four distinct strategies for building models of PROTAC complexes, three ligand-centric and one protein-centric (Figure 5.3). All four workflows were evaluated to determine which could best recapitulate the binding modes observed in publicly available crystal structures of PROTAC ternary complexes.

The first strategy, *Method 1*, initially builds the PROTAC with its linker in a fully extended conformation and then uses the coordinates of the warheads to add both proteins. The rotatable bonds in the linker are then varied one at a time, with each change in these dihedral angles propagated such that the bound proteins move in response to the changing PROTAC conformation. In *Method 2*, multiple conformations of the PROTAC alone are first sampled, without including the associated proteins. For each of the lowest energy conformations that are generated, the proteins are then added to yield the ternary complex; conceptually, this strategy assumes that the active conformation of the PROTAC in the ternary complex is also one of the most favorable in solution. *Method 3* builds up the pieces of the ternary complex sequentially, starting from the target (neosubstrate) protein. The functional group that binds this protein is added, along with the PROTAC linker, which is then energetically optimized. The E3-recruiting moiety is then added onto the linker and then the E3 ligase itself. Unfortunately, retrospective evaluation of *Methods 1–3* showed that in all the three cases, very few of the resulting models resembled the known crystal structures [68]. In retrospect, this difficulty likely arises from the ligand-centric sampling shared by these approaches: small changes in the rotatable bonds of the linker are exaggerated in the positioning of the warheads, which in turn lead to very large changes in the overall positioning of the two proteins. Put another way, it is exceedingly unlikely that the two proteins will robustly land with precisely complementary positioning relative to one another, given that their positioning relies in an extremely sensitive way on the linker conformation (which itself is generated without the proteins).

This hurdle is circumvented in *Method 4*, which is a protein-centric approach. Rather than focusing on the linker, sampling instead concentrates on docking the two proteins relative to one another. Each protein harbors the cognate piece of the PROTAC that recruits it, without any consideration of the linker that connects them. The resulting docked poses position the two proteins in orientations that are complementary to one another, but they cannot necessarily be connected by the linker. For this reason, the docked poses are then filtered to determine which are also compatible with the linker of interest. Gratifyingly, the retrospective benchmark showed that *Method 4* provided many more models that resembled known crystal structures of PROTAC complexes compared to the three earlier approaches [68].

Although many important details differ, and performance can vary widely, each of the contemporaneous and subsequent reports of pipelines for modeling PROTAC ternary complexes are essentially variations of *Method 4* (Figure 5.4). In a follow-up to their original study, Drummond et al. expanded *Method 4* by including restraints on PROTAC conformational freedom and clustering the output ternary models to recognize binding modes that emerge repeatedly; they termed this new approach *Method 4B* [70] (Figure 5.4, *orange*). To analyze the results, the authors clustered the protein components from the resulting models and separately clustered the PROTAC conformations. Any pairs of models in which the protein components resided in the same cluster, and the PROTAC conformations resided in the same cluster, were determined to share a "double cluster": thus, the models comprising a "double cluster" share a specific PROTAC conformation and a specific overall arrangement of the ternary complex. The authors then used the number of models in the largest "double cluster" as a proxy for how effectively a PROTAC would induce ternary complex formation, reasoning that this is an indication that the simulations have converged to a single solution [70].

In broad strokes, the authors found that having a highly populated "double cluster" did indeed provide some ability to distinguish between potent versus inactive PROTACs and also recapitulated the general selectivity trend of a PROTAC built using a pan-kinase warhead [70]. Some care must be taken, however, because they also found that a number of PROTAC conformations also seemed to correlate with the population of the largest double cluster [70]: that is to say, this method may be overly predisposed to predict that PROTACs with flexible linkers will have activity. The same general trend has also emerged for other variants of *Method 4*, suggesting that this indeed may be a consequence of the overall modeling strategy itself.

Fundamental to the success of protein-centric models (such as *Method 4*) is the expectation that favorable protein–protein interactions are critical to ternary complex formation: so much that their shape complementarity can be used to generate initial models (in the absence of the PROTAC) that will include the arrangement observed in the crystal structures of the ternary complex. Based on this assumption, Zaidman et al. developed the modeling pipeline PRosettaC [71] (Figure 5.4, *red*) that begins by using the PatchDock algorithm to generate initial docked poses. PatchDock works by first enumerating concave and convex patches on the surface of each protein and then by exhaustively trying to match every concave patch on one protein with every convex patch on the other [72]. Candidate poses are ranked based on the surface area of their buried interface, without being overly stringent if steric clashes are present [73]. To improve the detailed interactions before building ternary complex models, PRosettaC therefore refined the PatchDock poses using Rosetta [74, 75]. An important advantage of this two-step strategy for carrying out the initial protein docking step is that the PatchDock search is very fast, thus speeding up the computational demands of the docking stage.

To compare the performance of PRosettaC against *Method 4*, the authors evaluated how well ternary complexes already solved by crystallography could be reconstructed from their components using the same collection from Drummond and Williams' original study [68]. PRosettaC provided impressive performance in this experiment, with some models matching the corresponding crystal structures to exquisite detail [71]. Care must be taken not to overinterpret this seemingly promising outcome, although because the protein coordinates in this experiment were taken from the crystal structures of the ternary complexes. In effect, using the bound protein structures may provide strong clues as to the "correct" binding mode for the

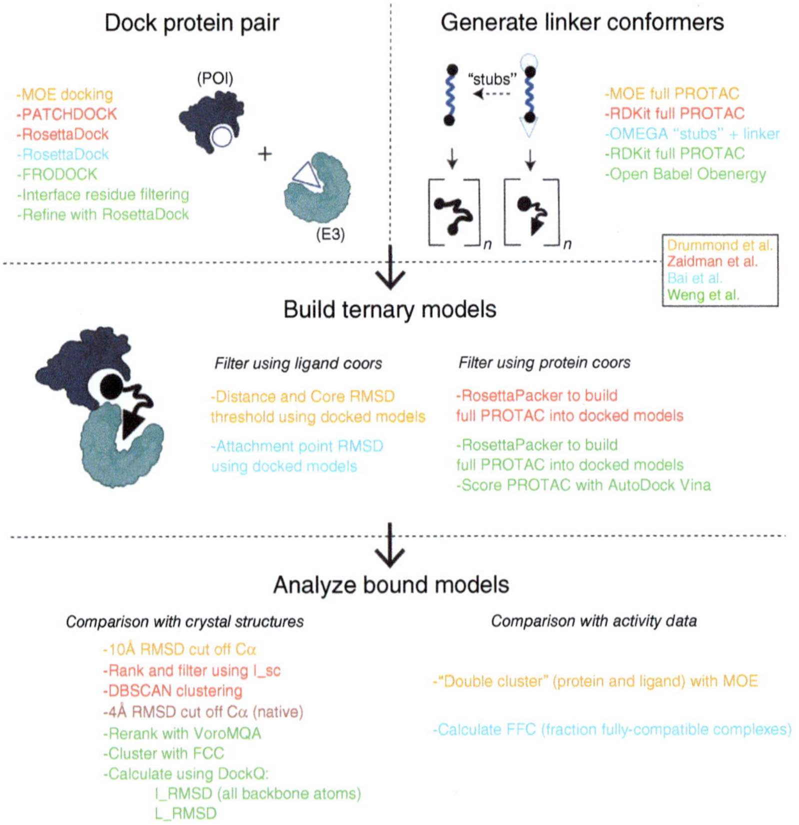

Figure 5.4 Comparison of related approaches for computational modeling of PROTAC ternary complexes. Several variants sharing the general strategy of *Method 4* (Figure 5.3) have been described. Differences have been explored at each step of the pipeline, with the approach used in each study indicated using different colors.

protein components; these would not be available in most "real" applications. Rather, prospective experiments will inevitably require using protein structures determined in the absence of their protein partner from the ternary complex, leaving as an open question the performance that one might expect in such scenarios. Importantly, to facilitate adoption and further benchmarking of their method, Zaidman et al. offer access to PRosettaC through a web server (accessible at https://prosettac.weizmann.ac.il/).

Another contemporaneous pipeline built upon the Rosetta software [75] was reported by Bai et al. [76] (Figure 5.4, *cyan*). Noting that an E3 ligase may recognize a given neosubstrate with more than one binding mode (as exemplified by the CRBN–dBET–BRD4 complexes described earlier [48]), these authors were concerned that ternary complexes in solution may comprise more diverse ensembles than can be reflected through static crystal structures (which themselves may be biased because of the artifacts of crystallography). Accordingly, the authors' analysis focused on comparing how well the *collection* of ternary complex models could explain PROTACs' degradation efficiency, rather than seeking to recapitulate crystal structures. As a proxy for a PROTAC's activity, Bai and colleagues calculated the fraction of all docked models that would be compatible with a given PROTAC (FFC, the "fraction of fully compatible complexes"). The authors reasoned that if protein docking mostly yielded poses that could not be joined by the linker of a given PROTAC (either because the preferred binding modes did not place the two proteins' active sites close to one another or the linker was too short/sterically incompatible), the FFC score would be low and this PROTAC would be unlikely to promote ternary complex formation. Conversely, a high FFC score could arise either because one distinct arrangement was found repeatedly (the same that would be found using the "double cluster" criterion [70]) or because the PROTAC could allow for multiple alternate arrangements with compelling protein–protein complementary.

Using this measure, the authors explored PROTACs built from the non-selective kinase inhibitor foretinib: depending on which E3-recuiting moiety is affixed to this warhead, a different subset of kinases was reported to be degraded [23]. Gratifyingly, Bai et al. found that FFC scores could correctly distinguish the degradation selectivity for each PROTAC, ostensibly through differences in the protein interactions for the underlying kinase/E3 pairings [76]. An additional capability demonstrated in this study – which presumably holds other *Method 4* variants as well – is that the (computationally expensive) protein–protein docking step is carried out agnostic of the specific PROTAC that will be studied; because of this, it is possible to rapidly screen many different candidate linkers (or attachment points) using an already-generated collection of docked structures and thus determine what linker length and composition are best suited to a given E3/neosubstrate pairing. Importantly, the *unbound* protein conformations were used throughout this study as there are (naturally) no crystal structures available for combinations that do not form observable ternary complexes or for large collections of PROTACs with varied linkers.

Returning to the challenge of building ternary complex models from unbound protein conformations (rather than simply reconstituting the pieces from a crystal structure of the ternary complex), Weng et al. developed an integrative modeling pipeline dubbed "PROTAC-Model" that applies stringent protein-based and chemistry-based filters at the early stages of the pipeline and extensive energy-based filters at the late stages [77] (Figure 5.4, *green*). Starting with model-building from bound conformations, the authors compared their results to the already-published data from the Drummond et al. [70] and Zaidman et al. [71] teams and found that PROTAC-Model yielded close matches to the crystal structures in more of the benchmark cases [77]. The authors went on to evaluate their method when starting from unbound conformations and found a modest deterioration in performance, which was unsurprisingly tied to the extent to which the protein conformation changes in response to ternary complex formation [77].

Historically, rebuilding protein structures from components provided in bound crystal structures has long been readily tractable, whereas accounting for conformational changes associated with binding has long proven challenging [78]. Determining the likely binding mode of protein pairs has also been much more straightforward than predicting their binding affinities [78]. In summary then, many of the conclusions from the studies highlighted here neatly reflect the state of protein–protein docking broadly.

Finally, we note that each of the methods described above focuses exclusively on modeling PROTAC ternary complexes. As pointed out in the preceding Section (5.2), however, ternary complex formation is necessary but not sufficient for inducing degradation [66, 67, 79]. Aiming to differentiate between productive versus unproductive complexes, recent studies have sought to build models of the complete ubiquitination complex, hypothesizing that the presence of absence of suitably placed lysine residues on the neosubstrate can explain why some potential targets are not degraded [67, 80]. These approaches face stark challenges not only because of the sheer size of the complexes (e.g. modeling CRBN/DDB1/CUL4A/Rbx1/NEDD8/E2/Ub instead of simply CRBN) but more importantly because of the key role played by these complexes' dynamics and flexibility [81–83]. Although daunting, moving toward the long-term goal of complete and predictive methods for designing effective degraders will ultimately require tackling these challenges.

5.4 PROTAC Design and Optimization

Starting from a warhead that binds the protein one seeks to degrade, there are potentially many ways to build it into a PROTAC (Figure 5.5). Using the bromodomain inhibitor JQ1 as a starting point, for example, the early PROTAC MZ1 was designed by appending a PEG linker and a VHL-recruiting moiety [20]. JQ1 is not a purely selective bromodomain binder: rather, it recognizes both bromodomains of Brd4 and also binds to both bromodomains of Brd2 and Brd3 [84]. Treating cells with PROTAC MZ1 at submicromolar concentrations surprisingly induced preferential degradation of Brd4 rather than Brd2 or Brd3 [20]; subsequent reporter assays ascribed this difference to MZ1 exhibiting a 10-fold preference for $Brd4_{BD2}$ over $Brd2_{BD2}$ and a 100-fold preference for $Brd4_{BD2}$ over $Brd3_{BD2}$ [48].

To test the hypothesis that recognizing both bromodomains of each protein diminished the selectivity of MZ1, the next-generation degrader macroPROTAC-1 replaced the PEG linker with a double linker that formed a macrocyclic structure and restricted the PROTAC's ability to stabilize multiple different binding modes [51]. This precluded cooperative ternary complex formation for the first bromodomain of Brd4 and Brd2, presumably requiring that degradation involves the second bromodomain of each protein; this new design enhanced the selectivity for Brd4 over Brd2 by about 10-fold compared to the selectivity of MZ1 [51]. Orthogonal efforts to improve the selectivity of MZ1 instead replaced its VHL-recruiting moiety with an alkyl-linked CRBN-recruiting group to yield ZXH-3-26; this compound effectively degraded Brd4 even below 10 nm, without any detectable effect on Brd2 or Brd3 at concentrations up to 10 μm [48]. A contemporaneous study focused on potency rather than selectivity and reported a similar design. This study uses a rigidified linker and a slightly different warhead than ZXH-3-26, leading to a PROTAC termed QCA570 that induces essentially complete degradation of Brd2/Brd3/Brd4 at 100 pm [85]. Thus, there can be many potential solutions for designing a potent

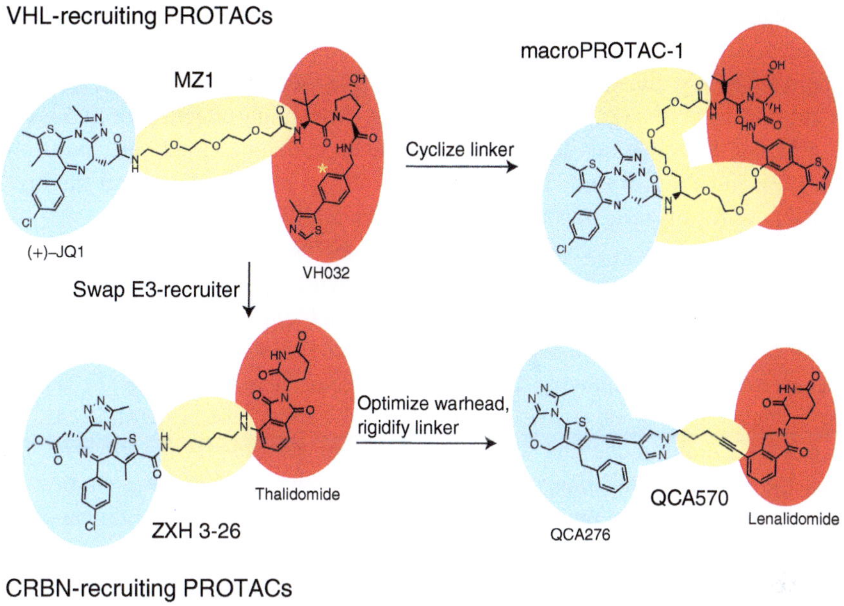

Figure 5.5 Many potent and selective degraders can be built from a given warhead. The bromodomain inhibitor (+)-JQ1 has emerged as a versatile warhead for PROTAC design. Its utility was first recognized with the development of MZ1 (*top left*), which used a PEG-linked VHL-recruiting moiety to induce degradation of BRD4. A crystal structure of the ternary complex inspired cyclization of the linker to a second attachment point (marked with *), yielding macroPROTAC-1 (*top right*). An orthogonal optimization path replaced VHL-recruiting group VH032 with classic CRBN recruiter thalidomide to obtain ZXH-3-26 (*bottom left*); another group used the closely related CRBN recruiter lenalidomide with a rigidified linker to build QCA570 (*bottom right*).

and selective PROTAC by elaborating a selected warhead, an appropriate linker, and an E3-recruiting moiety.

The human proteome is thought to include upward of 600 E3 ubiquitin ligases within the RING family alone [86]. Although the limited number of publicly disclosed warheads to use as recruiting moieties drastically reduces the set that can be immediately used for PROTACs design, already numerous pairings are possible for a given target protein – and the available pairings are certain to grow in future as more E3-recruiting warheads become available [87]. That said, emerging reports from the literature suggest that certain E3 ligases (specifically CRBN, VHL, MDM2, and IAP) may be more permissive for ubiquitinating non-native substrates, and certain other E3 ligases being much more restrictive [88, 89]. Because PROTACs inherently rely on E3 ligase promiscuity for ubiquitinating a non-native substrate, these differences – which may arise from protein flexibility of the ubiquitin ligase machinery – may guide which E3 ligases prove most useful in development of new PROTACs in future. As noted earlier, however, these broad preferences remain inextricably juxtaposed with the importance of adventitious protein–protein interactions between the E3 ligase and the specific neosubstrate of interest.

Recognizing that certain E3 ligases are better suited to degrade a given target than others, and that the linker length and composition play a critical role, an early study sought to rapidly diversify the warhead, the E3 ligase, and the linker in search of useful starting points [22]. This strategy proved exceedingly effective for BCR–ABL, as different combinations led to PROTACs with different target selectivity profiles [22], and another study also explored PROTACs built from some of the many available warheads targeting this fusion oncoprotein [90].

Similarly, it is now possible to rapidly access and test PROTACs built using many different E3 ligase ligands, and straightforward synthetic routes enable the use of multiple different attachment points for many of them [91]. Indeed, an atypical attachment point was used in a recently reported SMARCA2/SMARCA4/PBRM1 degrader ACBI1 by employing a phenolic exit vector near the middle of the VHL-recruiting moiety: a crystal structure of the ACBI1 ternary complex with SMARCA2 revealed a binding mode that would not have been possible from a PROTAC that used the conventional linkage for this warhead [49]. In subsequent studies, the authors then found that moving the exit vector to a slightly different non-canonical site led to adoption of a distinct binding mode in the ternary complex: through this "exit vector hopping" strategy, the authors ultimately enabled the development of an SMARCA2-selective degrader with an oral *in vivo* efficacy [92].

Nonetheless, the challenge of finding a potent degrader inevitably does eventually become distilled to the problem of identifying an appropriate linker to join the two "functional" components. Indeed, varying the linker chemistry and points of attachment has led to potent PROTACs even from starting points that did not look promising at their early stages [89]. Besides potency, the linker is also an important determinant of selectivity: as mentioned earlier, the same promiscuous kinase inhibitor could yield different PROTACs of diverse selectivity simply by varying the linker [66].

At its core, the challenge of finding a linker that results in potent target degradation (termed "linkerology") requires efficient sampling from a huge swath of chemical space. Click chemistry [93, 94] and custom one-pot synthetic routes [95] can facilitate combinatorial synthesis of large compound collections, but ultimately, the sheer magnitude of design combinations facing any new campaign remains daunting – and if anything, it continues to grow with the availability of more E3 ligase ligands, potential attachment points, and warheads to use [90, 91]. Tasks that require separately evaluating huge numbers of potential solutions are exceedingly well suited for computational approaches, as will be described below.

5.5 Emerging Methods for Computationally Designing and Optimizing PROTACs

To date, examples of a rational design of new PROTACs have been extremely limited because of the recency of modeling efforts. As summarized elsewhere [96], the notable successes so far have instead come from the inspection of crystal structures using early PROTAC candidates, inspiring derivatives that improved on serendipitous contacts made by the linker [49], rationally adjusted the linker length [48], or cyclized the linker [51].

The obvious low-hanging fruit with regard to incorporating computational design into linker design is to use the approaches described above for modeling ternary complex structures (Figure 5.4). By analogy to insights from crystal structures, one group recently built a model of their PROTAC targeting H-PGDS and found that the linker was predicted to be much longer than was needed: this led them to design shorter and shorter linkers, until ultimately arriving at a "linkerless" construct more potent than their earlier designs [97].

Taking a larger view, however, protein-centric methods begin with protein–protein docking, and thus, there is no real need to begin with an existing PROTAC. Rather, one could instead simply dock the two proteins (along with their cognate warheads) and then computationally search for appropriate linkers. Each of the studies aiming to model ternary complexes clearly lay out this path [68, 70, 71, 76, 77], with the expectation that one could (for example) sequentially test PEG or alkyl linkers of different lengths/attachment points, and determine which one(s) best bridge the warheads in the preferred binding mode(s). There has not yet been a published report of a PROTAC designed purely from this type of modeling, presumably because of the nascency of these methods.

Looking into the future, however, an important potential contribution from computational methods will be in facilitating the move away from PEG or alkyl linkers. Incorporating alkynes and/or cyclic structures into linkers has already been demonstrated as a means to confer rigidity (for example in QCA570, Figure 5.5), leading to improved activity [85, 98]. The selection of a linker also impacts the resulting PROTAC's physicochemical properties, which in turn strongly affect the activity by modulating cellular uptake, oral bioavailability, and pharmacokinetics [79, 99–102].

Rather than simply screening an existing collection of candidate linkers, an alternative approach is to design new linkers from scratch that will optimally fit the geometric requirements of the ternary complex. Methods to tackle this problem were originally inspired from fragment-based drug discovery (FBDD). Specifically, the need for "fragment linking" arises when two fragments occupy adjacent but non-overlapping binding modes and involves designing a chemical linker so that the resulting compound can make both fragments' interactions at once [103, 104]. Computational approaches have also been developed for fragment linking [105–112], although in practice designing productive linkers has proven challenging for the field so far: this may be due simply to the technical challenges in precise molecular design or because of more theoretical considerations [113]. Most recently, generative deep learning models have been developed to create entirely new structural motifs for ligand merging.

In broad terms, deep learning (DL) models are trained on prepared information to discover patterns in data; the resulting model can then be used to facilitate the extraction of patterns in unseen information. Various architectures are used to construct DL models, which differ mainly in the organization of neural layers and in the representation of input data. With respect to models that take chemical structures as their input or output, these are typically encoded in either graph notation

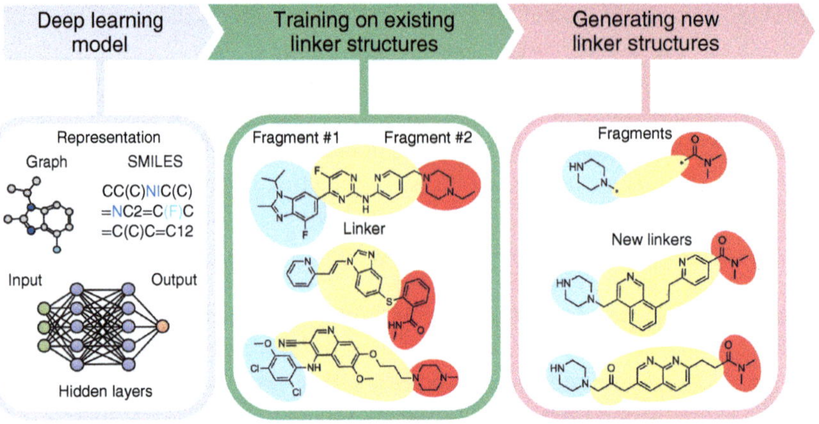

Figure 5.6 Schematic representation of workflow for building new linker structures by generative deep learning (DL). *Step 1 (purple):* First, a suitable structural representation and architecture of DL neural network architecture must be implemented. This typically entails using either graph-based or text-based encodings of chemical structures and a neural network that uses multiple hidden layers to connect the inputs to the outputs. *Step 2 (green):* Next, the model is trained on a pre-existing set of compounds with annotated linkers. *Step 3 (pink):* If successfully trained, the model will generalize from the training data, allowing it to produce new linkers (not seen in the training set) that connect the fragments.

(where atoms are nodes and bonds are edges) or as a string of characters (such as the SMILES format [114]) (Figure 5.6, *purple*). When training on a set of annotated merged fragments, such as PROTACs, the DL model is provided with a set of examples of how fragments can credibly be linked (Figure 5.6, *green*). Provided the model is appropriately trained, it will learn to generalize the connectivity principles in the training data, rather than the details specific to each example. If successful, the model can then be used in a "generative" context to produce novel linkers (i.e. not present in the training set), as a means for joining previously unseen fragments. Such a model will thus generate chemically valid structures where warheads and E3 recruiting moieties are merged into a PROTAC using novel chemical linkers (Figure 5.6, *pink*).

With respect to implementation, there are two complementary strategies for building linkers. The first strategy, as exemplified by DeLinker [109, 111] (Figure 5.7a), focuses directly on bridging the available 3D space between the two disassembled warheads, as captured by the distance and angles needed to span the gap. This graph-based generative neural network begins by adding a set of new nodes (corresponding to a free-floating atom in the linker region) and then adding edges to connect these nodes to one another and to the fixed warheads. The latter process is repeated until the fragments have been fully connected by the edges, representing a new candidate linker. Relative to textual molecular representations, an important advantage of the graph-based representation used here is that it allows for a more intuitive representation of the 3D structure [115–117]. Further, this

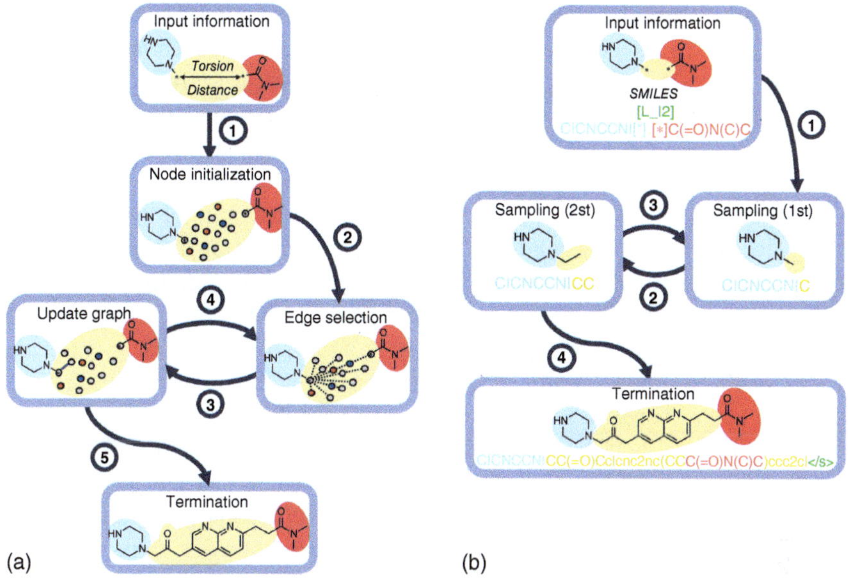

Figure 5.7 DeLinker and SyntaLinker workflows for generating novel linkers. (a) DeLinker uses a generative graph-based deep learning model. (1) As an input, the model takes a graph encoding of mergeable fragments, distance, and torsion angle between "grow" points of each fragment. The model then (2) initializes atom candidates (nodes) for linker construction, (3) selects a candidate for addition to an existing graph, (4) updates graph state and repeats several times until it is no longer possible to add a node to the graph, and then (5) terminates linker generation. (b) SyntaLinker uses a generative symbolic (text-based) deep learning model. (1) As an input, the model takes a collection of mergeable fragments in SMILES format and the desired length of the linker to build. The model then (2, 3) iteratively adds new symbols to the linker until (4) the stop-symbol (in this case <\s>) is generated to terminate the linker.

representation facilitates storage of richer information (i.e. the spatial coordinates of atoms), thus allowing focused generation of compounds tailored to capture the desired geometry needed for the PROTAC ternary complex. In a retrospective benchmark, the warheads from the ACBI1 PROTAC (drawn from the crystal structure of the ternary complex) [49] were supplied to DeLinker: this method then generated new structurally distinct linkers that happened to share remarkable 3D similarly with ACBI1 [109].

A second implementation strategy for designing linkers instead uses processive fragment building to merge the warheads, as exemplified by SyntaLinker [112] (Figure 5.7b). This method uses natural language processing (NLP) models to build strings in the SMILES format [114] that encode specific chemical structures. Although SyntaLinker uses a transformer model [118] at its core, other state-of-the-art NLP models (such as recursive neural networks (RNNs) [119] and variational autoencoders (VAEs) [120]) are also being actively used for generative modeling in drug development and could be applied for this task. Given the text-based representation that underlies the SMILES format, building a new linker is relatively straightforward: the approach starts with one warhead, then generates a string corresponding to the linker, and then adds the other warhead. While SyntaLinker has not explicitly been evaluated in the context of PROTAC linkers, a FBDD benchmark involving fragment linking confirmed that SyntaLinker could retrospectively generate the known (mature) compound, as well as others that scored even better [112].

Relative to DeLinker, an important limitation of SyntaLinker is that the geometry of the fragment endpoints is not explicitly considered at the generative stage. Thus, huge collections of linkers can be produced with a distribution of hydrogen bond donors/acceptors, rotatable bonds and rings, etc., that reflect the linkers in the training set, but the method includes no explicit design consideration that steers these linkers toward the specific geometry needed in a PROTAC ternary complex. For DeLinker and especially for SyntaLinker, then, an important final step is to build models of the proposed compounds in the ternary complex using the methods described earlier (Figure 5.4) to filter for those most likely to yield productive degraders. To date, both methods have been trained using generic linkers rather than those which have proven useful in PROTAC design specifically: with growing collections of PROTAC structures [46, 101], it may soon become possible to evaluate results from generative models trained exclusively on linkers from previously described PROTACs.

5.6 Looking into the Future

In many ways, development of computational tools to contribute to understanding and designing PROTACs follows naturally from developments in the field as a whole. Five years ago, experimental studies were focused primarily on finding combinations of warheads and linkers that would yield potent degraders, with little understanding of why certain constructs proved better than others. Now, drawing upon the important insights from biophysical and structural studies, structure-based modeling of ternary complexes is positioned to provide guidance into design and optimization of PROTACs.

At the same time, numerous contributions to PROTAC efficacy are still not well understood from a fundamental level and thus not yet ready for incorporation into computational pipelines. For example, studies using engineered E3 ligases for inducible proximity (via HaloTag) showed ubiquitination of multiple lysines on the model substrate (EGFP); these led primarily to polyubiquitination chains linked through K48 and K11 but also through K27 and K6 in certain cases [121]. Another analysis of one PROTAC series' structure–activity relationships showed that cellular permeability could frequently serve as a limiting determinant of activity but also that the most potent degrader in the set was neither the most effective at inducing ternary complex formation nor the most cell penetrant [79]. Although the existing computational methods focus primarily on predicting ternary complex formation, this is certainly insufficient to fully explain the extent to which certain PROTACs are more effective than others: this will undoubtedly require careful modeling of the structure and dynamics of the complete ubiquitination complex [67, 80]. Dynamics within the ternary complex are also not yet understood fully; this includes the inconvenient prospect that some PROTAC ternary complexes may occupy multiple binding modes, implying that the snapshots provided by crystal structures may be misleading in these cases. The kinetics of ternary complex formation and of ubiquitin transfer surely also play a key role in certain instances, alongside effects of cooperativity on each of these processes [122]. Finally, even as computational structure-based approaches can contribute to designing degraders with potent and selective cellular activity, the challenge of designing PROTACs that are additionally orally bioavailable and active *in vivo* will still loom ahead.

In summary, validated computational tools are already in place for structure-based modeling of ternary complexes and have begun to emerge for linker design as well. As further experiments continue to guide important design considerations for PROTACs moving forward, additional computational tools will no doubt emerge to include these insights and will accelerate the pipeline of new PROTACs to the clinic.

Acknowledgments

This contribution was written with support from the NIH/NCI Cancer Center Support Grant P30CA006927.

References

1 Callis, J. (2014). The ubiquitination machinery of the ubiquitin system. *Arabidopsis Book* 12: e0174.

2 Gao, H., Zheng, C., Du, J. et al. (2020). FAK-targeting PROTAC as a chemical tool for the investigation of non-enzymatic FAK function in mice. *Protein Cell.* 11: 534–539.

3 Cromm, P.M., Samarasinghe, K.T.G., Hines, J., and Crews, C.M. (2018). Addressing kinase-independent functions of Fak via PROTAC-mediated degradation. *J. Am. Chem. Soc.* 140: 17019–17026.

4 Burslem, G.M., Smith, B.E., Lai, A.C. et al. (2018). The advantages of targeted protein degradation over inhibition: an RTK case study. *Cell Chem. Biol.* 25: 67–77.e3.

5 Winter, G.E., Buckley, D.L., Paulk, J. et al. (2015). DRUG DEVELOPMENT. Phthalimide conjugation as a strategy for *in vivo* target protein degradation. *Science* 348: 1376–1381.

6 Bassi, Z.I., Fillmore, M.C., Miah, A.H. et al. (2018). Modulating PCAF/GCN5 immune cell function through a PROTAC approach. *ACS Chem. Biol.* 13: 2862–2867.

7 Edmondson, S.D., Yang, B., and Fallan, C. (2019). Proteolysis targeting chimeras (PROTACs) in 'beyond rule-of-five' chemical space: recent progress and future challenges. *Bioorg. Med. Chem. Lett.* 29: 1555–1564.

8 Wei, M., Zhao, R., Cao, Y. et al. (2021). First orally bioavailable prodrug of proteolysis targeting chimera (PROTAC) degrades cyclin-dependent kinases 2/4/6 *in vivo*. *Eur. J. Med. Chem.* 209: 112903.

9 Guo, W.H., Qi, X., Yu, X. et al. (2020). Enhancing intracellular accumulation and target engagement of PROTACs with reversible covalent chemistry. *Nat. Commun.* 11: 4268.

10 Bondeson, D.P., Mares, A., Smith, I.E. et al. (2015). Catalytic *in vivo* protein knockdown by small-molecule PROTACs. *Nat. Chem. Biol.* 11: 611–617.

11 Sakamoto, K.M., Kim, K.B., Kumagai, A. et al. (2001). Protacs: chimeric molecules that target proteins to the Skp1-Cullin-F box complex for ubiquitination and degradation. *Proc. Natl. Acad. Sci. U.S.A.* 98: 8554–8559.

12 Nishimura, K., Fukagawa, T., Takisawa, H. et al. (2009). An auxin-based degron system for the rapid depletion of proteins in nonplant cells. *Nat. Methods* 6: 917–922.

13 Itoh, Y., Ishikawa, M., Naito, M., and Hashimoto, Y. (2010). Protein knockdown using methyl bestatin-ligand hybrid molecules: design and synthesis of inducers of ubiquitination-mediated degradation of cellular retinoic acid-binding proteins. *J. Am. Chem. Soc.* 132: 5820–5826.

14 Itoh, Y., Ishikawa, M., Kitaguchi, R. et al. (2011). Development of target protein-selective degradation inducer for protein knockdown. *Bioorg. Med. Chem.* 19: 3229–3241.

15 Rodriguez-Gonzalez, A., Cyrus, K., Salcius, M. et al. (2008). Targeting steroid hormone receptors for ubiquitination and degradation in breast and prostate cancer. *Oncogene* 27: 7201–7211.

16 Wang, L., Guillen, V.S., Sharma, N. et al. (2018). New class of selective estrogen receptor degraders (SERDs): expanding the toolbox of PROTAC degrons. *ACS Med. Chem. Lett.* 9: 803–808.

17 Sakamoto, K.M., Kim, K.B., Verma, R. et al. (2003). Development of Protacs to target cancer-promoting proteins for ubiquitination and degradation. *Mol. Cell. Proteomics* 2: 1350–1358.

18 Lu, J., Qian, Y., Altieri, M. et al. (2015). Hijacking the E3 ubiquitin ligase cereblon to efficiently target BRD4. *Chem. Biol.* 22: 755–763.

19 Sun, B., Fiskus, W., Qian, Y. et al. (2018). BET protein proteolysis targeting chimera (PROTAC) exerts potent lethal activity against mantle cell lymphoma cells. *Leukemia* 32: 343–352.

20 Zengerle, M., Chan, K.H., and Ciulli, A. (2015). Selective small molecule induced degradation of the BET bromodomain protein BRD4. *ACS Chem. Biol.* 10: 1770–1777.

21 Nunes, J., McGonagle, G.A., Eden, J. et al. (2019). Targeting IRAK4 for degradation with PROTACs. *ACS Med. Chem. Lett.* 10: 1081–1085.

22 Lai, A.C., Toure, M., Hellerschmied, D. et al. (2016). Modular PROTAC design for the degradation of oncogenic BCR-ABL. *Angew. Chem. Int. Ed.* 55: 807–810.

23 Bondeson, D.P., Smith, B.E., Burslem, G.M. et al. (2018). Lessons in PROTAC design from selective degradation with a promiscuous warhead. *Cell Chem. Biol.* 25: 78–87.e5.

24 Huang, H.T., Dobrovolsky, D., Paulk, J. et al. (2018). A chemoproteomic approach to query the degradable kinome using a multi-kinase degrader. *Cell Chem. Biol.* 25: 88–99.e6.

25 Sun, Y., Zhao, X., Ding, N. et al. (2018). PROTAC-induced BTK degradation as a novel therapy for mutated BTK C481S induced ibrutinib-resistant B-cell malignancies. *Cell Res.* 28: 779–781.

26 Zorba, A., Nguyen, C., Xu, Y. et al. (2018). Delineating the role of cooperativity in the design of potent PROTACs for BTK. *Proc. Natl. Acad. Sci. U.S.A.* 115: E7285–E7292.

27 Robb, C.M., Contreras, J.I., Kour, S. et al. (2017). Chemically induced degradation of CDK9 by a proteolysis targeting chimera (PROTAC). *Chem. Commun. (Camb.)* 53: 7577–7580.

28 Zhang, C., Han, X.R., Yang, X. et al. (2018). Proteolysis targeting chimeras (PROTACs) of anaplastic lymphoma kinase (ALK). *Eur. J. Med. Chem.* 151: 304–314.

29 Crew, A.P., Raina, K., Dong, H. et al. (2018). Identification and characterization of Von Hippel-Lindau-recruiting proteolysis targeting chimeras (PROTACs) of TANK-binding kinase 1. *J. Med. Chem.* 61: 583–598.

30 Olson, C.M., Jiang, B., Erb, M.A. et al. (2018). Pharmacological perturbation of CDK9 using selective CDK9 inhibition or degradation. *Nat. Chem. Biol.* 14: 163–170.

31 Powell, C.E., Gao, Y., Tan, L. et al. (2018). Chemically induced degradation of anaplastic lymphoma kinase (ALK). *J. Med. Chem.* 61: 4249–4255.

32 Chen, H., Chen, F., Liu, N. et al. (2018). Chemically induced degradation of CK2 by proteolysis targeting chimeras based on a ubiquitin-proteasome pathway. *Bioorg. Chem.* 81: 536–544.

33 Buhimschi, A.D., Armstrong, H.A., Toure, M. et al. (2018). Targeting the C481S ibrutinib-resistance mutation in Bruton's tyrosine kinase using PROTAC-mediated degradation. *Biochemistry* 57: 3564–3575.

34 Hati, S., Zallocchi, M., Hazlitt, R. et al. (2021). AZD5438-PROTAC: A selective CDK2 degrader that protects against cisplatin- and noise-induced hearing loss. *Eur. J. Med. Chem.* 226: 113849.

35 Li, Z., Pinch, B.J., Olson, C.M. et al. (2020). Development and characterization of a wee1 kinase degrader. *Cell Chem. Biol.* 27: 57–65.e9.

36 Cao, S., Ma, L., Liu, Y. et al. (2021). Proteolysis-targeting chimera (PROTAC) modification of dovitinib enhances the antiproliferative effect against FLT3-ITD-positive acute myeloid leukemia cells. *J. Med. Chem.* 64: 16497–16511.

37 Pal, P., Thummuri, D., Lv, D. et al. (2021). Discovery of a novel BCL-XL PROTAC degrader with enhanced BCL-2 inhibition. *J. Med. Chem.* 64: 14230–14246.

38 Girardini, M., Maniaci, C., Hughes, S.J. et al. (2019). Cereblon versus VHL: hijacking E3 ligases against each other using PROTACs. *Bioorg. Med. Chem.* 27: 2466–2479.

39 Powell, C.E., Du, G., Bushman, J.W. et al. (2021). Selective degradation-inducing probes for studying cereblon (CRBN) biology. *RSC Med. Chem.* 12: 1381–1390.

40 Fu, D., Yuan, Y., Qin, F. et al. (2021). Design, synthesis and biological evaluation of tyrosinase-targeting PROTACs. *Eur. J. Med. Chem.* 226: 113850.

41 Xu, C., Meng, F., Park, K.S. et al. (2021). A NSD3-targeted PROTAC suppresses NSD3 and cMyc oncogenic nodes in cancer cells. *Cell Chem. Biol.* 29 (3): 386–397.

42 Chen, P., Wang, S., Cao, C. et al. (2021). alpha-naphthoflavone-derived cytochrome P450 (CYP)1B1 degraders specific for sensitizing CYP1B1-mediated drug resistance to prostate cancer DU145: structure activity relationship. *Bioorg. Chem.* 116: 105295.

43 Zhou, L., Chen, W., Cao, C. et al. (2020). Design and synthesis of alpha-naphthoflavone chimera derivatives able to eliminate cytochrome P450 (CYP)1B1-mediated drug resistance via targeted CYP1B1 degradation. *Eur. J. Med. Chem.* 189: 112028.

44 Hu, M., Zhou, W., Wang, Y. et al. (2020). Discovery of the first potent proteolysis targeting chimera (PROTAC) degrader of indoleamine 2,3-dioxygenase 1. *Acta Pharm. Sin. B* 10: 1943–1953.

45 Khan, S., He, Y., Zhang, X. et al. (2020). PROteolysis TArgeting Chimeras (PROTACs) as emerging anticancer therapeutics. *Oncogene* 39: 4909–4924.

46 Weng, G., Shen, C., Cao, D. et al. (2021). PROTAC-DB: An online database of PROTACs. *Nucleic Acids Res.* 49: D1381–D1387.

47 Gadd, M.S., Testa, A., Lucas, X. et al. (2017). Structural basis of PROTAC cooperative recognition for selective protein degradation. *Nat. Chem. Biol.* 13: 514–521.

48 Nowak, R.P., DeAngelo, S.L., Buckley, D. et al. (2018). Plasticity in binding confers selectivity in ligand-induced protein degradation. *Nat. Chem. Biol.* 14: 706–714.

49 Farnaby, W., Koegl, M., Roy, M.J. et al. (2019). BAF complex vulnerabilities in cancer demonstrated via structure-based PROTAC design. *Nat. Chem. Biol.* 15: 672–680.

50 Roy, M.J., Winkler, S., Hughes, S.J. et al. (2019). SPR-measured dissociation kinetics of PROTAC ternary complexes influence target degradation rate. *ACS Chem. Biol.* 14: 361–368.

51 Testa, A., Hughes, S.J., Lucas, X. et al. (2020). Structure-based design of a macrocyclic PROTAC. *Angew. Chem. Int. Ed.* 59: 1727–1734.

52 Posternak, G., Tang, X., Maisonneuve, P. et al. (2020). Functional characterization of a PROTAC directed against BRAF mutant V600E. *Nat. Chem. Biol.* 16: 1170–1178.

53 Chung, C.W., Dai, H., Fernandez, E. et al. (2020). Structural insights into PROTAC-mediated degradation of Bcl-xL. *ACS Chem. Biol.* 15: 2316–2323.

54 Law, R.P., Nunes, J., Chung, C.W. et al. (2021). Discovery and characterisation of highly cooperative FAK-degrading PROTACs. *Angew. Chem. Int. Ed.* 60: 23327–23334.

55 Yu, X., Li, D., Kottur, J. et al. (2021). A selective WDR5 degrader inhibits acute myeloid leukemia in patient-derived mouse models. *Sci. Transl. Med.* 13: eabj1578.

56 Imaide, S., Riching, K.M., Makukhin, N. et al. (2021). Trivalent PROTACs enhance protein degradation via combined avidity and cooperativity. *Nat. Chem. Biol.* 17: 1157–1167.

57 de Castro, G.V. and Ciulli, A. (2021). Estimating the cooperativity of PROTAC-induced ternary complexes using (19)F NMR displacement assay. *RSC Med. Chem.* 12: 1765–1770.

58 Adhikari, B., Bozilovic, J., Diebold, M. et al. (2020). PROTAC-mediated degradation reveals a non-catalytic function of AURORA-A kinase. *Nat. Chem. Biol.* 16: 1179–1188.

59 Petzold, G., Fischer, E.S., and Thoma, N.H. (2016). Structural basis of lenalidomide-induced CK1alpha degradation by the CRL4(CRBN) ubiquitin ligase. *Nature* 532: 127–130.

60 Bussiere, D.E., Xie, L., Srinivas, H. et al. (2020). Structural basis of indisulam-mediated RBM39 recruitment to DCAF15 E3 ligase complex. *Nat. Chem. Biol.* 16: 15–23.

61 Faust, T.B., Yoon, H., Nowak, R.P. et al. (2020). Structural complementarity facilitates E7820-mediated degradation of RBM39 by DCAF15. *Nat. Chem. Biol.* 16: 7–14.

62 Du, X., Volkov, O.A., Czerwinski, R.M. et al. (2019). Structural basis and kinetic pathway of RBM39 recruitment to DCAF15 by a sulfonamide molecular glue E7820. *Structure* 27: 1625–33.e3.

63 Maniaci, C., Hughes, S.J., Testa, A. et al. (2017). Homo-PROTACs: bivalent small-molecule dimerizers of the VHL E3 ubiquitin ligase to induce self-degradation. *Nat. Commun.* 8: 830.

64 Burslem, G.M., Song, J., Chen, X. et al. (2018). Enhancing antiproliferative activity and selectivity of a FLT-3 inhibitor by proteolysis targeting chimera conversion. *J. Am. Chem. Soc.* 140: 16428–16432.

65 Bai, L., Zhou, H., Xu, R. et al. (2019). A potent and selective small-molecule degrader of STAT3 achieves complete tumor regression *in vivo*. *Cancer Cell.* 36: 498–511.e17.

66 Donovan, K.A., Ferguson, F.M., Bushman, J.W. et al. (2020). Mapping the degradable kinome provides a resource for expedited degrader development. *Cell* 183: 1714–31.e10.

67 Lv, D., Pal, P., Liu, X. et al. (2021). Development of a BCL-xL and BCL-2 dual degrader with improved anti-leukemic activity. *Nat. Commun.* 12: 6896.

68 Drummond, M.L. and Williams, C.I. (2019). In silico modeling of PROTAC-mediated ternary complexes: validation and application. *J. Chem. Inf. Model.* 59: 1634–1644.

69 Molecular Operating Environment (MOE) CCGU (2022). 1010 Sherbooke St. West, Suite #910, Montreal, QC, Canada, H3A 2R7, https://www.chemcomp.com/Research-Citing_MOE.htm.

70 Drummond, M.L., Henry, A., Li, H., and Williams, C.I. (2020). Improved accuracy for modeling PROTAC-mediated ternary complex formation and targeted protein degradation via new in silico methodologies. *J. Chem. Inf. Model.* 60: 5234–5254.

71 Zaidman, D., Prilusky, J., and London, N. (2020). PRosettaC: Rosetta based modeling of PROTAC mediated ternary complexes. *J. Chem. Inf. Model.* 60: 4894–4903.

72 Duhovny, D., Nussinov, R., and Wolfson, H.J. (2002). Efficient unbound docking of rigid molecules. In: *Algorithms in Bioinformatics*, 185–200. Berlin, Heidelberg: Springer.

73 Schneidman-Duhovny, D., Inbar, Y., Polak, V. et al. (2003). Taking geometry to its edge: fast unbound rigid (and hinge-bent) docking. *Proteins* 52: 107–112.

74 Lyskov, S. and Gray, J.J. (2008). The RosettaDock server for local protein-protein docking. *Nucleic Acids Res.* 36: W233–W238.

75 Leman, J.K., Weitzner, B.D., Lewis, S.M. et al. (2020). Macromolecular modeling and design in Rosetta: recent methods and frameworks. *Nat. Methods* 17: 665–680.

76 Bai, N., Miller, S.A., Andrianov, G.V. et al. (2021). Rationalizing PROTAC-mediated ternary complex formation using Rosetta. *J. Chem. Inf. Model.* 61: 1368–1382.

77 Weng, G., Li, D., Kang, Y., and Hou, T. (2021). Integrative modeling of PROTAC-mediated ternary complexes. *J. Med. Chem.* 64: 16271–16281.

78 Vakser, I.A. (2020). Challenges in protein docking. *Curr. Opin. Struct. Biol.* 64: 160–165.

79 Riching, K.M., Vasta, J.D., Hughes, S.J. et al. (2021). Translating PROTAC chemical series optimization into functional outcomes underlying BRD7 and BRD9 protein degradation. *Curr. Res. Chem. Biol.* 1: 100009.

80 Bai, N., Riching, K.M., Makaju, A. et al. (2022). Modeling the CRL4A ligase complex to predict target protein ubiquitination induced by cereblon-recruiting PROTACs. *J. Biol. Chem.* 298 (4): 101653.

81 Qian, S.B., Waldron, L., Choudhary, N. et al. (2009). Engineering a ubiquitin ligase reveals conformational flexibility required for ubiquitin transfer. *J. Biol. Chem.* 284: 26797–26802.

82 Liu, J. and Nussinov, R. (2011). Flexible cullins in cullin-RING E3 ligases allosterically regulate ubiquitination. *J. Biol. Chem.* 286: 40934–40942.

83 Cardote, T.A.F., Gadd, M.S., and Ciulli, A. (2017). Crystal structure of the Cul2-Rbx1-EloBC-VHL ubiquitin ligase complex. *Structure* 25: 901–11.e3.

84 Filippakopoulos, P., Qi, J., Picaud, S. et al. (2010). Selective inhibition of BET bromodomains. *Nature* 468: 1067–1073.

85 Qin, C., Hu, Y., Zhou, B. et al. (2018). Discovery of QCA570 as an exceptionally potent and efficacious proteolysis targeting chimera (PROTAC) degrader of the bromodomain and extra-terminal (BET) proteins capable of inducing complete and durable tumor regression. *J. Med. Chem.* 61: 6685–6704.

86 Zheng, N. and Shabek, N. (2017). Ubiquitin ligases: structure, function, and regulation. *Annu. Rev. Biochem.* 86: 129–157.

87 Schapira, M., Calabrese, M.F., Bullock, A.N., and Crews, C.M. (2019). Targeted protein degradation: expanding the toolbox. *Nat. Rev. Drug Discovery* 18: 949–963.

88 Wei, J., Meng, F., Park, K.S. et al. (2021). Harnessing the E3 ligase KEAP1 for targeted protein degradation. *J. Am. Chem. Soc.* 143: 15073–15083.

89 Zoppi, V., Hughes, S.J., Maniaci, C. et al. (2019). Iterative design and optimization of initially inactive proteolysis targeting chimeras (PROTACs) identify VZ185 as a potent, fast, and selective von Hippel-Lindau (VHL) based dual degrader probe of BRD9 and BRD7. *J. Med. Chem.* 62: 699–726.

90 Yang, Y., Gao, H., Sun, X. et al. (2020). Global PROTAC toolbox for degrading BCR-ABL overcomes drug-resistant mutants and adverse effects. *J. Med. Chem.* 63: 8567–8583.

91 Bricelj, A., Steinebach, C., Kuchta, R. et al. (2021). E3 ligase ligands in successful PROTACs: an overview of syntheses and linker attachment points. *Front. Chem.* 9: 707317.

92 Kofink, C., Trainor, N., Mair, B. et al. (2022). A selective and orally bioavailable VHL-recruiting PROTAC achieves SMARCA2 degradation *in vivo*. *ChemRxiv* https://doi.org/10.26434/chemrxiv-2022-q63s3.

93 Roberts, B.L., Ma, Z.X., Gao, A. et al. (2020). Two-stage strategy for development of proteolysis targeting chimeras and its application for estrogen receptor degraders. *ACS Chem. Biol.* 15: 1487–1496.

94 Wurz, R.P., Dellamaggiore, K., Dou, H. et al. (2018). A "click chemistry platform" for the rapid synthesis of bispecific molecules for inducing protein degradation. *J. Med. Chem.* 61: 453–461.

95 Bemis, T.A., La Clair, J.J., and Burkart, M.D. (2021). Traceless Staudinger ligation enabled parallel synthesis of proteolysis targeting chimera linker variants. *Chem. Commun. (Camb.)* 57: 1026–1029.

96 Bemis, T.A., La Clair, J.J., and Burkart, M.D. (2021). Unraveling the role of linker design in proteolysis targeting chimeras. *J. Med. Chem.* 64: 8042–8052.

97 Yokoo, H., Shibata, N., Endo, A. et al. (2021). Discovery of a highly potent and selective degrader targeting hematopoietic prostaglandin D synthase via in silico design. *J. Med. Chem.* 64: 15868–15882.

98 Han, X., Wang, C., Qin, C. et al. (2019). Discovery of ARD-69 as a highly potent proteolysis targeting chimera (PROTAC) degrader of androgen receptor (AR) for the treatment of prostate cancer. *J. Med. Chem.* 62: 941–964.

99 Atilaw, Y., Poongavanam, V., Svensson Nilsson, C. et al. (2021). Solution conformations shed light on PROTAC cell permeability. *ACS Med. Chem. Lett.* 12: 107–114.

100 Ermondi, G., Garcia Jimenez, D., Rossi Sebastiano, M., and Caron, G. (2021). Rational control of molecular properties is mandatory to exploit the potential of PROTACs as oral drugs. *ACS Med. Chem. Lett.* 12: 1056–1060.

101 Ermondi, G., Garcia-Jimenez, D., and Caron, G. (2021). PROTACs and building blocks: the 2D chemical space in very early drug discovery. *Molecules* 26 (3): 672.

102 Sabnis, R.W. (2022). Novel compounds for targeted degradation of BRD9 and their use for treating cancer. *ACS Med. Chem. Lett.* 13: 17–18.

103 Lamoree, B. and Hubbard, R.E. (2017). Current perspectives in fragment-based lead discovery (FBLD). *Essays Biochem.* 61: 453–464.

104 Kirsch, P., Hartman, A.M., Hirsch, A.K.H., and Empting, M. (2019). Concepts and core principles of fragment-based drug design. *Molecules* 24 (23): 4309.

105 Bancet, A., Raingeval, C., Lomberget, T. et al. (2020). Fragment linking strategies for structure-based drug design. *J. Med. Chem.* 63: 11420–11435.

106 Chung, S., Parker, J.B., Bianchet, M. et al. (2009). Impact of linker strain and flexibility in the design of a fragment-based inhibitor. *Nat. Chem. Biol.* 5: 407–413.

107 Dey, F. and Caflisch, A. (2008). Fragment-based de novo ligand design by multiobjective evolutionary optimization. *J. Chem. Inf. Model.* 48: 679–690.

108 Hoffer, L., Renaud, J.P., and Horvath, D. (2013). In silico fragment-based drug discovery: setup and validation of a fragment-to-lead computational protocol using S4MPLE. *J. Chem. Inf. Model.* 53: 836–851.

109 Imrie, F., Bradley, A.R., van der Schaar, M., and Deane, C.M. (2020). Deep generative models for 3D linker design. *J. Chem. Inf. Model.* 60: 1983–1995.

110 Yuan, H., Lu, T., Ran, T. et al. (2011). Novel strategy for three-dimensional fragment-based lead discovery. *J. Chem. Inf. Model.* 51: 959–974.

111 Imrie, F., Hadfield, T.E., Bradley, A.R., and Deane, C.M. (2021). Deep generative design with 3D pharmacophoric constraints. *Chem. Sci.* 12: 14577–14589.

112 Yang, Y., Zheng, S., Su, S. et al. (2020). SyntaLinker: automatic fragment linking with deep conditional transformer neural networks. *Chem. Sci.* 11: 8312–8322.

113 Yu, H.S., Modugula, K., Ichihara, O. et al. (2021). General theory of fragment linking in molecular design: why fragment linking rarely succeeds and how to improve outcomes. *J. Chem. Theory Comput.* 17: 450–462.

114 Weininger, D. (1988). SMILES, a chemical language and information system. 1. Introduction to methodology and encoding rules. *J. Chem. Inf. Comput. Sci.* 28: 31–36.

115 Jiang, D., Wu, Z., Hsieh, C.Y. et al. (2021). Could graph neural networks learn better molecular representation for drug discovery? A comparison study of descriptor-based and graph-based models. *J. Cheminf.* 13: 12.

116 Li, Y., Zhang, L., and Liu, Z. (2018). Multi-objective de novo drug design with conditional graph generative model. *J. Cheminf.* 10: 33.

117 Mercado, R., Rastemo, T., Lindelöf, E. et al. (2021). Graph networks for molecular design. *Mach. Learn. Sci. Technol.* 2: 025023.

118 Vaswani A, Shazeer N, Parmar N, Uszkoreit J, Jones L, Gomez A, Kaiser L, Polosukhin I. Attention is all you need. 2017, https://doi.org/10.48550/arXiv.1706.03762.

119 Gupta, A., Muller, A.T., Huisman, B.J.H. et al. (2018). Generative recurrent networks for *De Novo* drug design. *Mol. Inform.* 37 (1–2): 1700111.

120 Gomez-Bombarelli, R., Wei, J.N., Duvenaud, D. et al. (2018). Automatic chemical design using a data-driven continuous representation of molecules. *ACS Cent Sci.* 4: 268–276.

121 Ottis, P., Toure, M., Cromm, P.M. et al. (2017). Assessing different E3 ligases for small molecule induced protein ubiquitination and degradation. *ACS Chem. Biol.* 12: 2570–2578.

122 Rodriguez-Rivera, F.P. and Levi, S.M. (2021). Unifying catalysis framework to dissect proteasomal degradation paradigms. *ACS Cent Sci.* 7: 1117–1125.

6

Molecular Glue Degraders: From Serendipity to Hunting and Design

Luis Nieto-Barrado, Ana Domostegui and Cristina Mayor-Ruiz

IRB Barcelona – Institute for Research in Biomedicine, Baldiri Reixac, 10, 08028, Barcelona, Spain
Luis Nieto-Barrado and Ana Domostegui are equal contributors

6.1 Introduction

The use of small-molecule drugs to modulate disease-relevant proteins continues to be the backbone of pharmacopeia. Classical efforts in drug development have followed an inhibitor-centric paradigm based on the occupancy of accessible pockets to block specific protein functions. Despite decades of outstanding progress, more than 80% of all human proteins remain beyond the reach of traditional inhibitors [1–3]. Novel approaches are required to target transcription factors, scaffolding proteins and other proteins central to diseases that typically lack catalytic activity and have remained recalcitrant to drug development [4]. New biological modalities, such as antibodies, have addressed some of these challenging targets. However, biologicals are hampered by issues such as poor cell permeability, chemical instability, lack of oral availability, and limited affordability for healthcare systems.

Recent innovations around targeted protein degradation (TPD) embody a fascinating new modality in pharmacotherapeutics. In this regard, the chemical ablation of proteins has emerged as an excellent alternative and complementation to occupancy-based strategies. This method builds on the (long considered impossible) concept of drug-induced proximity between proteins. To date, most work and progress on TPD has focused on hijacking the ubiquitin-proteasome system (UPS). However, additional approaches that involve other protein homeostasis machineries have been described, such as lysosome-targeting chimeras (LYTACs) [5], autophagosome-tethering compounds (ATTECs) [6, 7], autophagy-targeting chimeras (AUTACs) [8], and bacterial protease-targeting chimeras (BacPROTACs) [9]. Beyond protein degradation, further proximity-inducing small molecules that endow other neofunctions and outcomes to proteins are emerging [10–13].

The field of UPS-mediated TPD has experienced tremendous progress in recent years. This strategy is based on small molecules typically referred to as *degraders*.

Inducing Targeted Protein Degradation: From Chemical Biology to Drug Discovery and Clinical Applications, First Edition. Edited by Philipp Cromm.

These pharmacological agents induce proximity between an E3 ubiquitin ligase and a target protein of interest (sometimes referred to as "neosubstrate"). The formation of an E3:degrader:target ternary complex results in polyubiquitination and subsequent proteasomal degradation of the target. Degraders modulate protein abundance, hence affecting both enzymatic and non-enzymatic activities. Moreover, most degraders have a catalytic mechanism of action because of their successful dissociation after promoting target polyubiquitination and are thus typically efficacious at very low doses. On the contrary, the classical inhibitor process is a competitive- and occupancy-driven event [14, 15].

Degraders can be classified on the basis of various criteria. We here divide them into multivalent or monovalent depending on the number of targeting moieties in the compound (Figure 6.1). In the multivalent category, heterobifunctional molecules known as proteolysis targeting chimeras (PROTACs) have paved the way. In 2001, pioneering work with peptidic ligands by C. M. Crews and R. J. Deshaies showed that an E3 could be redirected to ubiquitinate a protein of interest, and the term PROTAC was coined [16]. Interest in these bivalent molecules grew when they progressed to fully synthetic compounds that simultaneously bind target and E3 with dedicated warheads connected by a linker [17–22]. Recently, trivalent PROTACs have also been described [23]. Due to their modular architecture, multivalent degraders can be adapted to a spectrum of targets by exchanging the targeting warhead. This versatility renders PROTACs of particular interest for pharmaceutical development. However, this modularity also poses potential challenges for the clinical use of PROTACs as they often have high molecular weights, ranging from 700 to 1200 Da, and poor permeability (PROTACs have been extensively reviewed elsewhere [14, 15, 24]).

Monovalent degraders are single linker-less scaffolds that induce the degradation of target proteins by (a) gluing them to E3 ubiquitin ligases (*molecular glue degraders*) or by (b) promoting a vulnerable protein state (*destabilizers*) (Figure 6.1):

(a) *Molecular glue degraders* strengthen or induce de novo E3–target interactions that are often highly cooperative. This mode of action is exemplified by the clinically approved thalidomide and its analogs (the immunomodulatory imide drugs – IMiDs). Molecular glue degraders offer an exciting path for therapeutic innovations and will be the focus of this chapter.
(b) *Destabilizers* induce indirect E3–target dimerization. With this term, we refer to a diverse group of drugs that drive the target protein to a susceptible state, which is then recognized by an E3, prompting subsequent degradation. Upon target binding, destabilizers induce a variety of phenomena (e.g. revealing a degron, increasing surface hydrophobicity, inducing polymerization, and preventing protective interactions, among others). Examples are the clinically approved fulvestrant, which induces degradation of the estrogen receptor (ERα), or some kinase inhibitors that also induce target destabilization [25–27].

Whereas multivalent degraders follow a rational generalizable design, the discovery of monovalent degraders has been driven mostly by serendipity. In the following sections, we discuss the "molecular glue" concept and we review known

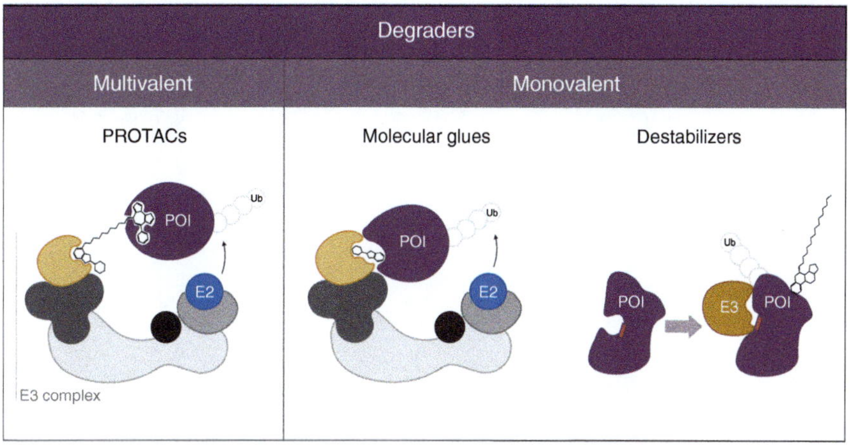

Figure 6.1 Types of degraders. Multivalent degraders (left, only bivalent PROTACs are depicted) bind E3 and target with dedicated warheads that are connected by a linker. Monovalent degraders (right) are small drug-like compounds and comprise: molecular glue degraders and destabilizers. Molecular glue degraders induce or stabilize direct protein–protein interactions between E3 and target. Destabilizers drive the target protein to a susceptible state via different phenomena (the exposure of a degron upon drug binding is shown). This susceptible state is then recognized by the degradation machinery (e.g. E3s). E3 schematics in PROTACs and molecular glue degraders represent an E3 of the cullin RING ligase (CLR) family. POI: protein of interest.

molecular glue degraders, with a special focus on (i) their accidental discovery and (ii) the progression toward more prospective strategies to identify and/or design them.

6.2 "Molecular Glue" Concept

6.2.1 Natural Compounds

6.2.1.1 Molecular Glues

Given that an estimated ~300,000 protein–protein interactions (PPIs) occur in human cells [28] and are involved in every physiological process, PPIs are an interesting, but arguably underexplored, target class. PPIs have recently become a major focus of investigation in drug discovery as the dysregulation of a number of PPIs has been linked to disease. Targeting PPI interfaces is challenging but not infeasible [29, 30]; however, inducing PPIs was long considered almost impossible. This view changed over the years with the discovery of a pool of natural compounds that cause protein associations and provide us with a wealth of inspiration and examples [31–34]. In particular, this capacity is well established for structurally complex natural products [35–40]. The concept of "molecular glue" was used in the early 1990s to describe the mechanism of action of the microbial macrolides FK506 and rapamycin (Figure 6.2a) and the cyclic peptide cyclosporin A. The former two bind to FKPB12, inducing neointeractions with calcineurin and mTOR, respectively

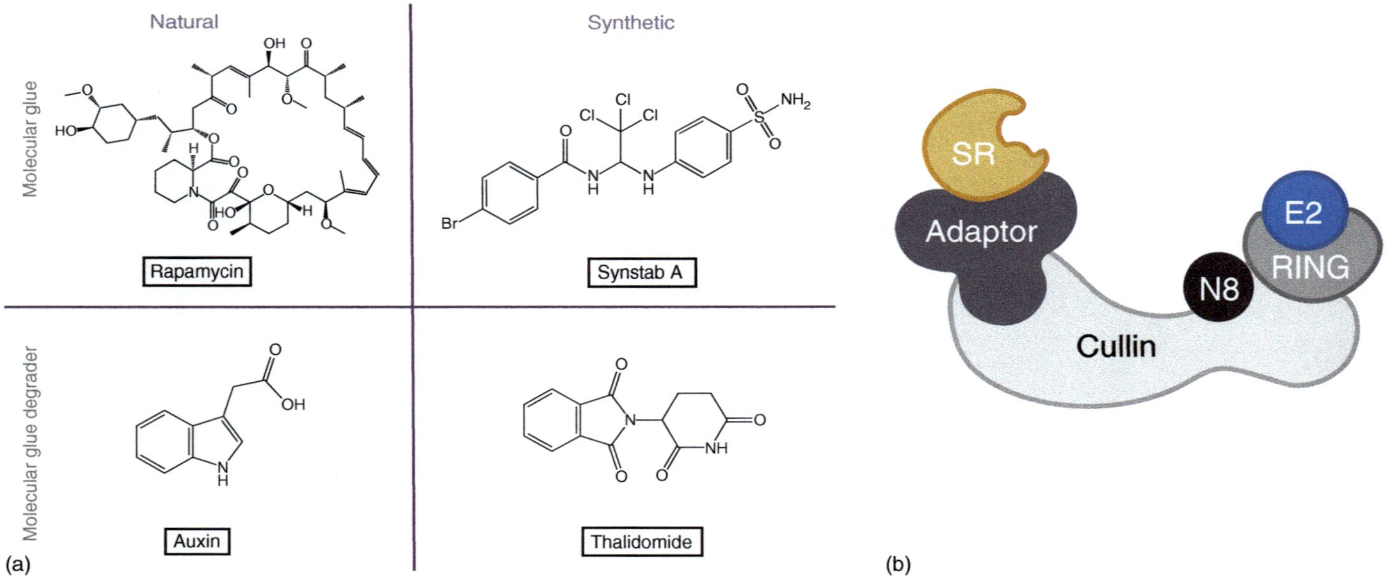

Figure 6.2 The "molecular glue" concept. (a) Selected natural and synthetic molecular glues and molecular glue degraders. (b) Schematic representation of the components of an E3 of the cullin-RING ligase (CRL) family. SR: substrate receptor. (c) Chemical properties of molecular glue degraders vs. bivalent PROTACs. Molecular weight, estimated topological polar surface area (TPSA), number of rotatable bonds, and octanol–water partition coefficient (logP) are shown. Molecular glue degraders: IMiDs ($n = 13$), aryl sulfonamides ($n = 5$) and cyclin K molecular glue degraders ($n = 20$). Bivalent degraders: VHL-based PROTACs ($n = 21$) and CRBN-based PROTACs ($n = 20$). Representative PROTACs were selected for the analysis (the 20 most cited PROTACs against the most common targets as reported in the open-access database PROTAC-DB) [41]. Chemical properties were either obtained from ChEMBL or calculated using ChemDraw v.20.1.0.112.

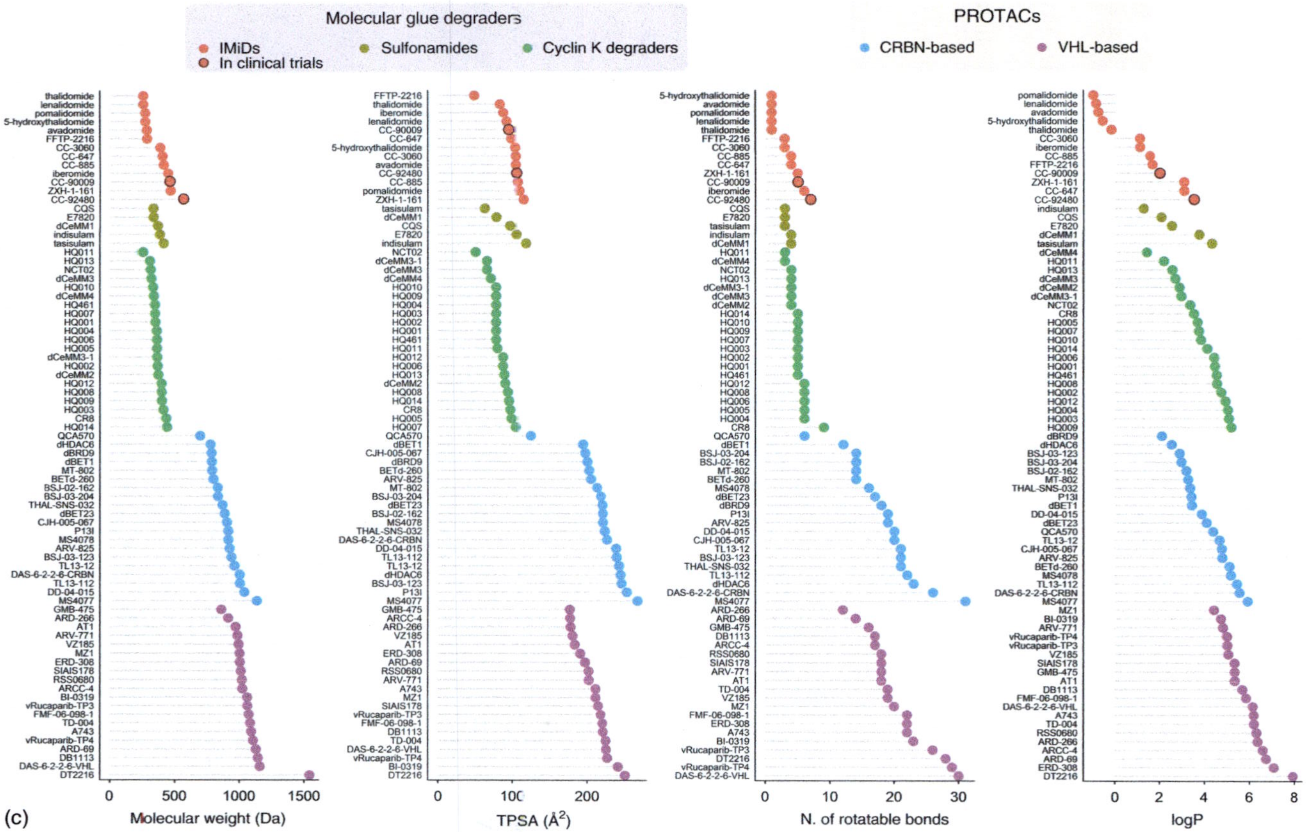

Figure 6.2 *(Continued)*

[37, 38]. Cyclosporin A induces dimerization between calcineurin and cyclophilin [36, 42]. These findings paved the way for the discovery of additional compounds with similar proximity-inducing properties. One example is sanglifehrin A, found to induce PPIs between cyclophilin and IMP [43]. The molecular glue-type mechanism is not a privilege of highly complex chemical structures [44]. The fungal metabolite brefeldin A, arguably simpler, is a macrocyclic lactone that selectively stabilizes the interaction of the complex formed by ARF–GDP and the guanine exchange factor ARNO, thereby preventing guanine release [45, 46]. In this case, brefeldin A is a PPI stabilizer rather than an inducer as it binds only to a site formed in the complex.

In plant biology, we also find examples of structurally simple molecules that induce the dimerization of proteins. Brassinosteroids are plant hormones that function as molecular glues to bring the membrane receptor kinase BRI1 and its co-receptors together [47, 48].

6.2.1.2 Molecular Glue Degraders

The concept of *molecular glue degrader* is used for molecules that, like the phytohormone auxin (Figure 6.2a), induce proximity to an E3 ubiquitin ligase. Auxin binds TIR1 (part of the E3 ligase SCF^{TIR1}) and facilitates its interaction with the transcriptional repressors AUX/IAA, resulting in their proteasomal degradation [49, 50]. Another example of a natural molecular glue degrader is methyl jasmonate, a phytohormone that recruits the E3 ligase SCF^{COI1} via binding to COI1 to trigger the degradation of JAZ repressor proteins [51]. Beyond plant biology, hijacking E3 ligases is used by many viruses to defend themselves against the host's response [52, 53]. Recently, the polyketide natural products asukamycin and manumycin A have been proposed to function as covalent molecular glue degraders [54].

We consider that the most compelling argument in favor of small-molecule modulation of PPIs stems from all the aforementioned natural products, which convey their physiological activity using this mode of action. Some of these molecules have been used for many years as therapeutic agents, such as the immunosuppressants FK506 (e.g. Prograf), rapamycin (Rapamune), and cyclosporin A (e.g. Sandimmun). Others, like auxin, are widely used tools in research.

As discussed in the next section, it was the discovery that simple synthetic compounds can also function as molecular glues (or molecular glue degraders) that drove greater interest in this seemly rare type of small molecules.

6.2.2 Synthetic Compounds

6.2.2.1 Molecular Glues

In 2000, synstab A (Figure 6.2a), a simple synthetic compound functioning as a molecular glue that promoted microtubule formation, was discovered [55] and followed by many other notable examples [56]. Of note, simple synthetic compounds can also function as intramolecular molecular glues, as exemplified by ET070 [57] which corrects the hyperactivation of mutant SHP2 [57]. All these synthetic molecular glues provided a proof of concept that simple, non-natural compounds can also induce PPIs.

6.2.2.2 Molecular Glue Degraders

The same pattern of events was true for molecular glue degraders. Episodic discoveries identified structurally simple synthetic compounds with anticancer activities and which were then shown to act as glue degraders. Prime examples are thalidomide (Figure 6.2a) and its analogs (IMiDs). Seminal studies uncovered that IMiD binding to the E3 $CRL4^{CRBN}$ leads to the recruitment and induced degradation of several targets (e.g. IZKF1/3) [58–61]. Similarly, aryl sulfonamides, such as indisulam or E7820, hijack $CRL4^{DCAF15}$ to degrade the splicing factor RBM39 and the paralog RBM23 [62, 63]. Importantly, all these molecular glue degraders, whether natural or synthetic, share a common feature, namely, their capacity to induce the degradation of target proteins considered *undruggable* according to conventional classifications (e.g. transcription factors). In addition, the E3 ubiquitin ligases hijacked belong to the cullin RING ligase (CRL) family. There are around 250 CRLs, which make up the largest family of E3s and account for almost 20% of all cellular UPS-dependent protein degradation. CRLs are modular assemblies formed by a cullin scaffold (in mammals Cul1, Cul2, Cul3, Cul4A/B, Cul5, Cul7, and Cul9), an adaptor protein, a substrate receptor that engages specific substrate proteins, and a RING protein subunit (RBX1 or RBX2) that recruits ubiquitin-loaded E2s to enable ubiquitin transfer onto the substrate (Figure 6.2b) [64, 65]. The E3 activity is tightly regulated, including activation by Nedd8 attachment, inhibition and substrate receptor exchange by Cand1, and inactivation with Nedd8 removal by the COP9 signalosome, among other regulatory layers. The substrate receptor governs endogenous substrate specificity and is typically the CRL component that is hijacked by molecular glue degraders. Most PROTACs also hijack the substrate receptors of CRLs, although additional E3s belonging to other families have also been utilized successfully (e.g. IAPs [66], MDM2 [67–69], RNF4 [70], and RNF114 [71]).

All the aforementioned discoveries have illustrated the great potential of molecular glue degraders. While these molecules share key features with PROTACs (e.g. modulation of protein abundance), they also have important advantages. For example, molecular glue degraders have favorable drug-like properties (e.g. molecular weight < 500 Da; Figure 6.2c). In addition, they have proven capacity to induce the degradation of seemingly unligandable proteins by strengthening and/or inducing de novo PPIs that are highly cooperative. Conversely, PROTACs are typically not designed to capitalize on cooperative interfaces, although there are examples that also prompt large PPIs [72–74]. In addition, molecular glue degraders have already provided clinical validation for the therapeutic concept of TPD [75–86]. A significant disadvantage of the glue degraders available is that most of them have been discovered unintentionally. In the following sections, we review known synthetic molecular glue degraders divided into two categories: serendipitous discoveries and the first examples of intentional findings.

6.3 Synthetic Molecular Glue Degraders: Serendipitous Discoveries

6.3.1 Molecular Glue Degraders Hijacking $CRL4^{CRBN}$ (IMiDs): Broad Target Accommodation

Thalidomide was used in the late 1950s to treat morning sickness in pregnant women but was withdrawn from the market soon after due to terrible teratogenic effects [78, 87]. Further studies revealed important therapeutic activities that led to the approval of thalidomide for the treatment of erythema nodosum leprosum (in 1998) and multiple myeloma (in 1999) [88]. This spurred the development of chemically similar analogs (IMiDs), first lenalidomide and then pomalidomide. The immunomodulatory and antiangiogenic properties of these analogs warranted clinical approval in 2006 for the treatment of relapsed or refractory myelomas [89]. Of note, IMiDs were approved before the elucidation of their mode of action. In 2010, over fifty years after thalidomide was first used in humans, Hiroshi Handa and colleagues found that this drug directly binds to the protein cereblon (CRBN), the substrate receptor of the E3 ligase $CLR4^{CRBN}$ [58]. By binding to CRBN, thalidomide was first thought to inhibit the activity of $CLR4^{CRBN}$, thus contributing to its teratogenicity. However, it was then shown that CRBN is necessary for the therapeutic effects of lenalidomide and pomalidomide [90, 91]. Soon after, several groups discovered that IMiDs do not inhibit the enzymatic activity of $CRL4^{CRBN}$ but instead confer neofunctions to this E3 ligase. In this regard, IMiDs induce CRBN-dependent proteasomal degradation of the C2H2-type zing-finger (ZF) transcription factors Ikaros (IKZF1) and Aiolos (IKZF3) [59–61]. Shortly after, lenalidomide was shown to also induce the degradation of the kinase CK1α, while the structurally similar thalidomide and pomalidomide do not [92]. This discovery reflected that small differences in the chemical structure could drive substantial differences in the specific set of proteins targeted for degradation. A plethora of additional targets of IMiDs have been identified since then [93].

These discoveries were key catalyzers in the field of TPD. In addition, decades of clinical experience have established thalidomide and its analogs as frontline agents in the treatment of some hematological malignancies, thus providing evidence that the induction of protein degradation via a glue-like mechanism can be an efficacious therapeutic strategy. Currently, thalidomide, lenalidomide, and pomalidomide are used in a variety of clinical settings, including the treatment of multiple myeloma, non-Hodgkin lymphoma, and myelodysplastic syndrome, as well as Kaposi sarcoma [78].

In 2014, the first crystal structures of IMiDs bound to CRBN in complex with the CRL adaptor DDB1 were published [94, 95]. They revealed that (i) the conserved glutarimide ring interacts with a hydrophobic pocket of CRBN made up of three tryptophan residues with a phenylalanine side chain as the base and (ii) the variable part of IMiDs (phthalimide or isoindolinone groups) was solvent exposed. ZF transcription factors are the biggest structural class of IMiD-induced targets. However, the first structures of ternary complexes, confirming that IMiDs are indeed molecular glue degraders, came in 2016 and involved two non-ZF targets: (i) CRBN in

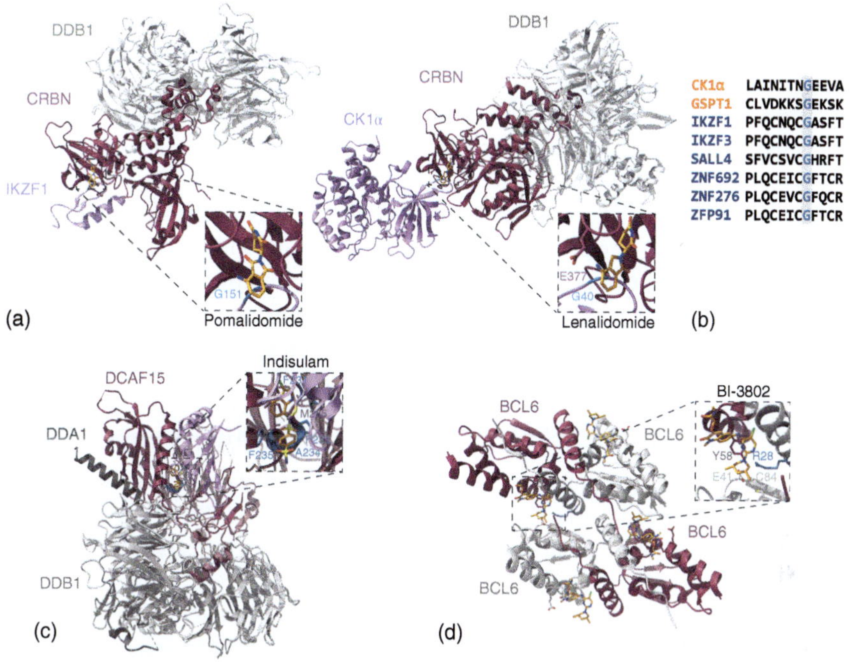

Figure 6.3 Overview of molecular glue degrader-induced protein–protein interfaces. (a) Selected IMIDs: DDB1–CRBN–lenalidomide–CK1α X-ray structure (PDB: 5FQD, right) [96] and DDB1–CRBN–pomalidomide–IKZF1 X-ray structure (PDB: 6H0F, left) [97]. (b) Sequence alignment of ZF targets of IMiDs (blue) and non-ZF targets (yellow). The key glycine of the β-hairpin loop is highlighted in blue (as in panel A). (c) Aryl sulfonamide example: DDB1–DDA1–DDCAF15–indisulam–RBM39 complex (PDB: 6Q0W). *Source:* Adapted from Faust et al. [98]. (d) BCL6–BI3802–BCL6 oligomers (PDB: 6XMX). *Source:* Adapted from Słabicki et al. [99].

complex with CK1α and lenalidomide (Figure 6.3a) [96] and (ii) CRBN in complex with the glue degrader CC-885 and the translation termination factor GSPT1 [100]. Subsequent studies showed IMiD-induced ternary complexes of CRBN and various ZF factors, namely, IKZF1 (Figure 6.3a) [97], ZNF692 [97], and SALL4 [101, 102]. These studies revealed common features in the degron of all these ZF targets. They all share a β-hairpin loop structure in one ZF domain, with a key glycine residue. The new IMiD derivatives CC-3060 and CC-647 target the ZF transcription factor ZBTB16 for degradation by primarily engaging distinct structural degrons on different ZF domains [103]. Similar structural features in proteins without ZF domains can also serve as IMiD degrons, as exemplified by GSPT1. This degron has little sequence homology to the known ZF targets of IMiDs but shares a β-hairpin loop containing a key glycine residue (Figure 6.3b) [96].

New thalidomide derivatives aiming to increase the selectivity and potency and that circumvent resistance to approved IMiDs have been developed, and some of them are approaching the clinic [104]. These next-generation CRBN modulators are based on modifications that alter the target–CRBN binding interface. These agents include the IKZF1/3 molecular glue degraders avadomide (CC-122) [105], iberdomide (CC-220) [106, 107], CC-92480 [108], CC-99282 [109], and CFT7455 [110, 111], among others.

Other chemical substituents have altered the recruitment of targets. Some of these pharmacologic agents are currently in clinical trials: CC-90009 (GSPT1 glue degrader) [112] and DKY709 (Helios degrader; NCT03891953).

Why are pharmaceutical companies investing so heavily in the development of thalidomide analogs? The prospect of having next-generation IMiD derivatives that might overcome therapeutic resistance or that, by altering the targets recruited to CRBN, have activity in new disease indications are highly appealing. With regard to potential revenue, lenalidomide was ranked the third top drug by global sales and the best-selling small-molecule drug worldwide both in 2019 [113] and in 2020 [114].

The downside of the broad target repertoire exhibited by IMiDs is the risk of toxicity, such as the tragic teratogenicity that occurred with thalidomide in the 1960s. Of note, the teratogenicity shown by thalidomide has recently been related to the degradation of SALL4 [101, 106, 115], PLZF [116], and p63 [117]. The potential of IMiDs other than thalidomide itself showing teratogenic effects has not been assessed (or reported).

Of note, IMiDs have also had a remarkable impact on the progression of PROTACs in recent years. The realization that IMiDs bind to CRBN fueled interest in heterobifunctional degraders by showing that IMiD-like molecules could be turned into CRBN-recruiting warheads. In 2015, Winter et al. reported the first *in vivo* compatible PROTAC (dBET1) by conjugation of an IMiD-like phthalimide moiety to the BET-bromodomain inhibitor JQ1 [20]. dBET1 induced fast and potent degradation of BRD2/3/4 both in cell lines and in xenograft models. The same year, Lu et al. reported IMiD-based PROTACs [118]. $CRL4^{CRBN}$, together with $CRL2^{VHL}$, have proven to be versatile E3 ligases that are ideally suited for PROTAC design. CRBN and VHL warheads are currently the most common moieties used in PROTACs. Of note, current VHL-based PROTACs did not evolve from molecular glue binders but initially relied on peptidic VHL ligands based on the natural substrate HIF1α. The subsequent design of small-molecule mimetics of the HIF1α peptide as VHL binders culminated in the first fully synthetic VHL-based PROTACs [21, 22].

While CRBN has shown broad IMiD-induced target accommodation, not all E3-based systems can be expected to exhibit similar flexibility. An example is DCAF15, which is hijacked by aryl sulfonamides and has a much more limited target spectrum, as discussed in the next section.

6.3.2 Molecular Glue Degraders Hijacking $CRL4^{DCAF15}$ (Aryl Sulfonamides): High Shape Complementarity

Anticancer aryl sulfonamides are the second class of synthetic molecular glue degraders described. A representative example is indisulam (E7070), initially identified in a phenotypic screen for small molecules with anticancer activity [119]. Its cytotoxic activity promotes G1-phase arrest and the death of human cancer cell lines [119, 120]. More than a decade later, the mechanism of action of indisulam and the related sulfonamides tasisulam, chloroquinoxaline sulfonamide (CQS), and E7820 was deciphered [62, 63]. They were found to promote the recruitment of the splicing factor RBM39 to the substrate receptor DCAF15 (part of the E3 ligase $CRL4^{DCAF15}$), leading to RBM39 polyubiquitination and proteasomal degradation. In addition to RBM39, subsequent studies identified the paralog RBM23 as an additional destabilized target [121]. Interestingly, the recently discovered aryl sulfonamide dCeMM1 displays exquisite selectivity for RBM39 degradation but not for RBM23 [122]. The pre-mRNA splicing factor PRPF39 [123] and HIF1-β [124] are additional targets of some aryl sulfonamides. The crystal structures of some ternary complexes have revealed that indisulam (Figure 6.3c) and E7820 interact with DCAF15 through the aryl sulfonamide moiety, which functionalizes a shallow, non-conserved cavity on DCAF15 [98, 125, 126]. This cavity establishes hydrophobic interactions with an α-helical degron motif on the RRM2 domain of RMB39, leading to its selective recruitment to DCAF15. RBM39 interacts both with DCAF15 and with the adaptor DDB1. The binding of DDB1 to an additional factor, DDA1, stabilizes the overall assembly (Figure 6.3c). Interestingly, IMiDs and sulfonamides show completely different binary binding affinities to the corresponding E3 substrate receptors. IMiDs display a strong nanomolar affinity for CRBN and their binding reshapes the E3 surface, promoting the recruitment of targets. In contrast, aryl sulfonamides present much lower binding affinities to DCAF15 alone. The low binary affinity is compensated by a large interaction surface between DCAF15 and RBM39, which almost doubles the area of CRBN–target interactions mediated by IMiDs. The large sulfonamide-dependent surface appears to be critical for overcoming an entropically unfavorable scenario: only when all three entities (DCAF15, aryl sulfonamide, and RBM39) come together does ternary complex formation occur. CRBN-bound IMiDs recruit a conserved β-hairpin loop, whereas DCAF15-bound sulfonamides recruit particular side chains from a helical scaffold.

While IMiDs are already a clinical reality, no aryl sulfonamide has merited approval to date. Earlier phase II clinical trials with indisulam and E7820 focused on patients with advanced-stage solid tumors but showed limited efficacy [127–134]. Current efforts to elucidate their mechanism of action may establish the bases for improved patient stratification.

Sulfonamide-based PROTAC design is not as straightforward as IMiD- or VHL ligand-based approaches [135]. The buried nature of aryl sulfonamides and the extensive DCAF15:RBM39 surface interface suggest a hard transition from a glue mechanism to a DCAF15-based PROTAC. Nevertheless, a novel DCAF15-based PROTAC against BRD4, named DP1, has recently been reported [136]. Conceptually, the sulfonamide-like mode of action suggests that non-ligandable E3s are also valuable for drug development campaigns, given that molecular glue degraders do not necessarily depend on high-affinity binding to the E3 in isolation.

6.3.3 BCL6 Degraders: Induction of Polymerization

Screens for novel BCL6 inhibitors by two independent groups led to the discovery of small molecules that, unexpectedly, induce the proteasomal degradation of BCL6, a transcriptional repressor and known oncogenic driver for lymphoma development [137, 138]. A recent study addressed the mechanism of action of one of these compounds: BI-3802 [99]. The authors revealed that BCL6 destabilization was elicited via compound-induced polymerization, with BI-3802 acting as a molecular glue between BCL6 proteins (Figure 6.3d). These filaments led to the enhanced ubiquitination by SIAH1, an E3 ligase of the RING family, and subsequent proteasomal degradation. To be precise, this mechanism of action is at the interface of both monovalent degrader subcategories (molecular glue degrader and destabilizer, Figure 6.1). BI-3802 does not directly glue an E3 to BCL6 and thus could be classified as a destabilizer. However, the glue-like mechanism prompting BCL6 polymerization and subsequent E3-dependent degradation supports the consideration of BI-3802 as a peculiar molecular glue degrader. Interestingly, and in contrast to all the aforementioned glue degraders, the E3 SIAH1 mediates the degradation of both endogenous and compound-dependent aggregated BCL6, the latter strongly facilitating SIAH1 ubiquitination and degradation. The concept of polymerization-dependent degradation induced by monovalent degraders offers interesting new opportunities for TPD. This mechanism of action may be shared with other monovalent degraders reported in the literature whose exact functioning has yet to be elucidated.

6.4 Synthetic Molecular Glue Degraders: Intentional Developments

The discovery of molecular glue degraders has been driven by fortuity, as outlined in the previous section, and strategies for their systematic development or identification are still lacking. Recently, we and others have challenged the "non-rational discovery" notion around this seemingly rare class of degraders. In this section, we discuss the first examples of rational strategies to develop molecular glue degraders, falling into binary combinations of the following categories: target agnostic, ligase agnostic, target driven, and ligase driven (Figure 6.4a).

6.4.1 β-Catenin Molecular Glue Degraders

In 2019, a target-driven and ligase-driven drug discovery effort by Simonetta et al. identified small molecules that enhanced the interaction between $CRL1^{\beta\text{-TrCP}}$ and mutant β-catenin [142]. They provided the first example of the intentional design of molecular glue degraders. Moreover, this was the first example of glue degraders that reinforce a native E3 ligase: substrate pair altered in cancer. β-catenin is often mutated at a phosphodegron recognized by $CRL1^{\beta\text{-TrCP}}$, leading to the stabilization of β-catenin with subsequent oncogenic consequences. A high-throughput biochemical screen based on fluorescence polarization was then coupled to structure-based lead optimization to identify several compounds, such as NRX-1532 or NRX-103094, able to re-enhance the binding and ubiquitination of mutant β-catenin (Figure 6.4b) [142]. This elegant study provides a blueprint for similar future endeavors toward the intentional development of molecular glue degraders.

6.4.2 Cyclin K Molecular Glue Degraders

In 2020, three groups reported the discovery of structurally divergent cyclin K (CycK) molecular glue degraders. Although all the studies converged on the identification of compounds with the same mechanism of action, they used distinct strategies as a starting point. Słabicki et al. and Mayor-Ruiz et al. developed target- and E3-agnostic approaches [122, 143]. Lv et al. executed a target-driven approach looking for NRF2 inhibitors, which then led to the identification of a molecular glue degrader against a different target (CycK) [139].

Słabicki et al. employed bioinformatic correlations of the transcriptional expression of E3 ligase components in cancer cell lines with pre-existing drug sensitivity data [143]. This exercise identified that DCAF15 expression correlated with aryl sulfonamide toxicity. In addition, the cytotoxicity of (*R*)-CR8, a known CDK inhibitor, correlated with the expression of the CRL adaptor DDB1. They showed that (*R*)-CR8 induces selective degradation of CycK in a DDB1-dependent manner. Mayor-Ruiz et al. developed a scalable chemical profiling strategy based on hyponeddylated models (UBE2M mutant cancer cells [144]) with widely impaired CRL function. The strategy was validated with the discovery of a novel RBM39 molecular degrader (dCeMM1) that hijacks $CRL4^{DCAF15}$. In addition, three small-molecule drugs, dCeMM2/3/4, identified as dependent on functional CRLs to exert their toxicity, proved to be CycK molecular glue degraders [122]. Finally, Lv et al. used a luciferase-based high-throughput screen in principle designed to identify NRF2 inhibitors, leading to the identification of yet another CycK molecular glue degrader, namely, HQ461 [139].

Deciphering the mechanisms of action of (*R*)-CR8, dCeMM2/3/4, and HQ461 was enabled by multi-omics campaigns to identify and validate the target and E3 involved. Importantly, all the studies converged on a unifying and unprecedented mechanism of action: drug binding to the active site of the usual CycK partner CDK12 (and, presumably, the paralog CDK13) strengthened the dimerization between CDK12:CycK and the CRL adaptor DDB1 in the absence of a dedicated substrate receptor. CDK12/13 act as non-native substrate receptors that position CycK in the ubiquitination zone accessible to the E2 loaded in the partial CRL4 complex. Extensive profiling, including a 6.5 Å structure solved by Słabicki et al., confirmed the DDB1–CR8–CDK12 complex formation and revealed a substantial protein–protein interface (Figure 6.4c). Of note, another group reported in 2021 the serendipitous discovery of yet another chemically distinct CycK glue degrader: NCT02. They conducted a screen for inhibitory compounds of colorectal cancer spheroids [145].

All these findings provided evidence of a novel mechanism in which a molecular glue degrader induces target degradation by a distant PPI rather than by directly reprogramming the target–E3 interface. In addition, these glue degraders showed that it is indeed possible to rewire a CRL adaptor instead of the substrate receptor as

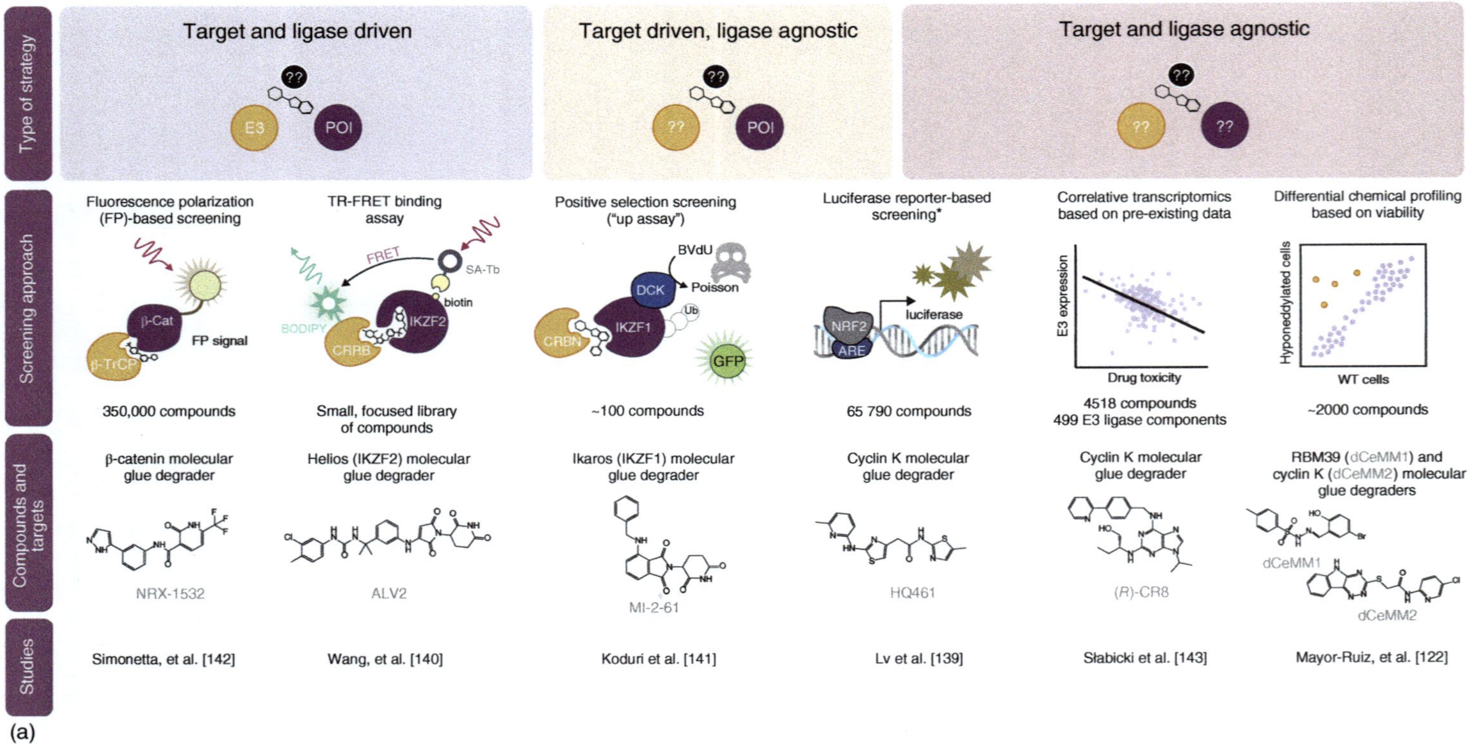

Figure 6.4 Prospective discovery of molecular glue degraders. (a) Strategies to intentionally discover molecular glue degraders. *The identification of the CycK degrader HQ461 is not categorized as a fully target-driven strategy as it was initially designed to identify NRF2 inhibitors. Source: Adapted from Lv et al. [139]. POI: protein of interest. **β**-Cat: **β**-catenin. CycK: Cyclin K. TR-FRET: Time-resolved fluorescence energy transfer. (b) Crystal structure of NRX-103094 bound to SKP1–**β**TrCP in complex with monophosphorylated Ser33 **β**-catenin (residues 16–48) (PDB: 6M91) [142]. (c) DDB1–CR8–CDK12:CycK (PDB: 6TD3). *Source:* Adapted from Słabicki et al. [143].

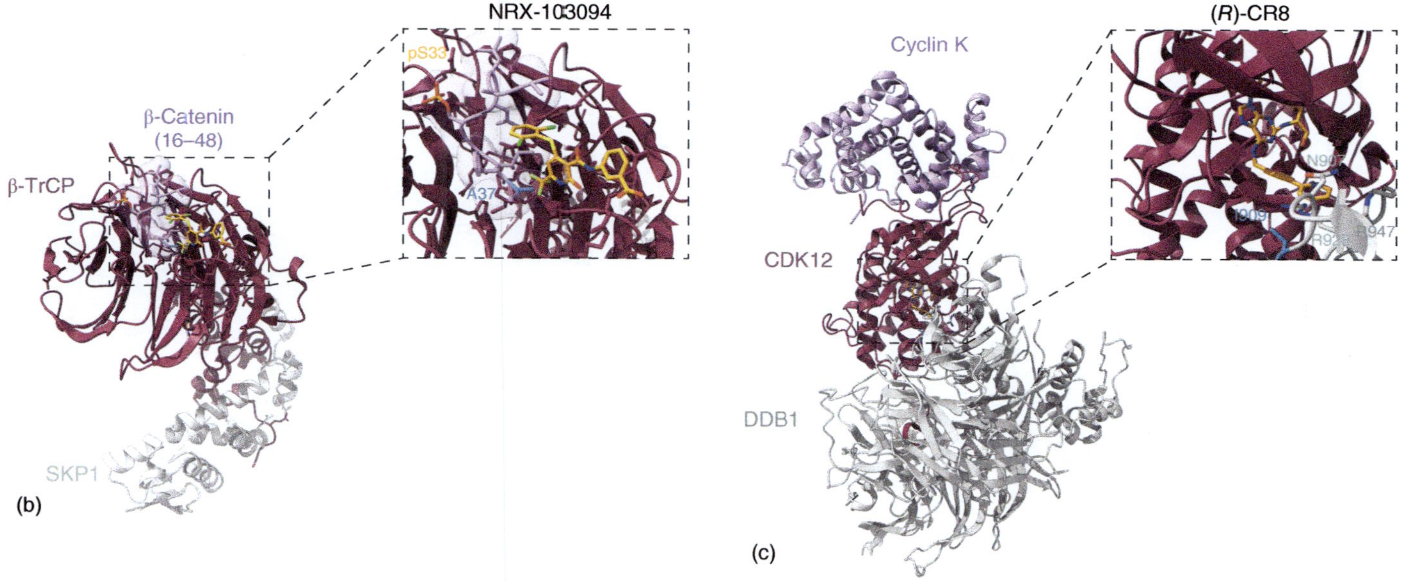

Figure 6.4 (*Continued*)

IMiDs and aryl sulfonamides do. As aryl sulfonamides showed with DCAF15, the CycK glue degraders recruit an E3 component (DDB1) considered unligandable. How the remarkable chemical diversity of CR8, dCeMM2/3/4, and HQ461 converges in the induced degradation of CycK remains unclear.

6.4.3 Prospective Discovery of IKZF1 Molecular Glue Degraders via "Up Assays"

Koduri et al. reported a target-driven E3-agnostic positive selection assay ("up assay") to identify novel monovalent degraders of IKZF1 [141]. This strategy makes use of the enzyme DCK fused to IKZF1. DCK converts a pro-drug (the non-natural nucleoside BVdU) into a toxic compound. Hence, degradation of the fusion protein prevents the DCK-mediated conversion of BVdU into a toxin. For the screening setup, they used a small library of several uncharacterized IMiD-like molecules described in the literature and approximately 100 newly synthesized analogs of pomalidomide. Chemical screens coupled to co-treatment with the BVdU allowed them to identify novel IMiD-like molecular glue degraders of IKZF1 via the concomitant resistance (e.g. MI-2-61). Although IMiD analogs were used for the screening, we have classified this strategy as "prospective" given the foreseen potential. Indeed, using a non-IMiD-like small library of compounds enriched in metabolic inhibitors, the same authors found that the small-molecule Spautin-1 degrades IKZF1 in a CRBN-independent manner. The exact mechanism of action of the direct/indirect compound-mediated IKZF1 degradation remains to be elucidated. Overall, this study provided proof of principle of how phenotypic "up assays" based on target fusion to suicide genes can be used to identify glue degraders.

6.4.4 Structure-Guided Development of Helios (IKZF2) Molecular Glue Degraders

In 2021, Wang et al. reported the structure-guided development of molecular glue degraders that recruit CRBN to the transcription factor Helios (IKZF2) involved in immunosuppression [140]. This study exemplified a target-driven, E3-driven approach to develop glue degraders.

Within the Ikaros family of ZF transcription factors, only Ikaros (IKZF1) and Aiolos (IKZF3) are degraded by canonical IMiDs. The presence of a glutamine residue in their second ZF domain enables IMiD-induced degradation [60], while the histidine residues in Helios (IKZF2) do not. Since the IMiD analog CC-885 can induce weak dimerization between CRBN and a mutant version of IKZF1 in which glutamine 146 is a histidine [100], they hypothesized that a more flexible CRBN-binding core could accommodate a key Helios histidine residue. They screened a small, focused library of analogs through a CRBN:Helios dimerization assay based on time-resolved fluorescence energy transfer (TR-FRET). Several rounds of medicinal chemistry optimization led to ALV1 and ALV2. The former induces CRBN-dependent degradation of both Ikaros and Helios, while the latter has relative selectivity for Helios over Ikaros/Aiolos. Of note, Eos (IKZF4), another member of the Ikaros transcription factor family, also encodes a histidine at the same position as Helios within the critical ZF domain that regulates the degradability of this family of proteins. As expected, ALV1 and ALV2 also induce Eos destabilization [140].

Although intentional, this strategy builds on the abundant structural information available for other members of the Ikaros family in complex with canonical IMiDs. Hence, it remains to be seen how similar strategies could be applied for different targets and E3 ligases. Nevertheless, similar structure-based efforts may yield molecular glue degraders for other previously unligandable targets by reprogramming E3 ligase substrate specificity.

6.4.5 Discovery of VHL-Binding Molecular Glue Degraders

VHL-focused approaches to discover molecular glue degraders, both in a target-agnostic and in a target-driven fashion, have been covered recently at several scientific events. Although not yet published, we provide a succinct description of these approaches.

Novartis (NIBR) has already disclosed a prototypical example of an E3-driven target-agnostic strategy based on *protein arrays* (unpublished). This strategy was used to screen for compound-induced interactions between the substrate receptor VHL and thousands of proteins. The small molecules “compound 4” and “compound 5” recruit VHL to CDO1, a critical regulator of cysteine metabolism, resulting in proteasomal degradation of the latter. Although the scalability of this approach is limited, it provides yet another valid avenue toward intended discoveries of molecular glue degraders.

Stuart Schreiber’s lab and colleagues have developed an unpublished strategy named diversity-oriented synthesis encoded by DNA oligonucleotides (DOSEDO) to synthesize DNA-barcoded compounds. The resulting DNA-encoded libraries (DELs) are incubated with tagged target proteins to advance the discovery of protein binders that can be “decoded” using DNA sequencing. They have also applied this strategy to molecular glue discovery for preselected targets by screening for cooperative binding. Differential screening using these DELs in the absence and presence of “presenter” proteins has brought about the discovery of presenter-dependent binders. As a proof-of-principle study, in collaboration with Novartis (NIBR), they used BRD4 as a preselected target and VHL as a presenter to find the molecular glue degrader FYI979 (unpublished).

The use of both protein arrays and DELs showcase exciting new possibilities to facilitate the intentional discovery of molecular glue degraders.

6.5 Conclusions and Outlook

Progress in the TPD field has brought us to exciting times on multiple fronts: approved drugs shown to act as molecular glue degraders, PROTACs in clinical phases, and a growing repertoire of new strategies to identify and design more of these pharmacological modalities. In this chapter, we aimed to summarize the discovery of molecular glue degraders, both by unintentional and by intentional endeavors. These examples, together with exhaustive mechanistic characterizations, have revealed that molecular glue degraders are more frequent than we anticipated, and they offer important lessons about compound-induced proximity for the development of efficient therapeutics. In addition, these molecules keep surprising us with new mechanisms of action. The pairing mechanisms by which molecular glue degraders may induce proximity between ~600 human E3 ligases (and potentially involving several core components in modular E3s) and > 20 000 protein targets seem virtually unlimited. We envisage that phenotypic screens will continue to be pivotal for the discovery of glue degraders, evolving toward more advanced and sophisticated target-driven approaches. It is also exciting to see the emergence of an increasing number of structural hypotheses on features that can determine the likelihood of a substrate being glued via this mechanism. Accordingly, structure-based drug design is also foreseen to pave the way toward more rational developments, together with in silico modeling tools and virtual screening assisted by artificial intelligence. Furthermore, critical technological progress in high-throughput proteomics will further help to accelerate drug discovery in this area. Finally, the advances made in TPD have fueled interest in other proximity-inducing pharmacological strategies, whose development will be fascinating to follow in the coming years.

Acknowledgments and Funding

We would like to thank the members of the Mayor-Ruiz group for helpful discussions. We apologize to the authors who could not be mentioned because of space restriction. The Mayor-Ruiz laboratory has received funding from the European Research Council (ERC) as a Starting Grant to C.M-R. (ERC-2021-StG-101040046 TrickE3), la Caixa Foundation, FERO-ASEICA, AECC, and the Spanish Ministry of Science and Innovation, among others. L.N-B. is supported by an FPI PhD fellowship (PRE2020-092066) and A.D. by a Juan de la Cierva postdoctoral fellowship (FJC2020-043715-I), both from the Spanish Ministry of Science and Innovation. The Mayor-Ruiz laboratory receives sponsored research support from Almirall and Aelin Therapeutics.

Conflict of Interest Statement

C.M-R. is part of the Scientific Advisory Board of Nostrum Biodiscovery. The remaining authors report no competing interests.

References

1 Finan, C. et al. (2017). The druggable genome and support for target identification and validation in drug development. *Sci. Transl. Med.* 9, https://doi.org/10.1126/scitranslmed.aag1166: eaag1166.

2 Kana, O. and Brylinski, M. (2019). Elucidating the druggability of the human proteome with eFindSite. *J. Comput. Aided Mol. Des.* 33: 509–519, https://doi.org/10.1007/s10822-019-00197-w.

3 Hopkins, A.L. and Groom, C.R. (2002). The druggable genome. *Nat. Rev. Drug Discov.* 1: 727–730, https://doi.org/10.1038/nrd892.

4 Dang, C.V., Reddy, E.P., Shokat, K.M., and Soucek, L. (2017). Drugging the 'undruggable' cancer targets. *Nat. Rev. Cancer* 17: 502–508, https://doi.org/10.1038/nrc.2017.36.

5 Banik, S.M. et al. (2020). Lysosome-targeting chimaeras for degradation of extracellular proteins. *Nature* 584: 291–297, https://doi.org/10.1038/s41586-020-2545-9.

6 Li, Z. et al. (2019). Allele-selective lowering of mutant HTT protein by HTT-LC3 linker compounds. *Nature* 575: 203–209, https://doi.org/10.1038/s41586-019-1722-1.

7 Li, Z., Zhu, C., Ding, Y. et al. (2020). ATTEC: a potential new approach to target proteinopathies. *Autophagy* 16: 185–187, https://doi.org/10.1080/15548627.2019.1688556.

8 Takahashi, D. et al. (2019). AUTACs: cargo-specific degraders using selective autophagy. *Mol. Cell* 76: 797–810 e710, https://doi.org/10.1016/j.molcel.2019.09.009.

9 Morreale, F.E. et al. (2022). BacPROTACs mediate targeted protein degradation in bacteria. *Cell* 185: 2338–2353.

10 Siriwardena, S.U. et al. (2020). Phosphorylation-inducing chimeric small molecules. *CellJ. Am. Chem. Soc.* 142: 14052–14057, https://doi.org/10.1021/jacs.0c05537.

11 Yamazoe, S. et al. (2020). Heterobifunctional molecules induce dephosphorylation of kinases-A proof of concept study. *J. Med. Chem.* 63: 2807–2813, https://doi.org/10.1021/acs.jmedchem.9b01167.

12 Dey, S.K. and Jaffrey, S.R. (2019). RIBOTACs: small molecules target RNA for degradation. *Cell Chem. Biol.* 26: 1047–1049, https://doi.org/10.1016/j.chembiol.2019.07.015.

13 Henning, N.J. et al. (2022). Deubiquitinase-Targeting Chimeras for Targeted Protein Stabilization. *Nat. Chem. Biol.* 18: 412–421, https://doi.org/10.1038/s41589-022-00971-2.

14 Burslem, G.M. and Crews, C.M. (2020). Proteolysis-targeting chimeras as therapeutics and tools for biological discovery. *Cell* 181: 102–114, https://doi.org/10.1016/j.cell.2019.11.031.

15 Mayor-Ruiz, C. and Winter, G.E. (2019). Identification and characterization of cancer vulnerabilities via targeted protein degradation. *Drug Discov. Today Technol.* 31: 81–90, https://doi.org/10.1016/j.ddtec.2018.12.003.

16 Sakamoto, K.M. et al. (2001). Protacs: chimeric molecules that target proteins to the Skp1-Cullin-F box complex for ubiquitination and degradation. *Proc. Natl. Acad. Sci. U. S. A.* 98: 8554–8559, https://doi.org/10.1073/pnas.141230798.

17 Schneekloth, J.S. Jr. et al. (2004). Chemical genetic control of protein levels: selective *in vivo* targeted degradation. *J. Am. Chem. Soc.* 126: 3748–3754, https://doi.org/10.1021/ja039025z.

18 Itoh, Y., Ishikawa, M., Naito, M., and Hashimoto, Y. (2010). Protein knockdown using methyl bestatin-ligand hybrid molecules: design and synthesis of inducers of ubiquitination-mediated degradation of cellular retinoic acid-binding proteins. *J. Am. Chem. Soc.* 132: 5820–5826, https://doi.org/10.1021/ja100691p.

19 Itoh, Y. et al. (2011). Development of target protein-selective degradation inducer for protein knockdown. *Bioorg. Med. Chem.* 19: 3229–3241, https://doi.org/10.1016/j.bmc.2011.03.057.

20 Winter, G.E. et al. (2015). Drug development. Phthalimide conjugation as a strategy for *in vivo* target protein degradation. *Science (New York, N.Y.)* 348: 1376–1381, https://doi.org/10.1126/science.aab1433.

21 Bondeson, D.P. et al. (2015). Catalytic *in vivo* protein knockdown by small-molecule PROTACs. *Nat. Chem. Biol.* 11: 611–617, https://doi.org/10.1038/nchembio.1858.

22 Zengerle, M., Chan, K.H., and Ciulli, A. (2015). Selective small molecule induced degradation of the BET bromodomain protein BRD4. *ACS Chem. Biol.* 10: 1770–1777, https://doi.org/10.1021/acschembio.5b00216.

23 Imaide, S. et al. (2021). Trivalent PROTACs enhance protein degradation via combined avidity and cooperativity. *Nat. Chem. Biol.* 17: 1157–1167, https://doi.org/10.1038/s41589-021-00878-4.

24 Farnaby, W., Koegl, M., McConnell, D.B., and Ciulli, A. (2021). Transforming targeted cancer therapy with PROTACs: a forward-looking perspective. *Curr. Opin. Pharmacol.* 57: 175–183, https://doi.org/10.1016/j.coph.2021.02.009.

25 Cornella-Taracido, I. and Garcia-Echeverria, C. (2020). Monovalent protein-degraders - insights and future perspectives. *Bioorg. Med. Chem. Lett.* 30: 127202, https://doi.org/10.1016/j.bmcl.2020.127202.

26 Hanan, E.J. et al. (2020). Monomeric targeted protein degraders. *J. Med. Chem.* 63: 11330–11361, https://doi.org/10.1021/acs.jmedchem.0c00093.

27 Kastl, J.M., Davies, G., Godsman, E., and Holdgate, G.A. (2021). Small-molecule degraders beyond PROTACs-challenges and opportunities. *SLAS Discov.* 26: 524–533, https://doi.org/10.1177/2472555221991104.

28 Zhang, Q.C. et al. (2012). Structure-based prediction of protein-protein interactions on a genome-wide scale. *Nature* 490: 556–560, https://doi.org/10.1038/nature11503.

29 Scott, D.E., Bayly, A.R., Abell, C., and Skidmore, J. (2016). Small molecules, big targets: drug discovery faces the protein–protein interaction challenge. *Nat. Rev. Drug Discov.* 15: 533–550, https://doi.org/10.1038/nrd.2016.29.

30 Arkin, M.R., Tang, Y., and Wells, J.A. (2014). Small-molecule inhibitors of protein-protein interactions: progressing toward the reality. *Chem. Biol.* 21: 1102–1114, https://doi.org/10.1016/j.chembiol.2014.09.001.

31 Stanton, B.Z., Chory, E.J., and Crabtree, G.R. (2018). Chemically induced proximity in biology and medicine. *Science (New York, N.Y.)* 359: eaao5902, https://doi.org/10.1126/science.aao5902.

32 Fischer, E.S., Park, E., Eck, M.J., and Thoma, N.H. (2016). SPLINTS: small-molecule protein ligand interface stabilizers. *Curr. Opin. Struct. Biol.* 37: 115–122, https://doi.org/10.1016/j.sbi.2016.01.004.

33 Andrei, S.A. et al. (2017). Stabilization of protein-protein interactions in drug discovery. *Expert Opin. Drug Discov.* 12: 925–940, https://doi.org/10.1080/17460441.2017.1346608.

34 Milroy, L.G., Grossmann, T.N., Hennig, S. et al. (2014). Modulators of protein-protein interactions. *Chem. Rev.* 114: 4695–4748, https://doi.org/10.1021/cr400698c.

35 Harding, M.W., Galat, A., Uehling, D.E., and Schreiber, S.L. (1989). A receptor for the immunosuppressant FK506 is a cis-trans peptidyl-prolyl isomerase. *Nature* 341: 758–760, https://doi.org/10.1038/341758a0.

36 Liu, J. et al. (1991). Calcineurin is a common target of cyclophilin-cyclosporin A and FKBP-FK506 complexes. *Cell* 66: 807–815.

37 Brown, E.J. et al. (1994). A mammalian protein targeted by G1-arresting rapamycin-receptor complex. *Nature* 369: 756–758, https://doi.org/10.1038/369756a0.

38 Sabatini, D.M., Erdjument-Bromage, H., Lui, M. et al. (1994). RAFT1: a mammalian protein that binds to FKBP12 in a rapamycin-dependent fashion and is homologous to yeast TORs. *Cell* 78: 35–43, https://doi.org/10.1016/0092-8674(94)90570 3.

39 Niu, T.K., Pfeifer, A.C., Lippincott-Schwartz, J., and Jackson, C.L. (2005). Dynamics of GBF1, a Brefeldin A-sensitive Arf1 exchange factor at the Golgi. *Mol. Biol. Cell* 16: 1213–1222, https://doi.org/10.1091/mbc.e04-07-0599.

40 Takeuchi, J. et al. (2014). Designed abscisic acid analogs as antagonists of PYL-PP2C receptor interactions. *Nat. Chem. Biol.* 10: 477–482, https://doi.org/10.1038/nchembio.1524.

41 Weng, G. et al. (2021). PROTAC-DB: an online database of PROTACs. *Nucleic Acids Res.* 49: D1381–D1387, https://doi.org/10.1093/nar/gkaa807.

42 Sabers, C.J. et al. (1995). Isolation of a protein target of the FKBP12-rapamycin complex in mammalian cells. *J. Biol. Chem.* 270: 815–822, https://doi.org/10.1074/jbc.270.2.815.

43 Fehr, T., Kallen, J., Oberer, L. et al. (1999). Sanglifehrins A, B, C and D, novel cyclophilin-binding compounds isolated from Streptomyces sp. A92-308110. II. Structure elucidation, stereochemistry and physico-chemical properties. *J. Antibiot. (Tokyo)* 52: 474–479, https://doi.org/10.7164/antibiotics.52.474.

44 Schreiber, S.L. (2019). A chemical biology view of bioactive small molecules and a binder-based approach to connect biology to precision medicines. *Isr. J. Chem.* 59: 52–59, https://doi.org/10.1002/ijch.201800113.

45 Chardin, P. and McCormick, F. (1999). Brefeldin A: the advantage of being uncompetitive. *Cell* 97: 153–155, https://doi.org/10.1016/s0092-8674(00)80724-2.
46 Peyroche, A. et al. (1999). Brefeldin A acts to stabilize an abortive ARF-GDP-Sec7 domain protein complex: involvement of specific residues of the Sec7 domain. *Mol. Cell* 3: 275–285, https://doi.org/10.1016/s1097-2765(00)80455-4.
47 Santiago, J., Henzler, C., and Hothorn, M. (2013). Molecular mechanism for plant steroid receptor activation by somatic embryogenesis co-receptor kinases. *Science (New York, N.Y.)* 341: 889–892, https://doi.org/10.1126/science.1242468.
48 Sun, Y. et al. (2013). Structure reveals that BAK1 as a co-receptor recognizes the BRI1-bound brassinolide. *Cell Res.* 23: 1326–1329, https://doi.org/10.1038/cr.2013.131.
49 Gray, W.M., Kepinski, S., Rouse, D. et al. (2001). Auxin regulates SCF(TIR1)-dependent degradation of AUX/IAA proteins. *Nature* 414: 271–276, https://doi.org/10.1038/35104500.
50 Tan, X. et al. (2007). Mechanism of auxin perception by the TIR1 ubiquitin ligase. *Nature* 446: 640–645, https://doi.org/10.1038/nature05731.
51 Sheard, L.B. et al. (2010). Jasmonate perception by inositol-phosphate-potentiated COI1-JAZ co-receptor. *Nature* 468: 400–405, https://doi.org/10.1038/nature09430.
52 Mahon, C., Krogan, N.J., Craik, C.S., and Pick, E. (2014). Cullin E3 ligases and their rewiring by viral factors. *Biomolecules* 4: 897–930, https://doi.org/10.3390/biom4040897.
53 Zhang, Y., Li, L.F., Munir, M., and Qiu, H.J. (2018). RING-domain E3 ligase-mediated host-virus interactions: orchestrating immune responses by the host and antagonizing immune defense by viruses. *Front. Immunol.* 9: 1083, https://doi.org/10.3389/fimmu.2018.01083.
54 Isobe, Y. et al. (2020). Manumycin polyketides act as molecular glues between UBR7 and P53. *Nat. Chem. Biol.* 16: 1189–1198, https://doi.org/10.1038/s41589-020-0557-2.
55 Haggarty, S.J. et al. (2000). Dissecting cellular processes using small molecules: identification of colchicine-like, taxol-like and other small molecules that perturb mitosis. *Chem. Biol.* 7: 275–286.
56 Schreiber, S.L. (2021). The rise of molecular glues. *Cell* 184: 3–9, https://doi.org/10.1016/j.cell.2020.12.020.
57 Zhu, G. et al. (2020). Phase separation of disease-associated SHP2 mutants underlies MAPK hyperactivation. *Cell* 183: 490–502 e418, https://doi.org/10.1016/j.cell.2020.03.038.
58 Ito, T. et al. (2010). Identification of a primary target of thalidomide teratogenicity. *Science (New York, N.Y.)* 327: 1345–1350, https://doi.org/10.1126/science.1177319.
59 Gandhi, A.K. et al. (2014). Immunomodulatory agents lenalidomide and pomalidomide co-stimulate T cells by inducing degradation of T cell repressors Ikaros and Aiolos via modulation of the E3 ubiquitin ligase complex CRL4(CRBN.). *Br. J. Haematol.* 164: 811–821, https://doi.org/10.1111/bjh.12708.
60 Kronke, J. et al. (2014). Lenalidomide causes selective degradation of IKZF1 and IKZF3 in multiple myeloma cells. *Science (New York, N.Y.)* 343: 301–305, https://doi.org/10.1126/science.1244851.

61 Lu, G. et al. (2014). The myeloma drug lenalidomide promotes the cereblon-dependent destruction of Ikaros proteins. *Science (New York, N.Y.)* 343: 305–309, https://doi.org/10.1126/science.1244917.

62 Han, T. et al. (2017). Anticancer sulfonamides target splicing by inducing RBM39 degradation via recruitment to DCAF15. *Science (New York, N.Y.)* 356 (6336): eaal3755, https://doi.org/10.1126/science.aal3755.

63 Uehara, T. et al. (2017). Selective degradation of splicing factor CAPERalpha by anticancer sulfonamides. *Nat. Chem. Biol.* 13: 675–680, https://doi.org/10.1038/nchembio.2363.

64 Petroski, M.D. and Deshaies, R.J. (2005). Function and regulation of cullin-RING ubiquitin ligases. *Nat. Rev. Mol. Cell Biol.* 6: 9–20, https://doi.org/10.1038/nrm1547.

65 Lydeard, J.R., Schulman, B.A., and Harper, J.W. (2013). Building and remodelling Cullin-RING E3 ubiquitin ligases. *EMBO Rep.* 14: 1050–1061, https://doi.org/10.1038/embor.2013.173.

66 Naito, M., Ohoka, N., and Shibata, N. (2019). SNIPERs-hijacking IAP activity to induce protein degradation. *Drug Discov. Today Technol.* 31: 35–42, https://doi.org/10.1016/j.ddtec.2018.12.002.

67 Schneekloth, A.R., Pucheault, M., Tae, H.S., and Crews, C.M. (2008). Targeted intracellular protein degradation induced by a small molecule: en route to chemical proteomics. *Bioorg. Med. Chem. Lett.* 18: 5904–5908, https://doi.org/10.1016/j.bmcl.2008.07.114.

68 Hines, J., Lartigue, S., Dong, H. et al. (2019). MDM2-recruiting PROTAC offers superior, synergistic antiproliferative activity via simultaneous degradation of BRD4 and stabilization of p53. *Cancer Res.* 79: 251–262, https://doi.org/10.1158/0008-5472.CAN-18-2918.

69 Zhao, Q., Lan, T., Su, S., and Rao, Y. (2019). Induction of apoptosis in MDA-MB-231 breast cancer cells by a PARP1-targeting PROTAC small molecule. *Chem. Commun. (Camb.)* 55: 369–372, https://doi.org/10.1039/c8cc07813k.

70 Ward, C.C. et al. (2019). Covalent ligand screening uncovers a RNF4 E3 ligase recruiter for targeted protein degradation applications. *ACS Chem. Biol.* 14: 2430–2440, https://doi.org/10.1021/acschembio.8b01083.

71 Spradlin, J.N. et al. (2019). Harnessing the anti-cancer natural product nimbolide for targeted protein degradation. *Nat. Chem. Biol.* 15: 747–755, https://doi.org/10.1038/s41589-019-0304-8.

72 Gadd, M.S. et al. (2017). Structural basis of PROTAC cooperative recognition for selective protein degradation. *Nat. Chem. Biol.* 13: 514–521, https://doi.org/10.1038/nchembio.2329.

73 Nowak, R.P. et al. (2018). Plasticity in binding confers selectivity in ligand-induced protein degradation. *Nat. Chem. Biol.* 14: 706–714, https://doi.org/10.1038/s41589-018-0055-y.

74 Chamberlain, P. (2018). Linkers for protein degradation. *Nat. Chem. Biol.* 14: 639–640, https://doi.org/10.1038/s41589-018-0057-9.

75 D'Amato, R.J., Loughnan, M.S., Flynn, E., and Folkman, J. (1994). Thalidomide is an inhibitor of angiogenesis. *Proc. Natl. Acad. Sci. U. S. A.* 91: 4082–4085, https://doi.org/10.1073/pnas.91.9.4082.

76 Dimopoulos, M. et al. (2007). Lenalidomide plus dexamethasone for relapsed or refractory multiple myeloma. *N. Engl. J. Med.* 357: 2123–2132, https://doi.org/10.1056/NEJMoa070594.

77 FDA (2020). *FDA Grants Accelerated Approval to Pomalidomide for Kaposi Sarcoma*. US Food & Drug Administration https://www.fda.gov/drugs/resources-informationapproved-drugs/fda-grants-accelerated-approvalpomalidomide-kaposi-sarcoma.

78 Jan, M., Sperling, A.S., and Ebert, B.L. (2021). Cancer therapies based on targeted protein degradation - lessons learned with lenalidomide. *Nat. Rev. Clin. Oncol.* 18 (7): 401–417, https://doi.org/10.1038/s41571-021-00479-z.

79 Kaur, I., Dogra, S., Narang, T., and De, D. (2009). Comparative efficacy of thalidomide and prednisolone in the treatment of moderate to severe erythema nodosum leprosum: a randomized study. *Australas. J. Dermatol.* 50: 181–185, https://doi.org/10.1111/j.1440-0960.2009.00534.x.

80 Leonard, J.P. et al. (2019). AUGMENT: a phase III study of lenalidomide plus rituximab versus placebo plus rituximab in relapsed or refractory indolent lymphoma. *J. Clin. Oncol.* 37: 1188–1199, https://doi.org/10.1200/JCO.19.00010.

81 List, A. et al. (2006). Lenalidomide in the myelodysplastic syndrome with chromosome 5q deletion. *N. Engl. J. Med.* 355: 1456–1465, https://doi.org/10.1056/NEJMoa061292.

82 Pearson, J.M. and Vedagiri, M. (1969). Treatment of moderately severe erythema nodosum leprosum with thalidomide--a double-blind controlled trial. *Lepr. Rev.* 40: 111–116, https://doi.org/10.5935/0305-7518.19690022.

83 Rajkumar, S.V. et al. (2006). Phase III clinical trial of thalidomide plus dexamethasone compared with dexamethasone alone in newly diagnosed multiple myeloma: a clinical trial coordinated by the eastern cooperative oncology group. *J. Clin. Oncol.* 24: 431–436, https://doi.org/10.1200/JCO.2005.03.0221.

84 Rajkumar, S.V. et al. (2002). Combination therapy with thalidomide plus dexamethasone for newly diagnosed myeloma. *J. Clin. Oncol.* 20: 4319–4323, https://doi.org/10.1200/JCO.2002.02.116.

85 Singhal, S. et al. (1999). Antitumor activity of thalidomide in refractory multiple myeloma. *N. Engl. J. Med.* 341: 1565–1571, https://doi.org/10.1056/NEJM199911183412102.

86 Weber, D.M. et al. (2007). Lenalidomide plus dexamethasone for relapsed multiple myeloma in North America. *N. Engl. J. Med.* 357: 2133–2142, https://doi.org/10.1056/NEJMoa070596.

87 Stephens, T. and Brynner, R. (2001). *Dark Remedy: The Impact of Thalidomide and its Revival as a Vital Medicine*. Basic Books.

88 Kim, J.H. and Scialli, A.R. (2011). Thalidomide: the tragedy of birth defects and the effective treatment of disease. *Toxicol. Sci.* 122: 1–6, https://doi.org/10.1093/toxsci/kfr088.

89 Bartlett, J.B., Dredge, K., and Dalgleish, A.G. (2004). The evolution of thalidomide and its IMiD derivatives as anticancer agents. *Nat. Rev. Cancer* 4: 314–322, https://doi.org/10.1038/nrc1323.

90 Zhu, Y.X. et al. (2011). Cereblon expression is required for the antimyeloma activity of lenalidomide and pomalidomide. *Blood* 118: 4771–4779, https://doi.org/10.1182/blood-2011-05-356063.

91 Lopez-Girona, A. et al. (2012). Cereblon is a direct protein target for immunomodulatory and antiproliferative activities of lenalidomide and pomalidomide. *Leukemia* 26: 2326–2335, https://doi.org/10.1038/leu.2012.119.

92 Kronke, J. et al. (2015). Lenalidomide induces ubiquitination and degradation of CK1alpha in del(5q) MDS. *Nature* 523: 183–188, https://doi.org/10.1038/nature14610.

93 Kozicka, Z. and Thoma, N.H. (2021). Haven't got a glue: protein surface variation for the design of molecular glue degraders. *Cell Chem. Biol.* 28: 1032–1047, https://doi.org/10.1016/j.chembiol.2021.04.009.

94 Chamberlain, P.P. et al. (2014). Structure of the human Cereblon-DDB1-lenalidomide complex reveals basis for responsiveness to thalidomide analogs. *Nat. Struct. Mol. Biol.* 21: 803–809, https://doi.org/10.1038/nsmb.2874.

95 Fischer, E.S. et al. (2014). Structure of the DDB1-CRBN E3 ubiquitin ligase in complex with thalidomide. *Nature* 512: 49–53, https://doi.org/10.1038/nature13527.

96 Petzold, G., Fischer, E.S., and Thoma, N.H. (2016). Structural basis of lenalidomide-induced CK1alpha degradation by the CRL4(CRBN) ubiquitin ligase. *Nature* 532: 127–130, https://doi.org/10.1038/nature16979.

97 Sievers, Q.L. et al. (2018). Defining the human C2H2 zinc finger degrome targeted by thalidomide analogs through CRBN. *Science (New York, N.Y.)* 362, https://doi.org/10.1126/science.aat0572.

98 Faust, T.B. et al. (2020). Structural complementarity facilitates E7820-mediated degradation of RBM39 by DCAF15. *Nat. Chem. Biol.* 16: 7–14, https://doi.org/10.1038/s41589-019-0378-3.

99 Słabicki, M. et al. (2020). Small-molecule-induced polymerization triggers degradation of BCL6. *Nature* 588: 164–168, https://doi.org/10.1038/s41586-020-2925-1.

100 Matyskiela, M.E. et al. (2016). A novel cereblon modulator recruits GSPT1 to the CRL4(CRBN) ubiquitin ligase. *Nature* 535: 252–257, https://doi.org/10.1038/nature18611.

101 Furihata, H. et al. (2020). Structural bases of IMiD selectivity that emerges by 5-hydroxythalidomide. *Nat. Commun.* 11: 4578, https://doi.org/10.1038/s41467-020-18488-4.

102 Matyskiela, M.E. et al. (2020). Crystal structure of the SALL4-pomalidomide-cereblon-DDB1 complex. *Nat. Struct. Mol. Biol.* 27: 319–322, https://doi.org/10.1038/s41594-020-0405-9.

103 Matyskiela, M.E. et al. (2020). Cereblon modulators target ZBTB16 and its oncogenic fusion partners for degradation via distinct structural degrons. *ACS Chem. Biol.* 15: 3149–3158, https://doi.org/10.1021/acschembio.0c00674.

104 Mullard, A. (2021). Targeted protein degraders crowd into the clinic. *Nat. Rev. Drug Discov.* 20 (4): 247–250, https://doi.org/10.1038/d41573-021-00052-4.

105 Hagner, P.R. et al. (2015). CC-122, a pleiotropic pathway modifier, mimics an interferon response and has antitumor activity in DLBCL. *Blood* 126: 779–789, https://doi.org/10.1182/blood-2015-02-628669.

106 Matyskiela, M.E. et al. (2018). A Cereblon modulator (CC-220) with improved degradation of Ikaros and Aiolos. *J. Med. Chem.* 61: 535–542, https://doi.org/10.1021/acs.jmedchem.6b01921.

107 Schafer, P.H. et al. (2018). Cereblon modulator iberdomide induces degradation of the transcription factors Ikaros and Aiolos: immunomodulation in healthy volunteers and relevance to systemic lupus erythematosus. *Ann. Rheum. Dis.* 77: 1516–1523, https://doi.org/10.1136/annrheumdis-2017-212916.

108 Hansen, J.D. et al. (2020). Discovery of CRBN E3 ligase modulator CC-92480 for the treatment of relapsed and refractory multiple myeloma. *J. Med. Chem.* 63: 6648–6676, https://doi.org/10.1021/acs.jmedchem.9b01928.

109 Lopez-Girona, A. et al. (2021). CC-99282 is a novel Cereblon E3 ligase modulator (CELMOD) agent with potent and broad antitumor activity in preclinical models of diffuse large b-cell lymphoma (DLBCL). *Hematol. Oncol.* 39: 315–316.

110 Henderson, J.A. et al. (2021). Abstract LB007: CFT7455: a novel, IKZF1/3 degrader that demonstrates potent tumor regression in IMiD-resistant multiple myeloma (MM) xenograft models. *Cancer Res.* 81 (13_Supplement): LB007. https://doi.org/10.1158/1538-7445.AM2021-LB007.

111 Perino, S. et al. (2021). CFT7455: a novel, IKZF1/3 degrader that demonstrates potent tumor regression in a spectrum of NHL xenograft models. *Hematol. Oncol.* 39: 316–317.

112 Surka, C. et al. (2021). CC-90009, a novel cereblon E3 ligase modulator, targets acute myeloid leukemia blasts and leukemia stem cells. *Blood* 137: 661–677, https://doi.org/10.1182/blood.2020008676.

113 Urquhart, L. (2020). Top companies and drugs by sales in 2019. *Nat. Rev. Drug Discov.* 19: 228, https://doi.org/10.1038/d41573-020-00047-7.

114 Urquhart, L. (2021). Top companies and drugs by sales in 2020. *Nat. Rev. Drug Discov.* 20: 253, https://doi.org/10.1038/d41573-021-00050-6.

115 Donovan, K.A. et al. (2018). Thalidomide promotes degradation of SALL4, a transcription factor implicated in Duane radial ray syndrome. *eLife* 7: e38430, https://doi.org/10.7554/eLife.38430.

116 Yamanaka, S. et al. (2021). Thalidomide and its metabolite 5-hydroxythalidomide induce teratogenicity via the cereblon neosubstrate PLZF. *EMBO J.* 40: e105375, https://doi.org/10.15252/embj.2020105375.

117 Asatsuma-Okumura, T. et al. (2019). p63 is a cereblon substrate involved in thalidomide teratogenicity. *Nat. Chem. Biol.* 15: 1077–1084, https://doi.org/10.1038/s41589-019-0366-7.

118 Lu, J. et al. (2015). Hijacking the E3 ubiquitin ligase Cereblon to efficiently target BRD4. *Chem. Biol.* 22: 755–763, https://doi.org/10.1016/j.chembiol.2015.05.009.

119 Owa, T. et al. (1999). Discovery of novel antitumor sulfonamides targeting G1 phase of the cell cycle. *J. Med. Chem.* 42: 3789–3799, https://doi.org/10.1021/jm9902638.

120 Supuran, C.T. (2003). Indisulam: an anticancer sulfonamide in clinical development. *Expert Opin. Investig. Drugs* 12: 283–287, https://doi.org/10.1517/13543784.12.2.283.

121 Ting, T.C. et al. (2019). Aryl sulfonamides degrade RBM39 and RBM23 by recruitment to CRL4-DCAF15. *Cell Rep.* 29: 1499–1510 e1496, https://doi.org/10.1016/j.celrep.2019.09.079.

122 Mayor-Ruiz, C. et al. (2020). Rational discovery of molecular glue degraders via scalable chemical profiling. *Nat. Chem. Biol.* 16: 1199–1207, https://doi.org/10.1038/s41589-020-0594-x.

123 Jia, X. et al. (2020). pSILAC method coupled with two complementary digestion approaches reveals PRPF39 as a new E7070-dependent DCAF15 substrate. *J. Proteome* 210: 103545, https://doi.org/10.1016/j.jprot.2019.103545.

124 Kim, S.A. et al. (2020). Aryl sulfonamides induce degradation of aryl hydrocarbon receptor nuclear translocator through CRL4(DCAF15) E3 ligase. *Mol. Cells* 43: 935–944, https://doi.org/10.14348/molcells.2020.0122.

125 Bussiere, D.E. et al. (2020). Structural basis of indisulam-mediated RBM39 recruitment to DCAF15 E3 ligase complex. *Nat. Chem. Biol.* 16: 15–23, https://doi.org/10.1038/s41589-019-0411-6.

126 Du, X. et al. (2019). Structural basis and kinetic pathway of RBM39 recruitment to DCAF15 by a sulfonamide molecular glue E7820. *Structure* 27: 1625–1633 e1623, https://doi.org/10.1016/j.str.2019.10.005.

127 Punt, C.J. et al. (2001). Phase I and pharmacokinetic study of E7070, a novel sulfonamide, given at a daily times five schedule in patients with solid tumors. A study by the EORTC-early clinical studies group (ECSG). *Ann. Oncol.* 12: 1289–1293.

128 Raymond, E. et al. (2002). Phase I and pharmacokinetic study of E7070, a novel chloroindolyl sulfonamide cell-cycle inhibitor, administered as a one-hour infusion every three weeks in patients with advanced cancer. *J. Clin. Oncol.* 20: 3508–3521, https://doi.org/10.1200/JCO.2002.09.030.

129 Dittrich, C. et al. (2003). Phase I and pharmacokinetic study of E7070, a chloroindolyl-sulfonamide anticancer agent, administered on a weekly schedule to patients with solid tumors. *Clin. Cancer Res.* 9: 5195–5204.

130 Terret, C. et al. (2003). Phase I clinical and pharmacokinetic study of E7070, a novel sulfonamide given as a 5-day continuous infusion repeated every 3 weeks in patients with solid tumours. A study by the EORTC Early Clinical Study Group (ECSG). *Eur. J. Cancer* 39: 1097–1104, https://doi.org/10.1016/s0959-8049(03)00128-x.

131 Haddad, R.I. et al. (2004). A phase II clinical and pharmacodynamic study of E7070 in patients with metastatic, recurrent, or refractory squamous cell carcinoma of the head and neck: modulation of retinoblastoma protein phosphorylation by a novel chloroindolyl sulfonamide cell cycle inhibitor. *Clin. Cancer Res.* 10: 4680–4687, https://doi.org/10.1158/1078-0432.Ccr-04-0229.

132 Smyth, J.F. et al. (2005). Phase II study of E7070 in patients with metastatic melanoma. *Ann. Oncol.* 16: 158–161, https://doi.org/10.1093/annonc/mdi016.

133 Yamada, Y. et al. (2005). Phase I pharmacokinetic and pharmacogenomic study of E7070 administered once every 21 days. *Cancer Sci.* 96: 721–728, https://doi.org/10.1111/j.1349-7006.2005.00109.x.

134 Talbot, D.C. et al. (2007). A randomized phase II pharmacokinetic and pharmacodynamic study of indisulam as second-line therapy in patients with advanced non-small cell lung cancer. *Clin. Cancer Res.* 13: 1816–1822, https://doi.org/10.1158/1078-0432.CCR-06-0249.

135 Zoppi, V. et al. (2019). Iterative design and optimization of initially inactive proteolysis targeting chimeras (PROTACs) identify VZ185 as a potent, fast, and selective von Hippel-Lindau (VHL) based dual degrader probe of BRD9 and BRD7. *J. Med. Chem.* 62: 699–726, https://doi.org/10.1021/acs.jmedchem.8b01413.

136 Li, L. et al. (2020). *in vivo* target protein degradation induced by PROTACs based on E3 ligase DCAF15. *Signal Transduct. Target. Ther.* 5: 129, https://doi.org/10.1038/s41392-020-00245-0.

137 Bellenie, B.R. et al. (2020). Achieving *in vivo* target depletion through the discovery and optimization of benzimidazolone BCL6 degraders. *J. Med. Chem.* 63: 4047–4068, https://doi.org/10.1021/acs.jmedchem.9b02076.

138 Kerres, N. et al. (2017). Chemically induced degradation of the oncogenic transcription factor BCL6. *Cell Rep.* 20: 2860–2875, https://doi.org/10.1016/j.celrep.2017.08.081.

139 Lv, L. et al. (2020). Discovery of a molecular glue promoting CDK12-DDB1 interaction to trigger cyclin K degradation. *eLife* 9: e59994, https://doi.org/10.7554/eLife.59994.

140 Wang, E.S. et al. (2021). Acute pharmacological degradation of Helios destabilizes regulatory T cells. *Nat. Chem. Biol.* 17: 711–717, https://doi.org/10.1038/s41589-021-00802-w.

141 Koduri, V. et al. (2021). Targeting oncoproteins with a positive selection assay for protein degraders. *Sci. Adv.* 7: eabd6263, https://doi.org/10.1126/sciadv.abd6263.

142 Simonetta, K.R. et al. (2019). Prospective discovery of small molecule enhancers of an E3 ligase-substrate interaction. *Nat. Commun.* 10: 1402, https://doi.org/10.1038/s41467-019-09358-9.

143 Słabicki, M. et al. (2020). The CDK inhibitor CR8 acts as a molecular glue degrader that depletes cyclin K. *Nature* 585: 293–297, https://doi.org/10.1038/s41586-020-2374-x.

144 Mayor-Ruiz, C. et al. (2019). Plasticity of the Cullin-RING ligase repertoire shapes sensitivity to ligand-induced protein degradation. *Mol. Cell* 75: 849–858 e848, https://doi.org/10.1016/j.molcel.2019.07.013.

145 Dieter, S.M. et al. (2021). Degradation of CCNK/CDK12 is a druggable vulnerability of colorectal cancer. *Cell Rep.* 36: 109394, https://doi.org/10.1016/j.celrep.2021.109394.

7

Targeted Protein Degradation as a Therapeutic Strategy in Neurodegenerative Diseases

Fleur M. Ferguson[1,2]

[1]*University of California San Diego, Department of Chemistry and Biochemistry, 9500 Gilman Dr. San Diego, CA, USA*
[2]*University of California San Diego, Skaggs School of Pharmacy and Pharmaceutical Sciences, 9500 Gilman Dr. San Diego, CA, USA*

7.1 Introduction

Targeted protein degradation (TPD) has been predominantly trialed in oncology, where it has enabled encouraging results in both pre-clinical and clinical studies [1]. For example, at least 15 heterobifunctional targeted protein degrader candidates are currently being tested, mainly in oncology clinical trails [1], and many others are currently in pre-clinical development. Approved anti-cancer drugs pomalidomide and lenalidomide act as molecular glue degraders to clear oncogenic transcription factors IKZF1/3 [2]. In addition to these serendipitously discovered drugs, rationally designed glues targeting GSPT1 [3] and IKZF2 [4] are now in Ph. I and Ph. II clinical trials. Innovation in expanding the number of E3 ligases that can be hijacked, the protein degradation pathways that can be hijacked (autophagy, lysosome, proteasome, etc.), and improvements to the small molecules that are used to do have allowed increased access to a wide array of protein targets [5].

These encouraging results have sparked interest in the application of TPD to other fields, where they may be able to overcome hurdles that traditional small-molecule drugs face. One of these areas is neurodegenerative diseases, which suffer from a lack of disease-modifying drugs, in particular for prevalent conditions such as Alzheimer's disease and related dementias. In this chapter, recent publications of degraders targeting proteins implicated in neurodegenerative diseases have been reviewed, and the challenges of translating these chemical tools into drug candidates is discussed.

Inducing Targeted Protein Degradation: From Chemical Biology to Drug Discovery and Clinical Applications, First Edition. Edited by Philipp Cromm.

7.2 Heterobifunctional Targeted Protein Degraders

Heterobifunctional degraders (also known as proteolysis targeting chimeras (PROTACs)) have been developed against neurodegenerative disease-relevant targets. Although only a small number of studies published to date have demonstrated both degradation and phenotypic activity in cellular or *in vivo* models of dementia, proof-of-concept degradation data for a broader range of therapeutically relevant targets have been described [6]. In this chapter, we focus on reported degraders of misfolded protein aggregates, kinases, and histone deacetylases (HDACs).

7.2.1 Misfolded Proteins

The accumulation of insoluble misfolded protein deposits concurrent with disease progression is a characteristic trait of diseases called proteinopathies [7]. Some examples of commonly occurring proteinopathies include Alzheimer's disease, characterized by extracellular amyloid aggregates and intracellular tau tangles [8]; frontotemporal dementia, characterized by misfolded tau [9]; Parkinsons' disease, characterized by intracellular misfolded alpha-synuclein [10]; and Huntingtons' disease characterized by accumulation of intracellular mutant Huntingtin protein [11]. Therefore, approaches to reduce these protein levels are of therapeutic interest. Although many of the reported approaches are in their infancy and lack the potency, stability, or selectivity of optimized chemical tools, they represent an interesting first step toward drugging these important targets (Figure 7.1).

The role of protein misfolding in driving and perpetuating neurodegeneration and their potential as therapeutic targets is controversial [12]. Given the stark differences between the 3D structures of the soluble and insoluble proteins, small-molecule binders that have selectivity for the misfolded conformer over the wild-type, healthy conformer have been developed as imaging agents and, in some cases, are approved as positron emission tomography (PET) tracers to aid in the diagnosis of proteinopathies [9]. Medicinal chemists have now begun to co-opt these selective binders and use them as "bait" in targeted protein degraders to selectively recruit disease-associated protein folds to the proteasome and clear them [13]. The hope is that these degrader chemical tools enable researchers to gain rapid, selective chemical control of these species, enabling experiments that can clarify the role of aggregates in driving disease progression and provide crucial pre-clinical validation (or invalidation) of them as therapeutic targets across different dementias.

7.2.1.1 Tau

Misfolded tau is observed in numerous dementias, including Alzheimer's disease, frontotemporal dementia, progressive supranuclear palsy, traumatic brain injury, and Parkinson's disease. Unlike amyloids, which are extracellular and surrounded in controversy regarding their potential as therapeutic targets [14], tau aggregates are intracellular and therefore amenable to TPD approaches, which may aid in target validation efforts. Therefore, identification of agents that can reduce or remove either total or misfolded tau is of high interest. Initial efforts at applying targeted

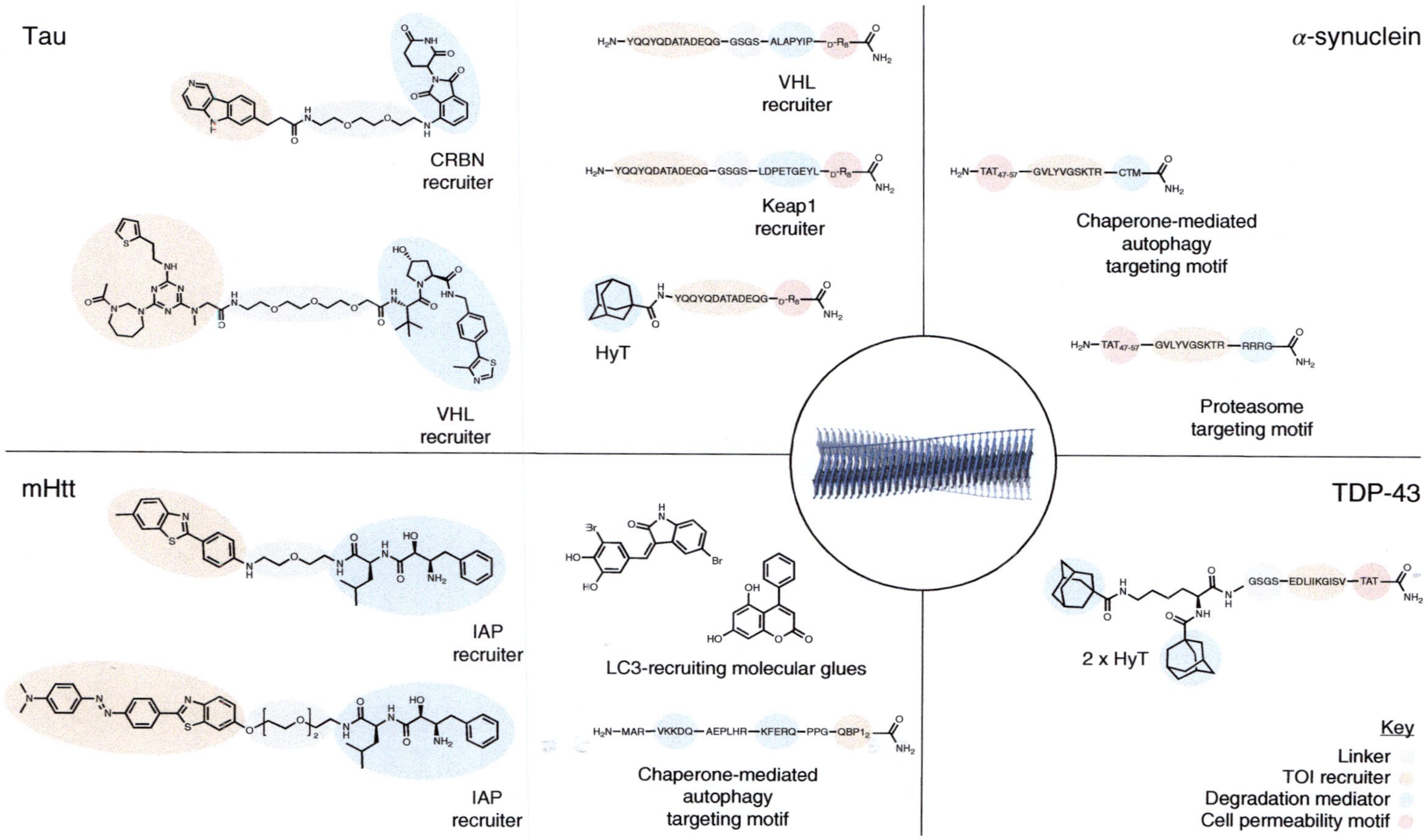

Figure 7.1 Reported targeted protein degraders of neurodegeneration-related misfolded proteins.

protein degradation toward this goal were reported in 2016 [15]. In this study, Chu et al. used a peptide-based approach to design a series of molecules that incorporated a tau binding sequence, a GSGS linker, a substrate motif to recruit either the Skp1 or VHL E3 ligase proteins, and a D-Arg_8 sequence to promote cell permeability. VHL-recruiting peptides were able to reduce fluorescence signals in Neuro2a cells overexpressing Tau-EGFP (enhanced green fluorescent protein) levels; however, high concentrations of peptide were required (50–100 μM, 24 hours treatment). These results were validated for lead peptide, TH006, in primary neuron cells derived from 3xTg-AD mice where it was able to mediate the toxicity of amyloid-β. Finally, TH006 was able to reduce tau levels in 3xTg-AD mice when administered at 15 mg/kg for 10 days using a combination of intravenous and intranasal dosing. Effects on phospho-tau or insoluble tau were not reported.

A second peptide-based tau degrader was reported by Lu et al. who used a similar peptide strategy, this time employing a recognition motif to recruit the KEAP1 E3 ligase [16]. Peptide 1 was able to reduce tau levels in three EGFP-Tau overexpressing cell lines, with maximal degradation observed following 48 hours of treatment with 20 μM peptide.

In a follow-up work, a hybrid approach that used tau-binding peptides functionalized with adamantane [17], known as hydrophobic tagging, to trigger recognition and degradation by the ubiquitin-proteasome system. These peptides were able to reduce EGFP-Tau levels following treatment of cells with 150 μM peptide for 24 hours, when co-treated with the translation inhibitor cycloheximide. Tau levels were also reduced in 3xTg-AD mice following i.v. dosing with 18 mg/kg of peptide for eight days. Together, their peptide-based approaches demonstrated that tau is amenable to induced degradation by TPD and paved the way for the development of small molecules.

Most recently, a small-molecule targeted protein degrader for misfolded-tau has been reported [13]. The clinical PET tracer T807, which binds to disease-associated tau, was linked via a PEG_2 linker to pomalidomide, which recruits CRBN, a component of the $CRL4^{CRBN}$ E3–ligase complex. Lead degrader QC-01-175 was able to degrade tau in frontotemporal dementia (FTD) patient iPSC-derived neurons following treatment with 1 μM for 24 hours and did not affect tau levels in healthy control neurons. Global proteomics analysis revealed a subset of iMiD targets, such as ZFP91, that are also degraded by QC-01-175. Finally, treatment of FTD neurons with 5 μM QC-01-175 was able to mediate the toxicity of amyloid-β. Advanced CRBN-recruiting tau degraders based on T807, and other tau binding scaffolds, have also been described in conference presentations and patents filed by Arvinas, Inc. Finally, Wang et al. used a triazole-based tau binder to develop a VHL-recruiting small-molecule degrader, which was reported to clear tau in HEK293 and SHSY-5Y cells overexpressing tau [18].

7.2.1.2 Alpha-Synuclein

Lewy body dementia (LBD), which encompasses dementia with Lewy bodies and Parkinson's disease (PD), is the third most common form of dementia after Alzheimer's disease and vascular dementia, yet no disease-modifying therapies have been discovered [13, 19, 20]. A hallmark of LBD is the accumulation of misfolded alpha-synuclein into intraneuronal deposits named Lewy bodies. Therefore, identification of agents that can reduce or remove either total or misfolded alpha-synnuclein is of high interest.

Peptide-based approaches have also been used to validate alpha-synuclein as a degradable target. Using a similar strategy to those described above, Qu et al. designed peptides to target alpha-synuclein for proteasomal degradation. These incorporated a cell-penetrating domain, an alpha-synuclein protein-binding domain, based on a motif in beta-synuclein (amino acids 36–45) reported to specifically and strongly interact with alpha-synuclein and a proteasome targeting motif (RRRG), also known as a peptide degron [21]. Treatment of SK-N-SH cells overexpressing alpha-synuclein with peptide, but not negative control peptide, resulted in loss of synuclein after four hours, with maximal degradation at 150 μM concentration. No cell toxicity or off target effects on DJ-1, APP, and tau were observed, although global proteomics evaluation of selectivity was not reported. Alpha-synuclein degradation in primary neurons was also observed [22].

Peptide-based approaches to hijack the chaperone-mediated autophagy system have also been utilized to degrade alpha-synuclein. Chaperone-mediated autophagy (CMA) is specific for protein substrates containing a pentapeptide targeting motif (KFERQ). Fan et al. used this motif to recruit the CMA system to non-endogenous substrates such as alpha-synuclein via a bifunctional peptide, containing a CMA-motif linked to the beta-synuclein peptide described above and a cell penetrating sequence. These molecules were able to successfully degrade alpha synuclein in primary neurons following a four hours treatment with 25 μM peptide [23].

Finally, small-molecule targeted protein degraders of misfolded alpha-synuclein have been reported in the patent literature by Arvinas Inc. [24] and Dana–Farber Cancer Institute/Massachusetts General Hospital (Patent citation: WO2021257650A1).

7.2.1.3 mHtt

Huntington's disease is an autosomal dominant neurodegenerative disease caused by polyQ expansions in the huntingtin protein (Htt) that leads to mutant huntingtin (mHtt) aggregation. As removal of toxic mHtt is expected to be a promising therapeutic approach, researchers have developed both peptide, small molecule, and molecular glue approaches to degrade mHtt.

Tomoshige et al. reported a mHtt degrading molecule that used pan-aggregate binding benzothiazole derivatives that recognize the beta-sheet secondary structure enriched in aggregated proteins, as mHtt recruiting bait [25]. These were conjugated via polyethylene glycol linkers to bestatin [26], a dipeptide containing natural product that functions as an aminopeptidase inhibitor and interacts with the E3 ligase cIAP. The resulting molecules were able to reduce mHtt in Huntington's disease patient-derived fibroblasts, following treatment with 10 μM degrader compound for 24 or 48 hours [25]. Under these conditions, they also cleared wtHtt from normal fibroblasts, which the authors attributed to the ability of wtHtt to form small ThT-binding aggregates based on studies of recombinant purified protein *in vitro* [27, 28]. In a follow-up paper by the same group, mHtt degraders were reported using the IAP antagonist MV1 as the E3 ligase recruiting component. However, these molecules were less potent that the bestatin-derived degraders and acted more slowly, requiring 72 hours for full degradation of mHtt to be observed following 10 μM compound concentration [29].

Peptide-based approaches for specific targeting of mHtt using the chaperone-mediated autophagy system described above have also been developed. This time, CMA-recruiting peptides able to recruit Hsc70 chaperone protein were fused to polyglutamine binding peptide 1, a sequence that binds to an expanded polyQ tract, but not to the polyQ motif found in normal Htt protein. Transfection of a plasmid encoding the degrader peptide (named RHQ), but not the controls, was able to reduce the levels of soluble and insoluble mHtt in Neuro2a cells. Intrastriatal injections of recombinant adeno-associated virus encoding RHQ were also able to reduce levels of both aggregated and soluble mHtt in the R6/2 murine model of Huntington's disease and ameliorate disease phenotypes such as weight loss, premature death, and performance on a rotarod test [30].

7.2.2 TDP-43

A hydrophobic tagging approach was used by Gao et al. to develop peptides able to degrade TDP-43 [31]. Specifically, peptides corresponding to the core aggregation domain of TDP-43 were used, linked to a cell penetrating peptide sequence, and two adamantane-derived hydrophobic tags. These molecules were able to reduce TDP-43 levels following treatment of Neuro2a or *Drosophila* overexpressing TDP-43 following treatment at 100 μM for 24 hours. Although these peptide degraders are not potent and induce incomplete degradation, they represent an early indication that TDP-43 may also be targetable by TPD approaches [31].

7.2.3 Kinases and HDACs

A number of kinases and HDACs have been reported to be desirable targets for combatting neurodegenerative diseases [32, 33]. However, inhibitor-based strategies have not yet afforded approved drugs. Targeted protein degradation strategies for a small number of these targets have been reported, and more still have been shown to be amenable to TPD.

Kinases have proven to be highly amenable to targeted protein degradation through chemoprotomic mapping approaches, allowing targeting of their scaffolding functions in addition to their enzyme activity. Among the kinases that have been reported to be promising targets for neurodegenerative diseases, targeted protein degraders have been reported for ABL1, GSK3-beta, MAPK14, RIPK1, and many others [34, 35]. Numerous attempts to develop a degrader of LRRK2, a large, multi-domain protein implicated in Parkinson's disease have been reported, including unsuccessful attempts, implying that this protein may be one of the more challenging targets to degrade with current degrader technologies [36, 37]. However, recent publications and patents have been published, indicating that that with enough perseverance, this challenge can be overcome. Liu et al. report in a preprint the discovery of brain-penetrant LRRK2 degraders, which may prove useful for future studies validating this as a therapeutic approach in Parkinson's Disease models [38].

HDACs 1-8 and HDAC10 have also been demonstrated to be accessible targets for degradation through systematic chemoproteomic screening approaches [39]. Although engineering in inhibitor selectivity among HDACs has historically been challenging, Xiong et al. were able to develop selective HDAC degraders from multitargeted inhibitors. Although these studies were performed in cancer cell lines, repurposing these degrader tools for neurodegenerative diseases may offer new avenues to validate them as targets. Class II HDACs have been reported as a promising target class for Parkinsons' disease [32], and Class III HDACs have been reported as putative therapeutic targets for tauopathies [40], whereas pan-HDAC inhibition promotes tau aggregation in models of Alzheimer's disease [41], indicating that selective HDAC degradation could be leveraged in these contexts.

7.3 Molecular Glues

Molecular glues are an attractive modality for degrading neurodegenerative disease targets, as they typically have physicochemical properties more closely aligned with those required for blood–brain barrier permeability [42]. However, identifying molecular glue degraders using targeted screening or rational design is challenging, and many of the known molecular glues were discovered serendipitously. To date, only one molecular glue developed against a neurodegenerative disease target, mHtt, has been reported [43]. Li et al. used small-molecule microarray oblique incidence reflectivity difference microscopy (OIRD) screening to detect compounds that interact with LC3, mHtt but not wtHtt recombinant proteins. They identified two hits and from focussed follow-up screens found an additional two analogs with the desired binding profile. These compounds lowered mHtt levels in primary cortical neurons from Huntington's disease (HD) mouse models, but not WT controls, and in addition reduced mHtt levels in HD patient fibroblasts [43]. However, the small molecules identified in this study have "PAINs (pan assay interference compounds)" compound pharmacophores [44]. Future work to validate these molecules and remove the problematic functional groups is needed.

7.4 Conclusion

TPD has provided an exciting opportunity to create small molecules targeting misfolded proteins, aiding target validation in a number of models. The limitation of the current progress is the availability of potent, selective binders or PET tracers for disease-associated protein conformations beyond tau. Another limitation is the translation of current findings into *in vivo* models because of the challenge of optimizing the stability and pharmacokinetics of these large molecules and peptides to permeate the blood–brain barrier. Advances in medicinal chemistry and TPD are poised to further enable the field.

Declaration of Interest

The authors claim the following competing financial interests: F.M.F. is a scientific co-founder and equity holder in Proximity Therapeutics, a scientific advisory board member (SAB) and equity holder in Triana Biomedicines. Fleur Ferguson is or was recently a consultant or received speaking honoraria from RA Capital, Tocris BioTechne, Eli Lilly and Co, and Plexium Inc. The Ferguson lab receives or has received research funding from Ono Pharmaceutical Co. Ltd.

References

1 Mullard, A. (2021). Targeted protein degraders crowd into the clinic. *Nat. Rev. Drug Discov.* 20 (4): 247–250.

2 Kronke, J., Udeshi, N.D., Narla, A. et al. (2014). Lenalidomide causes selective degradation of IKZF1 and IKZF3 in multiple myeloma cells. *Science* 343 (6168): 301–305.

3 Hansen, J.D., Correa, M., Alexander, M. et al. (2021). CC-90009: a cereblon E3 ligase modulating drug that promotes selective degradation of GSPT1 for the treatment of acute myeloid leukemia. *J. Med. Chem.* 64 (4): 1835–1843.

4 Wang, E.S., Verano, A.L., Nowak, R.P. et al. (2021). Acute pharmacological degradation of Helios destabilizes regulatory T cells. *Nat. Chem. Biol.* 17 (6): 711–717.

5 Ng, C.S.C. and Banik, S.M. (2022). Recent advances in induced proximity modalities. *Curr. Opin. Chem. Biol.* 67: 102107.

6 Tao, A.J., Gadbois, G.E., Buczynski, S.A., and Ferguson, F.M. (2022). Targeted protein degradation: emerging concepts and protein state-specific targeting principles. *Curr. Opin. Chem. Biol.* 67: 102114.

7 Bayer, T.A. (2015). Proteinopathies, a core concept for understanding and ultimately treating degenerative disorders? *Eur. Neuropsychopharmacol.* 25 (5): 713–724.

8 Atri, A. (2019). The Alzheimer's disease clinical spectrum: diagnosis and management. *Med. Clin. North Am.* 103 (2): 263–293.

9 Tsai, R.M., Bejanin, A., Lesman-Segev, O. et al. (2019). (18)F-flortaucipir (AV-1451) tau PET in frontotemporal dementia syndromes. *Alzheimers Res. Ther.* 11 (1): 13.

10 Hayes, M.T. (2019). Parkinson's disease and parkinsonism. *Am. J. Med.* 132 (7): 802–807.

11 McColgan, P. and Tabrizi, S.J. (2018). Huntington's disease: a clinical review. *Eur. J. Neurol.* 25 (1): 24–34.

12 Musiek, E.S., Gomez-Isla, T., and Holtzman, D.M. (2021). Aducanumab for Alzheimer disease: the amyloid hypothesis moves from bench to bedside. *J. Clin. Invest.* 131 (20): E154889.

13 Silva, M.C., Ferguson, F.M., Cai, Q. et al. (2019). Targeted degradation of aberrant tau in frontotemporal dementia patient-derived neuronal cell models. *eLife* 8: e45457.

14 Gallardo, G. and Holtzman, D.M. (2019). Amyloid-beta and tau at the crossroads of Alzheimer's disease. *Adv. Exp. Med. Biol.* 1184: 187–203.

15 Chu, T.T., Gao, N., Li, Q.Q. et al. (2016). Specific knockdown of endogenous tau protein by peptide-directed ubiquitin-proteasome degradation. *Cell Chem. Biol.* 23 (4): 453–461.

16 Lu, M., Liu, T., Jiao, Q. et al. (2018). Discovery of a Keap1-dependent peptide PROTAC to knockdown tau by ubiquitination-proteasome degradation pathway. *Eur. J. Med. Chem.* 146: 251–259.

17 Choi, S.R., Wang, H.M., Shin, M.H., and Lim, H.S. (2021). Hydrophobic tagging-mediated degradation of transcription coactivator SRC-1. *Int. J. Mol. Sci.* 22 (12): 6407.

18 Wang, W., Zhou, Q., Jiang, T. et al. (2021). A novel small-molecule PROTAC selectively promotes tau clearance to improve cognitive functions in Alzheimer-like models. *Theranostics* 11 (11): 5279–5295.

19 Lee, V.M. and Trojanowski, J.Q. (2006). Mechanisms of Parkinson's disease linked to pathological alpha-synuclein: new targets for drug discovery. *Neuron* 52 (1): 33–38.

20 Trigo-Damas, I., Del Rey, N.L., and Blesa, J. (2018). Novel models for Parkinson's disease and their impact on future drug discovery. *Expert Opin. Drug Discov.* 13 (3): 229–239.

21 Bonger, K.M., Chen, L.C., Liu, C.W., and Wandless, T.J. (2011). Small-molecule displacement of a cryptic degron causes conditional protein degradation. *Nat. Chem. Biol.* 7 (8): 531–537.

22 Qu, J., Ren, X., Xue, F. et al. (2020). Specific knockdown of alpha-Synuclein by peptide-directed proteasome degradation rescued its associated neurotoxicity. *Cell Chem. Biol.* 27 (6): 751–762 e4.

23 Fan, X., Jin, W.Y., Lu, J. et al. (2014). Rapid and reversible knockdown of endogenous proteins by peptide-directed lysosomal degradation. *Nat. Neurosci.* 17 (3): 471–480.

24 Kargbo, R.B. (2020). PROTAC compounds targeting alpha-Synuclein protein for treating neurogenerative disorders: Alzheimer's and Parkinson's diseases. *ACS Med. Chem. Lett.* 11 (6): 1086–1087.

25 Tomoshige, S., Nomura, S., Ohgane, K. et al. (2017). Discovery of small molecules that induce the degradation of huntingtin. *Angew. Chem. Int. Ed.* 56 (38): 11530–11533.

26 Umezawa, H., Aoyagi, T., Suda, H. et al. (1976). Bestatin, an inhibitor of aminopeptidase B, produced by actinomycetes. *J. Antibiot. (Tokyo)* 29 (1): 97–99.

27 Scherzinger, E., Sittler, A., Schweiger, K. et al. (1999). Self-assembly of polyglutamine-containing huntingtin fragments into amyloid-like fibrils: implications for Huntington's disease pathology. *Proc. Natl. Acad. Sci. U. S. A.* 96 (8): 4604–4609.

28 Matsuoka, S., Murai, M., Yamazaki, T., and Inoue, M. (2012). Short polyglutamine peptide forms a high-affinity binding site for thioflavin-T at the N-terminus. *Org. Biomol. Chem.* 10 (30): 5787–5790.

29 Tomoshige, S., Nomura, S., Ohgane, K. et al. (2018). Degradation of huntingtin mediated by a hybrid molecule composed of IAP antagonist linked to phenyldiazenyl benzothiazole derivative. *Bioorg. Med. Chem. Lett.* 28 (4): 707–710.

30 Bauer, P.O., Goswami, A., Wong, H.K. et al. (2010). Harnessing chaperone-mediated autophagy for the selective degradation of mutant huntingtin protein. *Nat. Biotechnol.* 28 (3): 256–263.

31 Gao, N., Huang, Y.P., Chu, T.T. et al. (2019). TDP-43 specific reduction induced by Di-hydrophobic tags conjugated peptides. *Bioorg. Chem.* 84: 254–259.

32 Mazzocchi, M., Collins, L.M., Sullivan, A.M., and O'Keeffe, G.W. (2020). The class II histone deacetylases as therapeutic targets for Parkinson's disease. *Neuronal. Signal.* 4 (2): NS20200001.

33 Benn, C.L. and Dawson, L.A. (2020). Clinically precedented protein kinases: rationale for their use in neurodegenerative disease. *Front. Aging Neurosci.* 12: 242.

34 Donovan, K.A., Ferguson, F.M., Bushman, J.W. et al. (2020). Mapping the degradable Kinome provides a resource for expedited degrader development. *Cell* 183 (6): 1714–1731 e10.

35 Bondeson, D.P., Smith, B.E., Burslem, G.M. et al. (2018). Lessons in PROTAC design from selective degradation with a promiscuous warhead. *Cell Chem. Biol.* 25 (1): 78–87 e5.

36 Konstantinidou, M., Oun, A., Pathak, P. et al. (2021). The tale of proteolysis targeting chimeras (PROTACs) for leucine-rich repeat kinase 2 (LRRK2). *ChemMedChem* 16 (6): 959–965.

37 Kargbo, R.B. (2020). Degradation of LRRK2 in the treatment of Parkinson's disease. *ACS Med. Chem. Lett.* 11 (11): 2070–2071.

38 Liu, X., Kalogeropulou, A., Domingos, S. et al. (2022). Discovery of XL01126: A Potent, Fast, Cooperative, Selective, Oral bioavailable and Blood Brain Barrier Penetrant PROTAC Degrader of Leucine Rich Repeat Kinase 2 (LRRK2). *ChemRxiv.* Cambridge: Cambridge Open Engage.

39 Xiong, Y., Donovan, K.A., Eleuteri, N.A. et al. (2021). Chemo-proteomics exploration of HDAC degradability by small molecule degraders. *Cell Chem. Biol.* 28 (10): 1514–1527 e4.

40 Yeong, K.Y., Berdigaliyev, N., and Chang, Y. (2020). Sirtuins and their implications in neurodegenerative diseases from a drug discovery perspective. *ACS Chem. Neurosci.* 11 (24): 4073–4091.

41 Jeong, H., Shin, S., Lee, J.S. et al. (2019). Pan-HDAC inhibitors promote tau aggregation by increasing the level of acetylated tau. *Int. J. Mol. Sci.* 20 (17): 4283.

42 Wager, T.T., Hou, X., Verhoest, P.R., and Villalobos, A. (2016). Central nervous system multiparameter optimization desirability: application in drug discovery. *ACS Chem. Neurosci.* 7 (6): 767–775.

43 Li, Z., Wang, C., Wang, Z. et al. (2019). Allele-selective lowering of mutant HTT protein by HTT-LC3 linker compounds. *Nature* 575 (7781): 203–209.

44 Baell, J.B. and Holloway, G.A. (2010). New substructure filters for removal of pan assay interference compounds (PAINS) from screening libraries and for their exclusion in bioassays. *J. Med. Chem.* 53 (7): 2719–2740.

8

Insights and Future Perspectives of Covalent Protein Degraders

Xiaoyu Zhang[1,2]

[1]*Northwestern University, Department of Chemistry, 2145 Sheridan Road, Evanston, IL, 60208, USA*
[2]*The Scripps Research Institute, Department of Chemistry, 10550 N Torrey Pines Road, La Jolla, CA, 92037, USA*

8.1 Introduction

Targeted protein degradation (TPD) is an emerging field in chemical biology and drug discovery. Compared with conventional small-molecule drugs that typically function through occupancy-driven mechanism, small molecules for TPD, or protein degraders, hijack the cellular recycling machinery to destroy the protein of interest (POI). This mechanism is referred to as "event-driven" pharmacology [1] and has been proven to overcome some of the limitations faced by conventional drug discovery efforts. For instance, proteins that have multiple functional domains, such as IRAK4 bearing both kinase and scaffolding domains [2], are considered challenging to be targeted with conventional small-molecule inhibitors, as inhibiting one of those domains may not fully disrupt protein functions. Protein degraders, on the other hand, chemically "knock-out" the target protein and simultaneously remove all the associated functions. In addition, protein degraders function as catalytic drugs and have also been demonstrated to target historically "undruggable" proteins, such as transcription factors and RNA splicing factors [1, 3, 4]. All these merits make protein degraders a rapidly evolving therapeutic modality that attracts attention from both academia and the industry. Lenalidomide, an FDA-approved drug for treating multiple myeloma and myelodysplastic syndromes, has been demonstrated to function as a degrader for transcriptional factors IKZF1, IKZF3, and CK1α [5–7]. To date, four protein degraders have entered phase II clinical trial, and more than a dozen protein degraders are under phase I clinical trial [8]. On the academic side, more than 1600 heterobifunctional protein degraders targeting over 100 proteins have been reported in the literature [9].

Protein degraders can be divided into two main categories based on the cellular machinery hijacked. The first category hijacks the ubiquitin-proteasome system (UPS). Proteolysis targeting chimeras (PROTACs), the key technology that opens up

Inducing Targeted Protein Degradation: From Chemical Biology to Drug Discovery and Clinical Applications, First Edition. Edited by Philipp Cromm.

the whole TPD field, belong to this category and degrade POI through inducing its proximity with an E3 ubiquitin ligase [10]. Other technologies include specific and non-genetic IAP-dependent protein erasers (SNIPERs) [11], Trim-away [12], hydrophobic tagging [13], cereblon modulators (CELMoDs) [14], and transcription factor targeting chimeras (TRAFTACs) [15]. The second category hijacks the lysosome system for extracellular and cell surface TPD and has been reported to pharmacologically engage diverse receptors involved in the lysosome-mediated protein degradation pathway. Technologies in this category include autophagy-targeting chimeras (AUTACs) [16], lysosome-targeting chimeras (LYTACs) [17], autophagosome-tethering compound (ATTEC) [18], antibody-based PROTACs (AbTACs) [19], molecular degraders of extracellular proteins through the asialoglycoprotein receptor (MoDE-As) [20], and covalently engineered nanobody chimeras (GlueBody) [21]. By far, the main focus of academic and industrial efforts has been on protein degraders that hijack the UPS. Therefore, this chapter will mainly discuss covalent protein degraders in this category.

Protein degraders can also be divided into heterobifunctional and monofunctional molecules based on the nature of their chemical structures. Heterobifunctional degraders contain two chemical moieties that engage both effector proteins (E3 ubiquitin ligases or certain receptors involved in lysosome-mediated protein degradation) and POIs for TPD. The two chemical moieties are connected via a chemical linker, another critical component of heterobifunctional degraders that has been shown to affect target/effector engagement, ternary complex stability, and ligand–protein interaction kinetics [22–24]. On the other hand, monofunctional degraders, or molecular glue degraders [25, 26], alter the surface patches of E3 ubiquitin ligases and induce neo protein–protein interactions (PPIs) or stabilize otherwise low-affinity PPIs. Monofunctional degraders may not show high-affinity interactions with the isolated E3 ligase and POI but can efficiently induce the formation of ternary complex when both proteins are present [27, 28].

Since the first reported PROTAC molecule [10], attention has been largely focused on non-covalent small molecules – part of the reason is that the ligands for the two most commonly used E3 ubiquitin ligases in PROTAC design, CRBN and VHL, are both non-covalent [29]. Therefore, it is conceptually straightforward to couple these non-covalent ligands to another molecule binding the POI. Some well-known examples are ARV-110 (androgen receptor degrader) [30], dBET1 (BRD4 degrader) [31], and SD-36 (STAT3 degrader) [32]. More recently, covalent protein degraders started emerging in the literature. Drugs that covalently attach to POIs have been used in a clinical setup for more than a century [33]. Since 1990, more than 35 drugs that function via covalent mechanism have been approved by the FDA. One recent phenomenal example is AMG510 that was approved by the FDA for treating KRAS G12C-mutated non-small-cell lung cancer (NSCLC). Mechanistically, AMG510 covalently engages cysteine 12 (Cys12) on KRAS G12C, a notoriously undruggable cancer target [34]. For covalent TPD, the covalent interaction can occur on either the E3 ubiquitin ligase or the substrate side (Figure 8.1). Initial efforts were focused on converting well-established covalent ligands for POI into PROTACs. One of the remarkable features for degraders that covalently engage POIs is that they have the

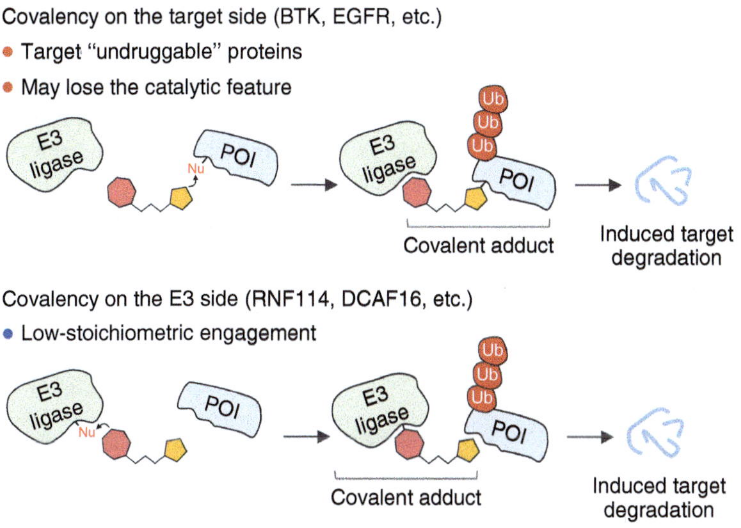

Figure 8.1 Schematic representation of strategies of leveraging covalent chemistry for TPD. Nu, nucleophilic amino acids; Ub, ubiquitination.

potential to target "undruggable" proteins, as those proteins that normally lack well-defined pockets for non-covalent ligand development might be targeted through covalent mode of action [35]. On the other hand, covalency on the POI side requires stoichiometric target engagement and therefore makes catalytic turnover almost impossible, which is a drawback of those molecules. More recent studies started exploring covalent engagement of E3 ubiquitin ligases by electrophiles, which has led to a number of discoveries in which covalent ligand–E3 ubiquitin ligase interactions can be leveraged to support TPD [36–39] (Figure 8.1). Protein degraders that covalently engage E3 ligases would presumably maintain the catalytic feature and have been demonstrated to function in a low-stoichiometry manner – a crucial feature that can avoid perturbing the native functions of the hijacked E3 ligases [37, 39]. Protein degraders that covalently engage E3 ubiquitin ligases also reduce the ternary complex model into a pseudo-binary complex model, which may improve the durability of induced TPD. In this chapter, we will review protein degraders that covalently engage either POI or E3 ubiquitin ligase and discuss the key technologies that have been used for covalent protein degrader discovery.

8.2 Protein Degraders that Covalently Interact with the Substrate Proteins

8.2.1 HaloPROTAC

Given the unique feature of covalent interaction, such as engaging shallow surface pockets, targeting proteins that lack non-covalent binders, high occupancy on the target protein, and improved pharmacodynamics [40], significant efforts have been made in recent years to covalently interact with and degrade target proteins. One of the earliest examples is the HaloPROTAC system developed by the Crews lab, in which a Halo tag is fused with the target of interest, so that an E3 recruiter coupled with chloroalkane can rapidly degrade the Halo tag-fused proteins (Figure 8.2a) [41]. The advantage of using a HaloPROTAC for targeted degradation is that this approach is not limited by the availability of POI ligands. Moreover, the Halo tag ligand chloroalkane enables selective interaction with the Halo tag-fused protein [42], which leads to selective target degradation by the HaloPROTAC. In one study, Tovell et al. employed clustered regularly interspaced short palindromic repeats (CRISPR)/Cas9 genome editing technology and fused an Halo tag to two endogenous proteins, SGK3 and VPS34 [43]. They showed that HaloPROTAC-E (Figure 8.2b) that tethers the chloroalkane to VHL binder VH298 induced rapid degradation of SGK3 and VPS34 [43]. The degradation of kinase SGK3 further blocked phosphorylation of its substrate NDRG1 [43]. Untargeted proteomic analysis revealed that the HaloPROTAC-E-induced VPS34 degradation is remarkably selective [43]. In parallel, the degradation tag (dTAG) [44] and the BromoTag [45] are two systems that fuse POI to engineered tags for non-covalent PROTAC-induced target degradation, which enables the usage of a single compound for the degradation of a variety of protein targets (dTAG-13 for dTAG system [44] and AGB1 for BromoTag system [45]).

8.2.2 METAP2 and BTK

The first PROTAC's substrate binding moiety, ovalicin, covalently modifies His231 of methionine aminopeptidase-2 (METAP2) [10, 46]. Incubating METAP2 with the PROTAC molecule resulted in two bands in Western blot analysis – with the upper band representing the covalently modified METAP2 [10]. Bruton's tyrosine kinase (BTK) is one well-studied example for which a number of covalent PROTACs have been developed, mainly owing to the success of covalent BTK inhibitors in treating chronic lymphocytic leukemia (CLL) [47]. In one study, the authors conjugated ibrutinib, an acrylamide-bearing BTK inhibitor, to lenalidomide [48] and found that this PROTAC (covalent PROTAC 4, Figure 8.3) did not reduce BTK protein level.

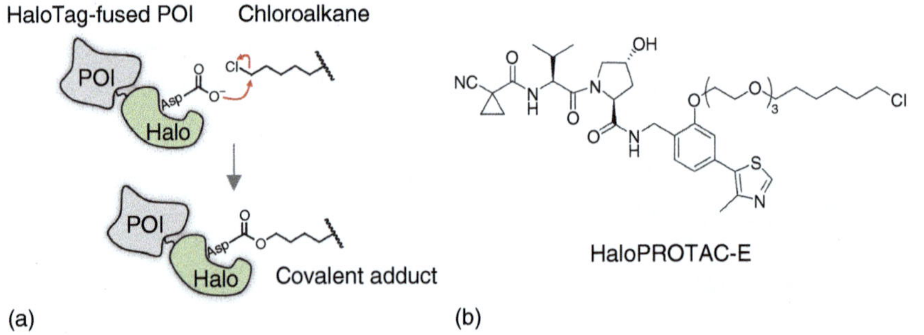

Figure 8.2 HaloPROTAC as a strategy to covalently engage and degrade POI. (a) Scheme showing the covalent bond formation between a Halo tag-fused POI and a compound bearing the chloroalkane moiety. (b) Chemical structure of HaloPROTAC-E that was used to degrade Halo tag-fused SGK3 and VPS34.

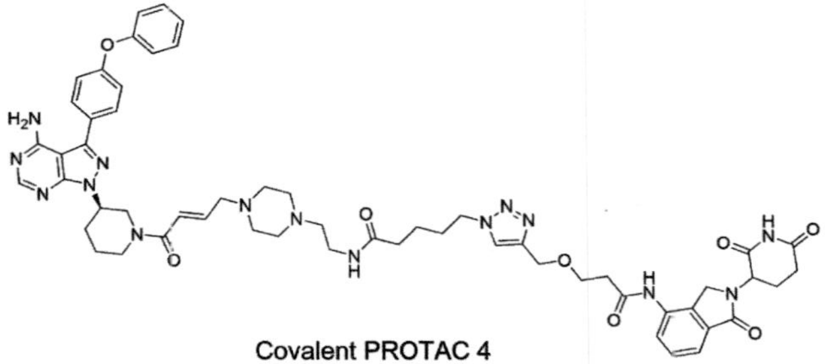

Covalent PROTAC 4

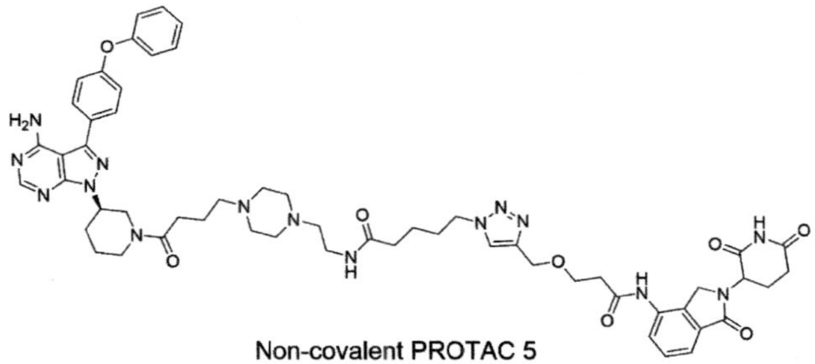

Non-covalent PROTAC 5

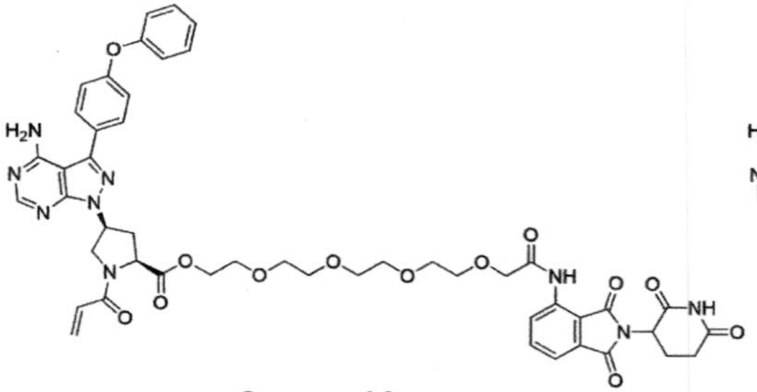

Compound 3c

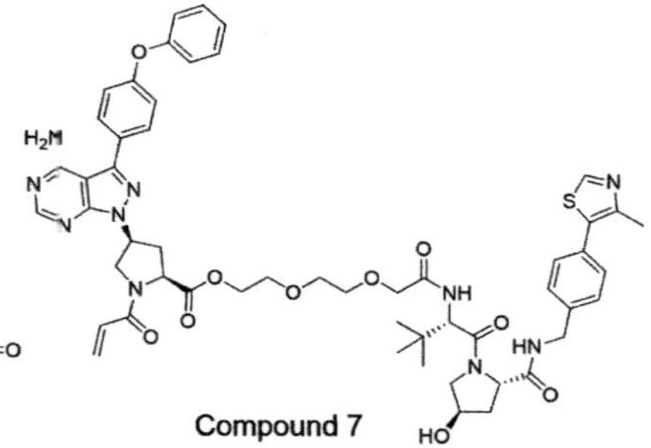

Compound 7

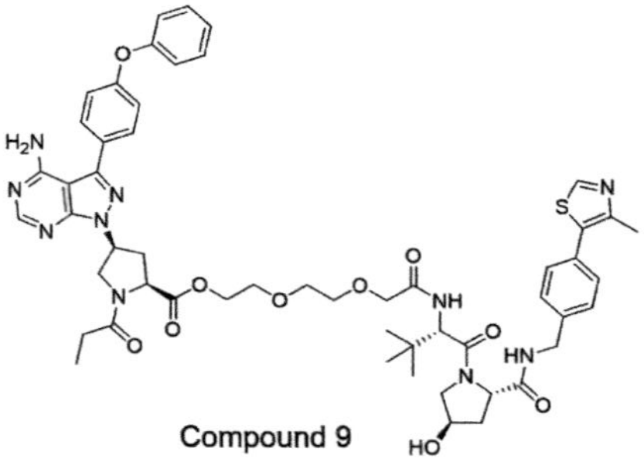

Compound 9

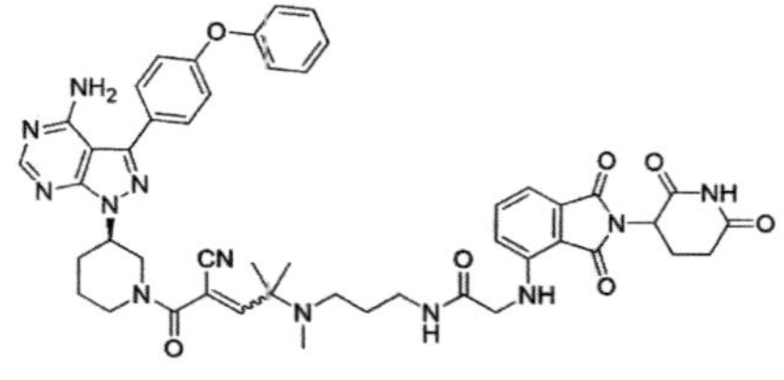

RC-1

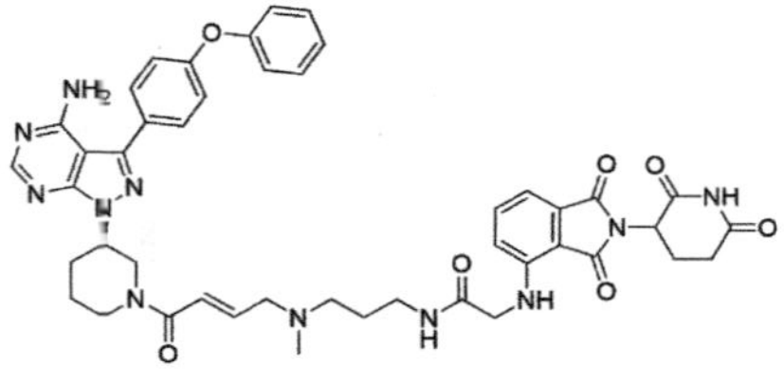

IRC-1

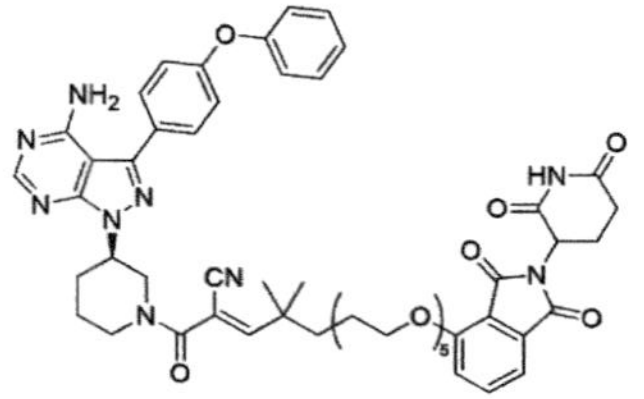

RC-3

Figure 8.3 Chemical structures of covalent and non-covalent BTK PROTACs.

In parallel, they synthesized another non-covalent PROTAC by replacing the acrylamide warhead with propenamide (non-covalent PROTAC 5, Figure 8.3) and found that this reversible PROTAC induced degradation of BTK. Interestingly, the covalent PROTAC 4 induced degradation of two SRC kinases, CSK and LYN, which had been shown to bind ibrutinib in a non-covalent manner [49]. These data suggest that in certain cases, covalent interaction with the target protein may compromise the induced degradation. One potential explanation is that for proteins with fast turnover rate, sufficient engagement on newly synthesized proteins may not be achieved with covalent interaction. Another possibility is that covalent binding of the compound may hinder ubiquitin transfer to the target protein, thereby extenuating degradation.

In another study, Xue et al. developed two covalent PROTACs, one bearing the CRBN recruiter pomalidomide and the other bearing the VHL recruiter VH032 (compounds 3c and 7, Figure 8.3), that both degraded endogenous BTK in K562 cells [50]. The authors also synthesized the corresponding non-covalent PROTACs (compound 9, Figure 8.3) and found that they maintained the capability to degrade BTK but are less potent than the covalent versions. Compared with covalent PROTAC 4 in which the linker is attached to the β carbon of acrylamide, compounds 3c and 7 use a different strategy where the linker is attached to the pyrrolidine ring of ibrutinib, which may explain the difference in the efficacy of BTK degradation. This work indicates that degraders converted from covalent protein inhibitors may retain high target engagement required for efficient degradation, but the position where the linker is introduced could affect the efficiency of target degradation.

Recently, reversible covalent warheads have been explored for ibrutinib-based PROTACs [51, 52]. In one work, Guo et al. reported a cyanoacrylamide derivative of ibrutinib-thalidomide PROTAC, RC-1 (Figure 8.3), and found that this compound degraded BTK in MOLM-14 cells [51]. They also synthesized an irreversible ibrutinib-based PROTAC, IRC-1 (Figure 8.3), and found that BTK engagement of RC-1 is threefold higher than that of IRC-1, indicating the unique dual function of reversible covalent BTK PROTAC as both inhibitor and degrader. Encouragingly, RC-1 is *in vivo* active as a BTK degrader and also showed desirable pharmacokinetics in a mouse model. In another independent work, Gabizon et al. reported a similar cyanoacrylamide-based BTK PROTAC, RC-3 (Figure 8.3), that degraded BTK in Mino cells and patient-derived CLL cells with nanomolar potency [52]. Interestingly, RC-3 does not affect the abundance of CSK and LYN, which was observed as off-targets of BTK degraders in other studies [48, 51], indicating the improved selectivity by installing a reversible covalent warhead on ibrutinib.

8.2.3 KRAS G12C

Another example of covalent PROTAC targets KRAS^{G12C}, a KRAS mutant found in ~13% of lung adenocarcinomas [53]. KRAS was historically considered as "undurggable" [34, 54], but several recent breakthrough studies have successfully targeted KRAS^{G12C} [34, 54–57]. In one study, by conjugating the KRAS^{G12C}

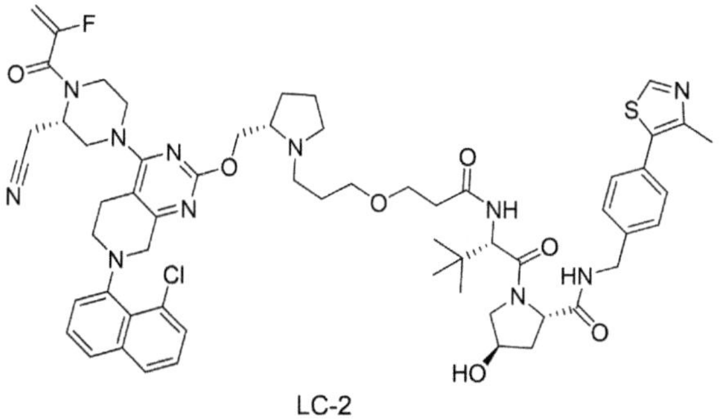

LC-2

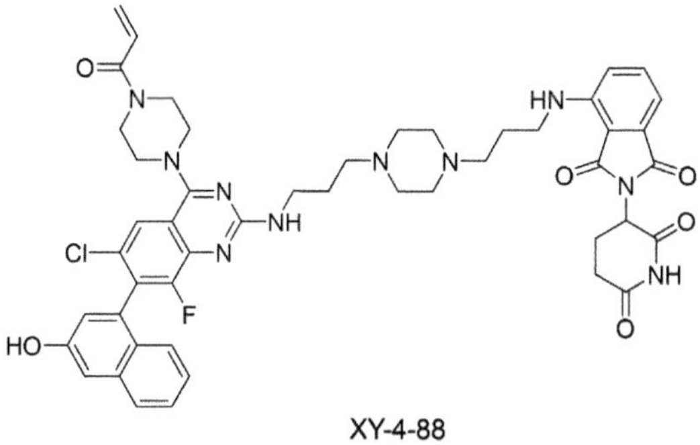

XY-4-88

Figure 8.4 Chemical structures of covalent $KRAS^{G12C}$ PROTACs LC-2 and XY-4-88.

inhibitor MRTX849 to the VHL ligand VH032, Crews and coworkers showed that this PROTAC molecule (LC-2, Figure 8.4) induced degradation of endogenous $KRAS^{G12C}$ in five $KRAS^{G12C}$-expressing cell lines (NCI-H2030, MIA PaCa-2, SW1573, NCI-H23, and NCI-H358) [58]. Interestingly, another study from the Gray lab showed that by conjugating another $KRAS^{G12C}$ covalent ligand, ARS1620 [56], to CRBN ligand thalidomide, the PROTAC molecule (XY-4-88, Figure 8.4) degraded GFP-fused $KRAS^{G12C}$ but not the endogenous $KRAS^{G12C}$ in MIA PaCa2 and NCI-H358 cells [59]. One possibility for this result is that in the presence of XY-4-88, CRBN may not work in a cooperative way and dimerize with endogenous $KRAS^{G12C}$. This challenge may be overcome by hijacking VHL as demonstrated by the Crews lab [58]. These studies also highlight the need for uncovering additional E3 ligases that can be pharmacologically controlled to promote target degradation.

8.2.4 EGFR, ERK1/2, and ERRα

Burslem et al. reported a PROTAC that conjugates afatinib, a covalent inhibitor for epidermal growth factor receptor (EGFR), to a VHL ligand (PROTAC 4, Figure 8.5) and showed that the resulting PROTAC degraded EGFR in H1975 cells [60], a cell

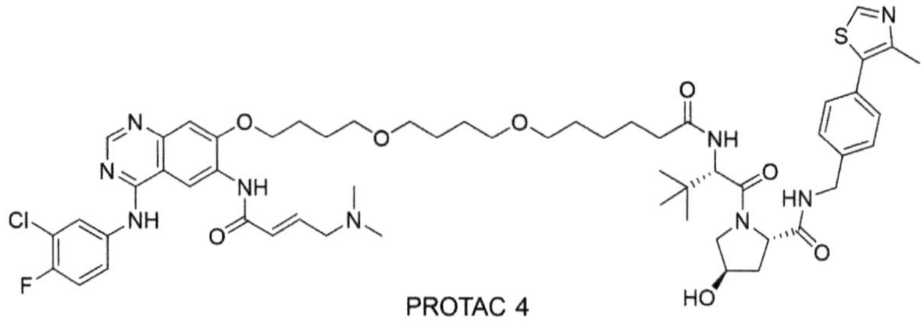

PROTAC 4

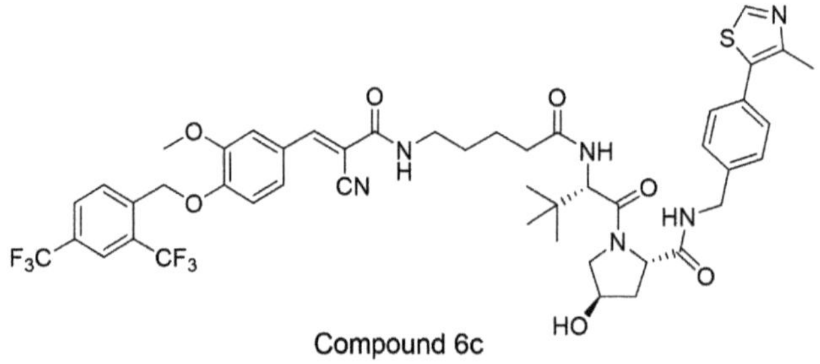

Compound 6c

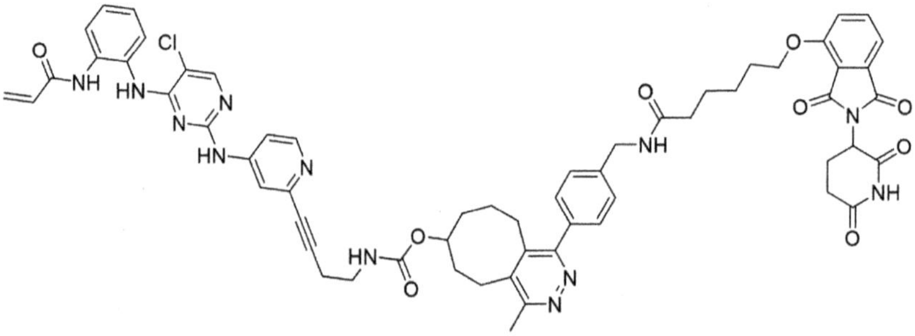

ERK CLIPTAC

Figure 8.5 Chemical structures of covalent EGFR PROTAC (PROTAC 4), ERK1/2 PROTAC (ERK CLIPTAC), and ERRα PROTAC (compound 6c).

model expressing EGFR L858R/T790M double mutant that is resistant to the non-covalent EGFR inhibitor gefitinib [61]. Another study by Lebraud et al. reported a PROTAC that covalently engages and degrades ERK1/2 kinases in HCT116 cells [62]. Interestingly, they used an in-cell bio-orthogonal click approach [63] by employing trans-cyclooctene and tetrazine functional groups. This approach enables the formation of a heterobifunctional PROTAC molecule in cells (ERK click-formed proteolysis targeting chimeras [CLIPTAC], Figure 8.5), which may exhibit improved degradation efficiency as the two individual ligands may better follow Lipinski's rule of 5 than the conjugated heterobifunctional molecule. Another study by Peng et al. developed a reversible covalent binder bearing cyanoacrylamide warhead for estrogen-related receptor alpha (ERRα) [64] and conjugated it to the VHL ligand

VH032. They further showed that the resultant PROTAC is a highly potent degrader for ERRα in MDA-MB-231 cells (compound 6c, Figure 8.5) [64].

8.2.5 Monofunctional Protein Degraders

In addition to heterobifunctional PROTAC molecules, monofunctional molecules that covalently engage POI have also been demonstrated to promote TPD. In one study, Vinogradova et al. reported a compound, EV-3 (Figure 8.6), that promoted the proteasomal degradation of baculoviral IAP repeat containing 2 (BIRC2) and baculoviral IAP repeat containing 3 (BIRC3) in primary human T cells [65]. Mutating BIRC2 Cys45 and BIRC3 Cys28 to alanine fully blocked EV-3-mediated BIRC2 and BIRC3 degradation, which reflects a mechanism of action involving covalent engagement of BIRC2 Cys45 and BIRC3 Cys28 by EV-3. In the same study, the authors reported another compound, EV-96 (Figure 8.6), that promoted proteasomal degradation of tyrosine-protein kinase ITK in stimulated human T cells. In this case, the mechanism of action may involve covalently engaging ITK Cys442 by the compound [65]. Interestingly, in another study by Seixas et al., compound JS25 (Figure 8.6) covalently engaged Cys496 of the bone marrow tyrosine kinase in chromosome X (BMX) and induced its degradation [66]. For both studies, covalently engaging POI may expose a hydrophobic moiety on protein surface and subsequently trigger the cellular quality control for target degradation. The ligand-substrate adduct may also recruit an E3 ubiquitin ligase that functions independent of the quality control machinery. In either case, identifying the E3 ubiquitin ligases that drive the target degradation could provide more insights into the mechanism of action of these monofunctional degraders. Compared with heterobifunctional degraders, monofunctional degraders may better follow Lipinski's rule of 5 and have ideal pharmacokinetic properties. However, the challenge is that the approach to discover such molecules may not be generalizable, as each degrader may have unique mechanism of action to induce the imperative ternary complex formation.

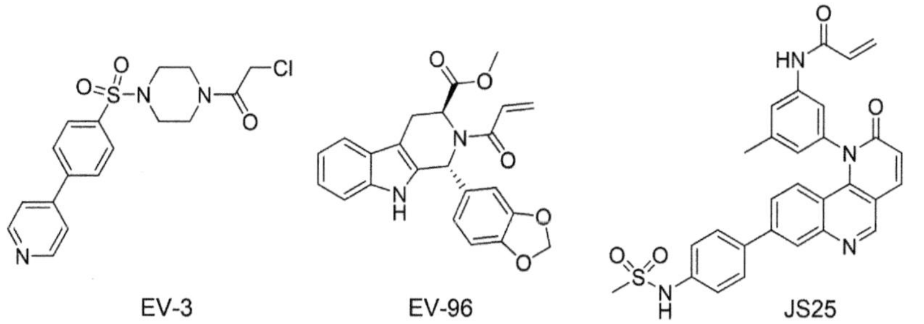

Figure 8.6 Chemical structures of monofunctional degraders EV-3 (BIRC2 and BIRC3 degrader), EV-96 (ITK degrader), and JS25 (BMX degrader).

8.3 Protein Degraders that Covalently Interact with E3 Ubiquitin Ligases

As mentioned above, diverse proteins have been demonstrated to undergo ligand-induced degradation in cells. Despite these successful case studies, only a handful of over 600 human E3 ubiquitin ligases have been found to support TPD [10, 67–71], with most studies harnessing established ligands for CRBN and VHL. Importantly, these E3 ubiquitin ligases have been found to show restricted substrate specificities, which are not yet easily controlled or predicated [72, 73]. These limitations underscore the need for discovering additional hijackable E3 ubiquitin ligases, especially the ones with differentiated properties, to expand the substate scope of TPD.

In recent years, many groups reported additional E3 ubiquitin ligases and the paired ligands that can be co-opted to promote TPD. Interestingly, many of these discoveries employ covalent chemistry. Compared with the previously well-established non-covalent E3 binders, covalent ligands for E3 ubiquitin ligase may offer several advantages in developing effective protein degraders. First, the covalent interaction between the electrophilic ligand and the E3 ubiquitin ligase has been found to facilitate ligand-induced protein degradation at low fractional engagement of E3 ubiquitin ligase [37–39], indicating that covalent protein degraders may support TPD while minimally perturbing the endogenous substrates of E3 ubiquitin ligase, leaving the endogenous substrates to be degraded by the predominantly unmodified E3 ligase. Second, the covalent interaction enables ligand-induced protein degradation to proceed via a pseudo-binary complex between the substrate and the ligand-E3 adduct. This is different from the mechanism of action of non-covalent PROTACs, which form ternary complexes that must accommodate two reversible interaction interfaces to support TPD. Third, the covalent interaction may also improve the durability of target degradation in biological systems, as loss of degradation activity should correlate with turnover of the E3 ubiquitin ligase versus clearance of the covalent degrader. In this section, we will summarize the E3 ubiquitin ligases that can be covalently engaged by small molecules to support TPD.

8.3.1 RNF4

Ward et al. found that RNF4, an E3 ubiquitin ligase that recognizes SUMOylated proteins and promotes their ubiquitination and subsequent degradation [74, 75], possessed reactive cysteines that were labeled by tetramethylrhodamine-5-iodoacetamide *in vitro* [36]. They further employed gel-based activity-based protein profiling (ABPP) to screen for compounds that engage RNF4-reactive cysteines, leading to the identification of TRH 1-23 (Figure 8.7). Mass spectrometry analysis further revealed that TRH 1-23 engaged one of the two zinc-coordinating cysteines Cys132 and Cys135 on RNF4. Next, the authors employed a medicinal chemistry campaign and identified CCW16 (Figure 8.7) that exerts improved potency

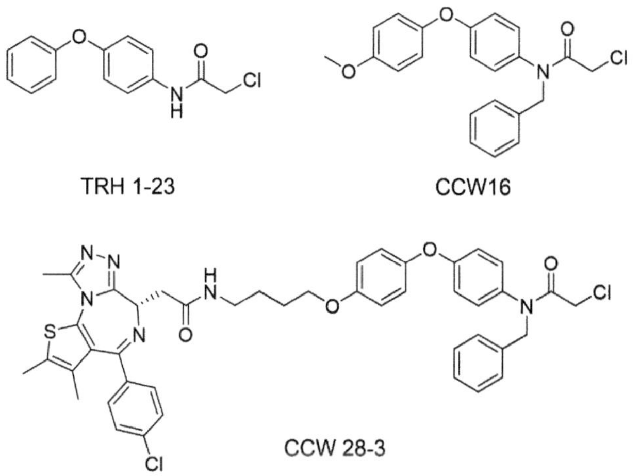

Figure 8.7 Chemical structures of ligands for RNF4 (TRH 1-23 and CCW16) and the PROTAC (CCW 28-3) that covalently engages RNF4 for BRD4 degradation.

against RNF4. Prompted by these results, they synthesized a PROTAC molecule (CCW 28-3, Figure 8.7) by conjugating CCW 16 to JQ1, an inhibitor for BET bromodomain family [76], and demonstrated that it degraded BRD4 in a RNF4-dependent manner in HeLa cells [36].

8.3.2 RNF114

In another work, Spradlin et al. initially aimed at identifying the protein targets of the electrophilic natural product, nimbolide (Figure 8.8), that shows anti-cancer activity [77, 78]. By employing an ABPP-based chemical proteomic approach, they identified the E3 ubiquitin ligase RNF114 as the target that is directly engaged by nimbolide and plays a critical role in nimbolide-mediated anti-proliferation in breast cancer cells [38]. Mechanistically, nimbolide modifies Cys8 in the intrinsically disordered region of RNF114. This covalent interaction disrupts the binding between RNF114 and its native protein substrate p21, a well-established tumor suppressor [79], leading to its stabilization. The authors then utilized nimbolide as an RNF114 recruiter and generated a heterobifunctional PROTAC targeting BRD4 (XH2, Figure 8.8). By Western blotting and mass spectrometry-based whole proteome analyses, they showed that XH2 degraded BRD4 in a RNF114-dependent manner [38].

Nimbolide is a complex natural product that presents a high bar for chemical synthesis. To translate this functional natural product into fully synthetic small molecules that would facilitate the application of RNF114 for PROTAC development, in a follow-up work, the authors identified a fully synthetic ligand for RNF114 (EN219, Figure 8.8) and used it to degrade two oncogenic proteins, BRD4 (ML 2-14) and BCR-ABL (ML 2-23) (Figure 8.8) [80].

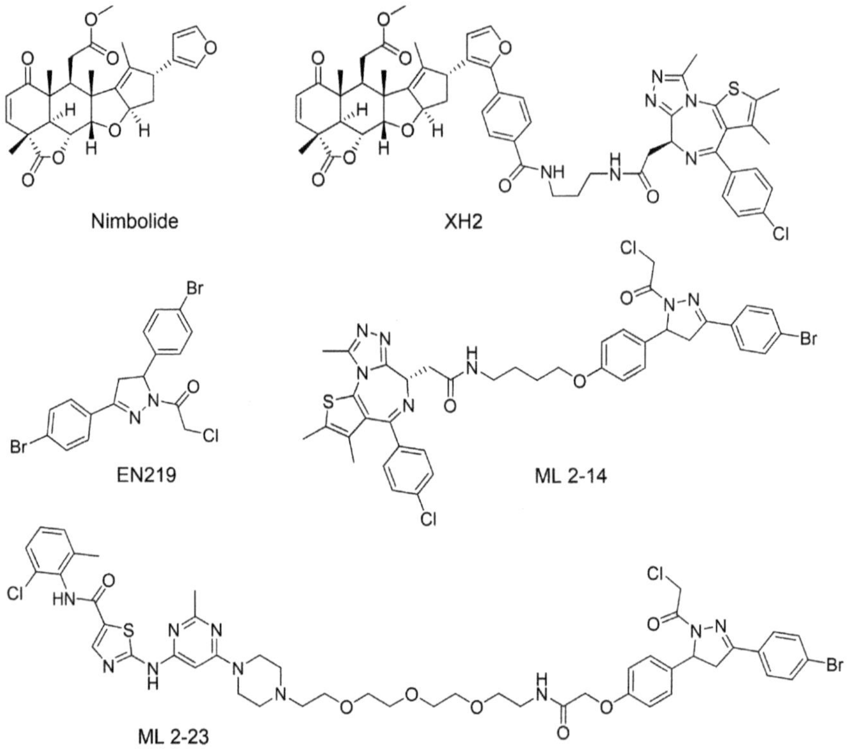

Figure 8.8 Chemical structures of natural product (nimbolide) and the synthetic ligand (EN219) for RNF114 and their corresponding PROTACs (XH2 is a BRD4 degrader bearing nimbolide, and ML 2-14 and ML 2-23 are BRD4 and BCR-ABL degraders, respectively, that bear EN219 as RNF114 recruiter).

8.3.3 KEAP1

KEAP1 is best recognized as the E3 ubiquitin ligase targeting transcription factor NRF2 for proteasomal degradation [81–83]. KEAP1 contains a number of reactive cysteines (Cys151, Cys226, Cys273, Cys288, and Cys613) and serves as an oxidative stress sensor. Covalent modification of KEAP1 by various endogenous electrophiles, such as 4-hydroxynonenal (4-HNE) and 15-deoxy-Δ12,14-prostaglandin J2 (15d-PGJ2), blocks NRF2 degradation, leading to the nuclear accumulation and activation of NRF2 [84]. From PROTAC development perspective, KEAP1 has been demonstrated to promote target degradation when recruited by a peptide sequence [85] or a non-covalent binder [86]. Based on the triterpene derivative bardoxolone methyl (CDDO-Me, Figure 8.9), an electrophilic natural product targeting KEAP1 [87], Tong et al. developed a PROTAC by conjugating CDDO-Me to JQ1 and showed that CDDO-JQ1 (Figure 8.9) degraded BRD4 in 231MFP cells [88]. Notably, at 1 and 5 μM, CDDO-JQ1 also destabilizes KEAP1, while at lower concentrations (0.2 and 0.05 μM), CDDO-JQ1 induces robust BRD4 degradation without affecting KEAP1 abundance. These findings suggest that extra cautions need to be taken

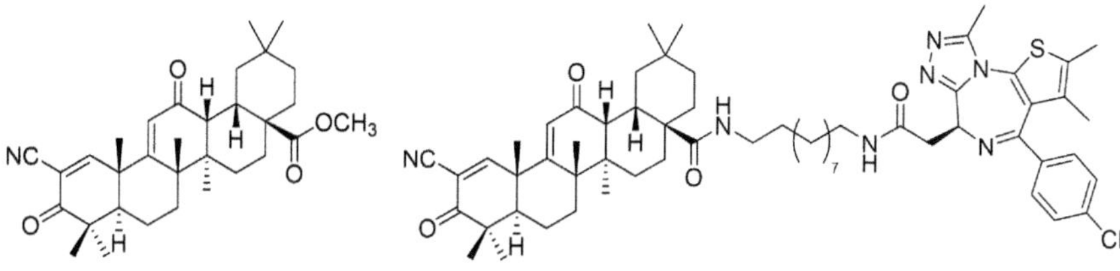

Figure 8.9 Chemical structures of the natural product CDDO-Me as a ligand for KEAP1 and the CDDO-Me-based KEAP1 recruiter for BRD4 PROTAC (CDDO-JQ1) development.

when employing KEAP1 for target degradation; thus, KEAP1 would stay in the catalytic cycle without being degraded by the PROTAC molecule.

8.3.4 FEM1B

FEM1B is an E3 ubiquitin ligase that was recently identified as a critical regulator for cellular reductive stress [89]. Cys186 plays an essential role in FEM1B-mediated substrate recognition, pointing to a possibility of using small molecules to engage FEM1B Cys186 for TPD. To this end, Henning et al. screened a focused library containing 566 cysteine-reactive electrophiles and identified EN106 as a hit compound that engaged FEM1B Cys186 (Figure 8.10) [90]. Inspired by this discovery, the authors further synthesized a PROTAC molecule, NJH-01-106 (Figure 8.10), by conjugating EN106 to JQ1 and showed that NJH-01-106 degraded BRD4 in HEK293T cells in a FEM1B-dependent manner. Whole proteome analysis further revealed that NJH-01-106-induced degradation was BRD4 selective, with only one off-target identify (PNMAL1) [90].

8.3.5 SPSB2

A recent study by Pinch et al. reported a platform, named covalent functionalization followed by E3 electroporation into live cells (COFFEE), that bypasses the ligand discovery step and allows direct evaluation of selected E3 ubiquitin ligases for their degradative activity [91]. In this approach, the authors coupled a ligand for a POI to maleimide, a cysteine-reactive handle, and used this PROTAC precursor to

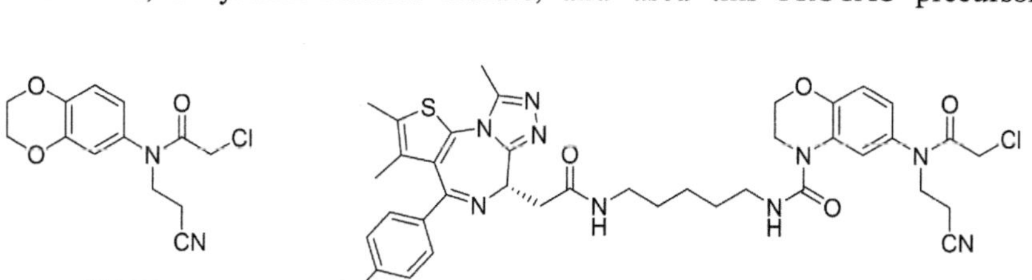

Figure 8.10 Chemical structures of ligand for FEM1B (EN106) and FEM1B-based BRD4 PROTAC (NJH-01-106).

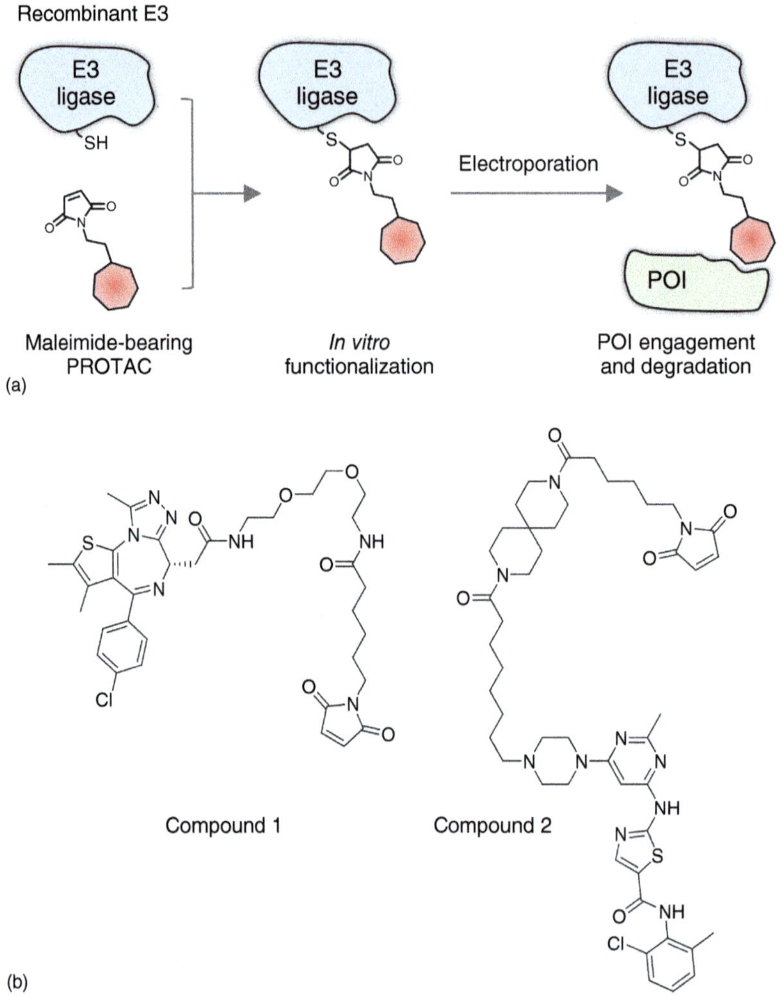

Figure 8.11 Covalent functionalization followed by E3 electroporation into live cells (COFFEE) is a platform that leverages covalent chemistry to identify E3 ubiquitin ligases that support TPD. (a) Scheme showing the concept of COFFEE. (b) Chemical structures of compounds 1 and 2 as JQ1- and dasatinib-based PROTACs, respectively.

covalently engage the recombinantly purified E3 of interest *in vitro* (Figure 8.11a). This "functionalized" E3-ligand adduct was then electroporated into cells to recruit POI for TPD (Figure 8.11a). This approach not only allows potent ligand engagement on the E3 ubiquitin ligase of interest but also achieves a E3-ligand selective interaction, thereby providing a powerful avenue to evaluate individual E3s for their ability to support TPD. As a proof of concept, they showed that by functionalizing VHL Cys77, they could degrade BRD4 and multiple kinases by using JQ1 and dasatinib as the substrate recruiters, respectively (Figure 8.11b). Next, by using the same dasatinib-based compound, the authors found that a SOCS box E3 ligase, SPSB2, can be chemically controlled to degrade ABL1 and Lyn kinases. Although cellularly active ligands for the E3 ubiquitin ligase are still to be identified, this platform provides valuable information regarding whether a certain E3 ubiquitin ligase is hijackable for TPD. Functionalizing other nucleophilic amino acids on selected E3 ubiquitin ligases for TPD could be an interesting direction for further investigation.

8.3.6 DCAF16

The discovery of the E3 ubiquitin ligases (RNF4, RNF114, KEAP1, FEM1B, and SPSB2) for TPD utilizes a target-based approach, in which ligand–E3 interaction is first evaluated, followed by the examination of whether such interaction leads to target degradation. Recently, we developed a "function-first" approach to discover novel E3 ubiquitin ligases that can be pharmacologically controlled for TPD. In one study [39], we generated three heterobifunctional PROTACs (Figure 8.12) bearing a selective ligand for FKBP12, synthetic ligand of FKBP12 (SLF), coupled to a broadly cysteine-reactive electrophilic fragment (KB02, KB03, or KB05) that engages a number of E3 ubiquitin ligases [92] and measured if any compound degraded cytosolic- or nuclear-localized FKBP12. We found that one compound, KB02-SLF (Figure 8.12), degraded nuclear but not cytosolic FKBP12. Further evidence revealed that this degradation was mediated by cullin-RING ubiquitin ligases (CRLs), as the neddylation inhibitor MLN4924 [93] that inhibits CRL activity fully blocked KB02-SLF-induced FKBP12 degradation. We initially attempted to identify KB02-SLF-engaged E3 ubiquitin ligase(s) by a mass spectrometry-based method isoTOP-ABPP (isotopic tandem orthogonal proteolysis-activity-based protein profiling) [92, 94] but did not find any CRL(s) that were strongly engaged (>75%) on cysteines. One possibility is that KB02-SLF engages a CRL in a low stoichiometry manner, which can be catalytically active for TPD but is challenging to be mapped by competition-based methods such as isoTOP-ABPP. We then employed an affinity purification mass spectrometry (AP-MS) approach to capture low stoichiometrically engaged proteins, in which substrate FKBP12 enrichment was performed to identify ligand-dependent associated proteins. This approach identified two CRLs, DCAF16 and DTL, that were enriched (>5-fold) in KB02-SLF-treated cells compared to DMSO-treated cells. Using small-hairpin RNA (shRNA)-mediated knockdown and CRISPR-mediated knockout, we confirmed that DCAF16, but not DTL, mediated KB02-SLF-induced FKBP12 degradation. By employing mass spectrometry and mutagenesis approaches, we found that KB02-SLF covalently modified one of the three consecutive cysteines (Cys177, 178, and 179) on DCAF16 and further showed that the engagement on these sites plays an essential role in promoting FKBP12 degradation. We then synthesized another PROTAC by conjugating KB02 to JQ1 and found that KB02-JQ1 degraded BRD4 in HEK293T cells (Figure 8.12) [39]. Finally, by using a multiplexing and quantitative ABPP method, we found that KB02-SLF and KB02-JQ1 produced ~10% and 40% engagement, respectively, of the DCAF16 peptide containing the three

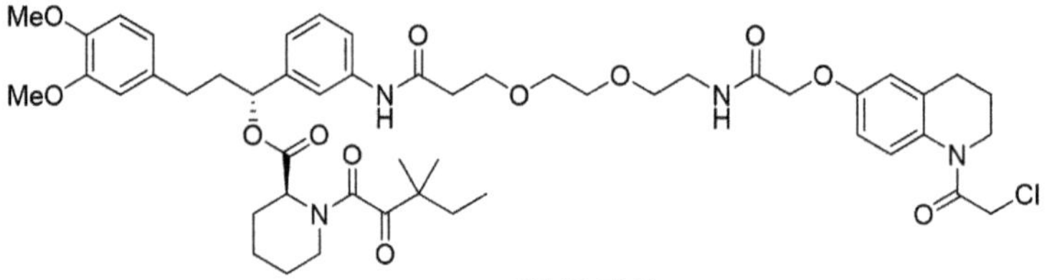

KB02-SLF

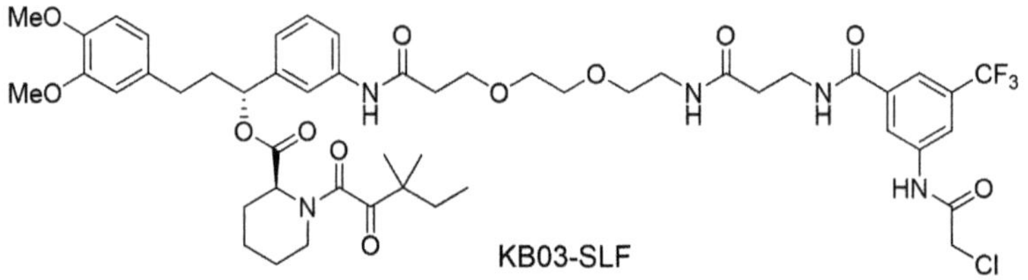

KB03-SLF

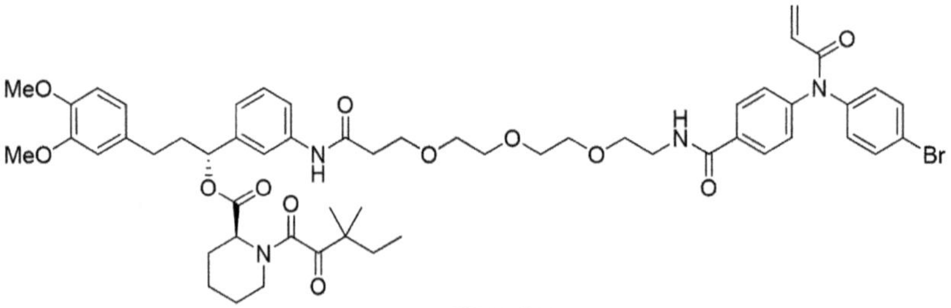

KB05-SLF

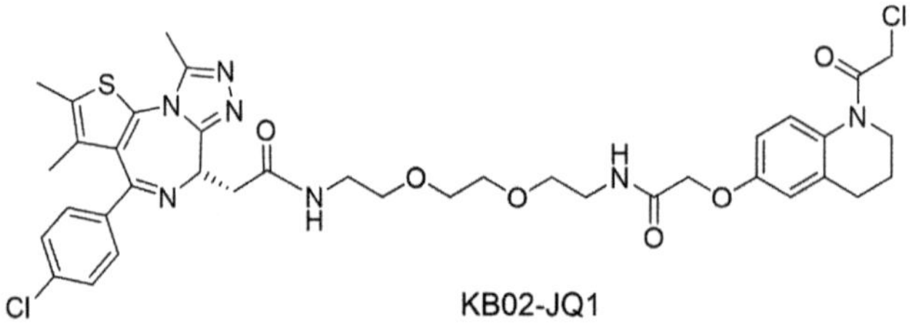

KB02-JQ1

Figure 8.12 Leveraging PROTACs bearing a selective substrate-bound ligand (SLF for FKBP12 and JQ1 for BRD4) and a fragment-based "scout" ligand (KB02, KB03, or KB05) to discover E3 ubiquitin ligases that support TPD.

consecutive cysteines. This finding indicates that low stoichiometric engagement on DCAF16 is sufficient to drive efficient target degradation. The low fractional engagement of DCAF16 may also minimally perturb endogenous substrates of DCAF16, as those substrates could be degraded by the unmodified DCAF16. This study not only underscores the value of using broadly reactive scout fragments to discover ligandable and functional sites on poorly characterized proteins, but also shows the feasibility of using "function-first" approach to simultaneously discover novel E3 ubiquitin ligases with the paired ligands that can be co-opted to promote target degradation. One caveat is that the PROTACs bearing scout fragments in this study still modify a number of other proteins in cells, which may limit the application of these early-stage compounds in biological studies. Therefore, developing advanced DCAF16 ligands with improved potency and selectivity should be a fertile area of future investigation.

8.3.7 DCAF11

Encouraged by the discovery of DCAF16 as a ligandable E3 ubiquitin ligase for TPD, we hypothesized that by expanding the library of electrophilic heterobifunctional compounds and measuring the target degradation across a broader panel of cell lines, we may identify additional E3 ubiquitin ligases and their ligands for TPD. To this end, we synthesized a focused library of 26 candidate electrophilic PROTACs bearing a ligand for FKBP12 coupled to a structurally varied electrophilic group and screened them in four human cancer cell lines (H1975, H2122, 22Rv1, and BxPC-3) expressing cytosolic or nuclear localized FKBP12 fused to luciferase (Figure 8.13a) [37]. A hit compound, 21-SLF (Figure 8.13b), was found to degrade both cytosolic and nuclear localized FKBP12 in prostate cancer cell line 22Rv1. 21-SLF-induced FKBP12 degradation was mediated by a CRL, as the neddylation inhibitor MLN4924 fully blocked the degradation. We next employed a similar proteomic approach as described in the DCAF16 story to identify proteins that were associated with FKBP12 in the presence of 21-SLF. This experiment led to the identification of a single CRL – DCAF11. Knocking out DCAF11 in 22Rv1 cells abolished 21-SLF-induced FKBP12 degradation, indicating an essential role of DCAF11 in 21-SLF-mediated FKBP12 degradation. In order to identify DCAF11 cysteines involved in 21-SLF-induced FKBP12 degradation, we used mutagenesis approach and found that 21-SLF may promote FKBP12 degradation through engaging multiple cysteines, as none of the single cysteine mutants completely blocked the degradation. It turns out that mutating three cysteines in DCAF11 (Cys443, Cys460, and Cys485) completely blocked 21-SLF-induced degradation of FKBP12. By comparing DCAF11 with the U5 subunit of human spliceosome, a homolog that shares a similar WD40-repeat (WDR) domain to DCAF11, we hypothesized that Cys443, Cys460, and Cys485 on DCAF11 are in proximity, and engaging any of them by 21-SLF could lead to FKBP12 degradation. Nevertheless, C460A single mutant partially blocked 21-SLF-induced FKBP12 degradation, while C443A/C485A double mutant showed similar degradation activity to wild type (WT) DCAF11. This indicates that C460 is likely the preferred liganded cysteine in WT DCAF11. From ligand discovery perspective, developing advanced ligand targeting DCAF11 Cys460 might be sufficient for TPD. Finally, we synthesized another PROTAC (21-ARL, Figure 8.13b) bearing the DCAF11 recruiter and an androgen receptor (AR) ligand [95, 96] and showed that 21-ARL degraded AR in 22Rv1 DCAF11 WT but not knockout (KO) cells. Interestingly, 21-SLF induced FKBP12 degradation in 22Rv1 but not the other tested cell lines. Although DCAF11 is expressed in all these cell

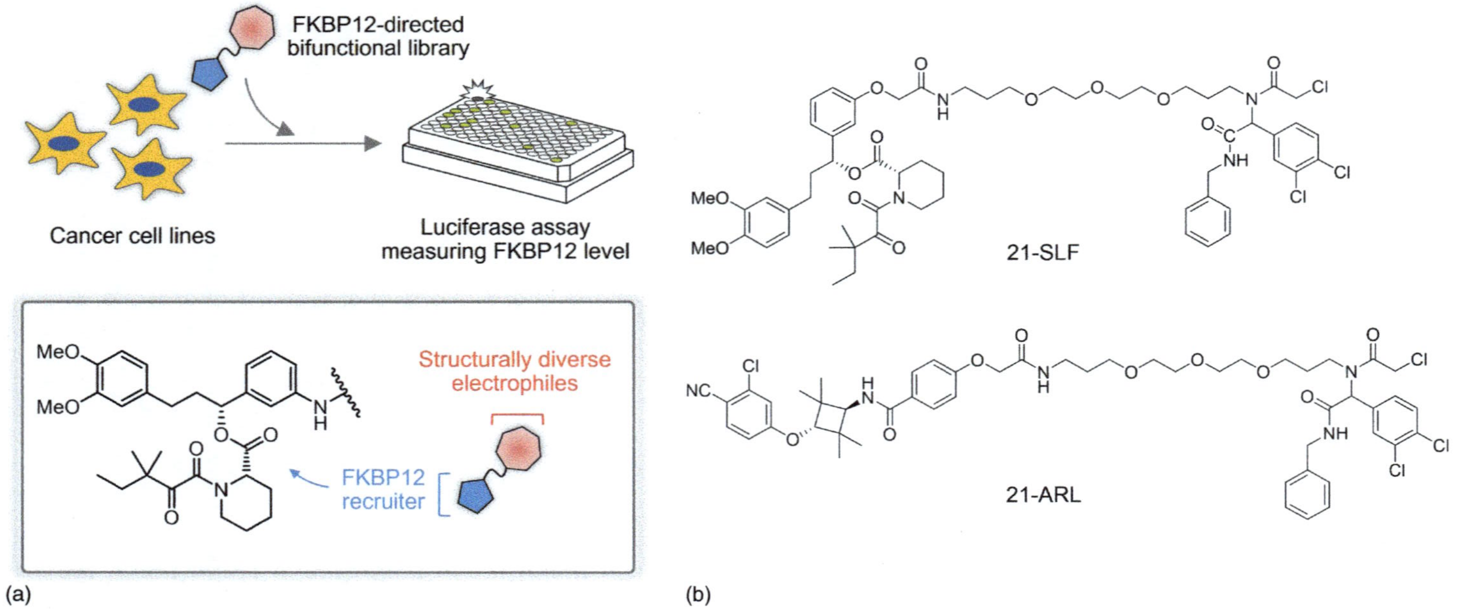

Figure 8.13 Discovery of DCAF11 as a ligandable E3 ubiquitin ligase for TPD. (a) Scheme showing the platform that integrates a focused electrophilic heterobifunctional compound library and luciferase assay to discover E3 ubiquitin ligases for TPD. (b) Chemical structures of 21-SLF (FKBP12 degrader) and 21-ARL (AR degrader).

lines, it has higher abundance in 22Rv1 than other tested cell lines [97], leading to a hypothesis that DCAF11 might be a privileged E3 ubiquitin ligase in prostate cancer cells for TPD. Moreover, the integrated functional assay and chemical proteomic platform described in this study can be further expanded in order to discover additional E3 ubiquitin ligases with differential properties. Another future direction is to employ a medicinal chemistry campaign to improve the potency and selectivity of electrophilic PROTACs acting through DCAF11.

8.4 Technologies for Covalent Protein Degrader Discovery

Isotopic tandem orthogonal proteolysis-activity-based protein profiling (isoTOP-ABPP) is a method that quantitatively and site specifically identifies protein targets of covalent ligands on a proteome-wide scale [94, 98]. This method facilitates the identification of ligands that covalently engage E3 ubiquitin ligases. These ligands can be subsequently converted into bifunctional PROTACs by conjugating with a second ligand for POI. This method can also identify ligands covalently engaging substrate proteins. Those ligands, regardless of their effect on target function, can be converted into functional PROTAC degraders by conjugating with an E3 recruiter. A typical isoTOP-ABPP setup is to pretreat intact cells or cell lysates with cysteine reactive electrophiles, followed by labeling with a broad-spectrum cysteine-reactive probe, such as iodoacetamide (IA)-alkyne (Figure 8.14). Proteins labeled with IA-alkyne on cysteine residues are conjugated with isotopically labeled azide-biotin tags (heavy and light, Figure 8.14) by copper-mediated "click" chemistry [99]. Next, "Heavy"- and "light"-labeled samples are combined, enriched by streptavidin, and proteolytically digested to yield isotopic peptides that are analyzed by liquid chromatography–mass spectrometry (LC–MS). MS1 chromatographic peaks are quantified for the comparison of "heavy"- and "light"-labeled peptides. IsoTOP-ABPP performed on a proteome-wide scale can simultaneously provide quantitation and selectivity information. By using this technology, the Nomura lab identified E3 ubiquitin ligase RNF114 as the target of electrophile nimbolide and further demonstrated that the interaction between nimbolide and RNF114 can be exploited to promote TPD [38].

With multiplexing mass spectrometry technology [100], a tandem mass tag (TMT)-ABPP-based method has been reported to study ligand–cysteine interaction on a proteome-wide scale [65]. Compared with isoTOP-ABPP for pairwise comparison, TMT-ABPP uses isobaric labeling approach and can multiplex up to 18 samples in a single MS run (Figure 8.15). The maximum number for multiplexing is still growing [101]. Multiplexing mass spectrometry increases the throughput of covalent ligand discovery [37, 39, 65]. On the one hand, isoTOP-ABPP and TMT-ABPP can be employed to identify protein targets of electrophilic compounds [38, 65].

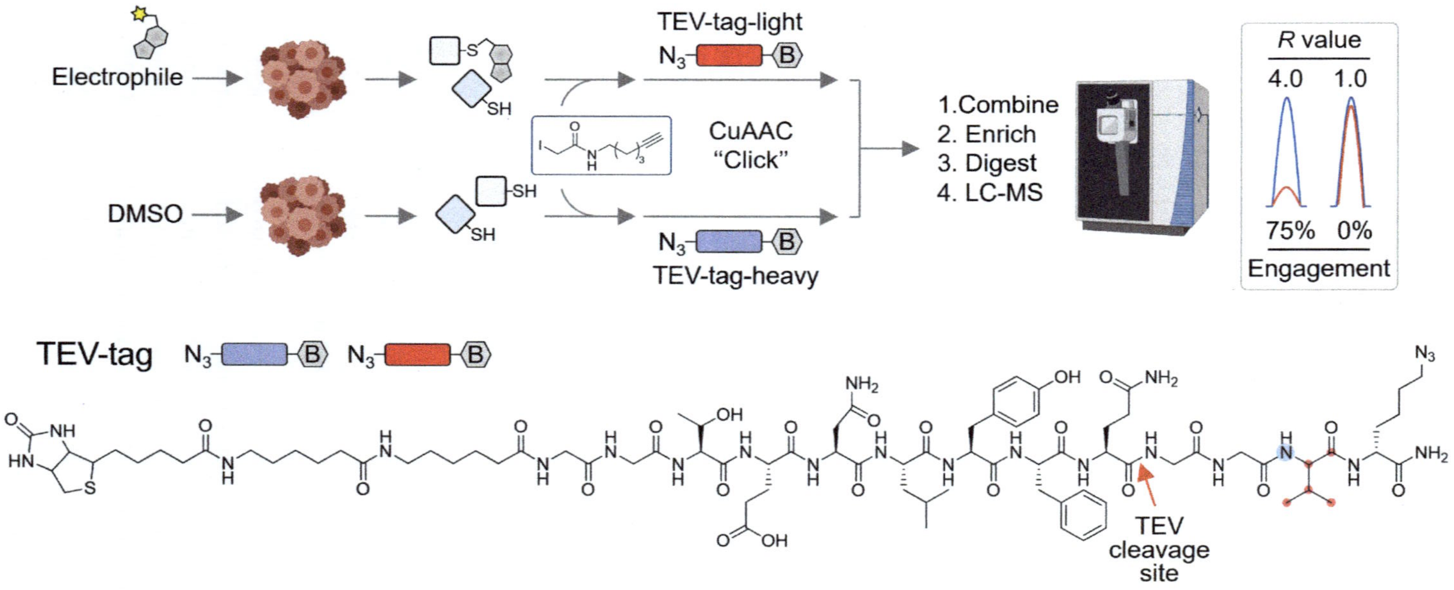

Figure 8.14 IsoTOP-ABPP technology for covalent binder discovery on a proteome-wide scale.

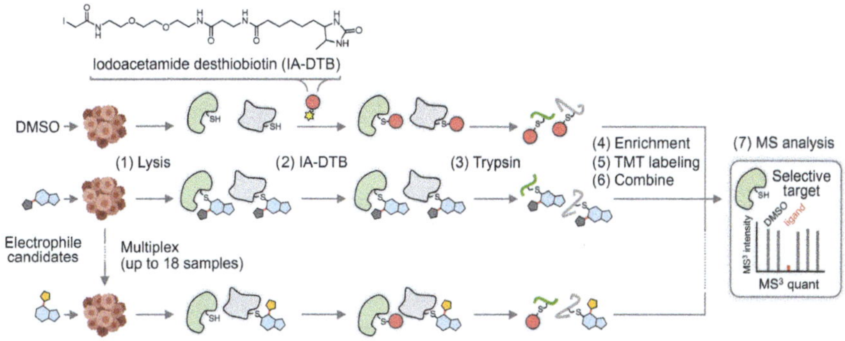

Figure 8.15 TMT-ABPP technology for covalent binder discovery on a proteome-wide scale.

One the other hand, they can quantitatively measure ligand engagement on E3 ubiquitin ligases and POIs, thereby providing stoichiometry information. Two DCAF16-based PROTACs have been shown to engage 10% and 40% engagement of the DCAF16 peptide containing Cys177-179 at pharmacologically relevant concentrations [39]. In the case of DCAF11, the PROTAC 21-SLF also shows modest (~10%) engagement of DCAF11 Cys460 at the concentration that induces FKBP12 degradation [37].

Another technology for covalent ligand-target discovery has been developed in which a focused electrophile library is screened against purified proteins. A mass shift on an intact protein indicates a covalent ligand-target adduct [102]. In the same study, the authors focused on one deubiquitinase OTUB2 and one pyrophosphatase NUDT7, suggesting the applicability of this approach to diverse proteins. Going forward, this platform can be applied to discover ligands against E3 ubiquitin ligases and POIs. Those ligands can be further converted into bifunctional protein degraders.

The COFFEE platform is a powerful approach to discover functional E3 ligases with reactive cysteines that support TPD [91]. With this information, one can further employ rational drug design or high-throughput screening (HTS) approach to identify elaborated ligands that engage E3 ubiquitin ligases in cells. Converting these ligands into bifunctional degraders for TPD would facilitate the application of these ligands in biological studies and therapeutics.

If "function-first" approach is used to identify the functional degraders, followed by the deconvolution of degrader-engaged E3 ligases, the E3 ligases that show low stoichiometric ligand engagement may not be identified using competition based approaches such as isoTOP-ABPP and TMT-ABPP [39]. This limitation can be overcome by an enrichment-based approach, as we described above for DCAF16 and DCAF11 [37, 39]. In both cases, low fractional engagement is sufficient to promote target degradation; therefore, this enrichment-based approach would serve as a powerful alternative approach to discover ligand-engaged E3 ubiquitin ligases.

8.5 Outlook of Leveraging Covalent Chemistry for Targeted Protein Degradation

As of date, all covalent E3 recruiters and most covalent substrate binders target cysteine, an intrinsically reactive amino acid [103] that tends to react with various electrophilic reactive groups [104]. A study by the Cravatt lab in 2016 [92] used a fragment-based covalent ligand discovery approach and identified 700+ ligandable cysteines in the human proteome. Their more recent study has expanded this number to 3000+ on functionally and structurally diverse proteins in human T cells [65]. These studies point to a large space to be explored to identify covalent ligands that target cysteine residues. In addition, chemical probes that selectively target other nucleophilic non-cysteine amino acids, including lysine [105, 106], serine [107], tyrosine [108], histidine [109], aspartate [110], and glutamate [110], have been reported, indicating the possibility of covalently engaging additional amino acids for protein degrader development. For instance, in two recent studies that aim at profiling proteome-wide lysine reactivity by lysine reactive probes [105, 106], the authors identified several E3 ubiquitin ligases that were engaged by lysine-reactive probes (for example, TRIM28 K377, TRIM25 K335, and RNF40 K420). Investigating whether these lysine reactive binders can be converted into functional degraders would be a fertile future direction. On the target side, these novel covalent interactions could facilitate expanding the ligandable and degradable proteome by conjugating these ligands to well-established E3 recruiters.

Covalent ligands have the potential to engage non-functional binding sites on previously intractable proteins [92, 105]. Such "silent" binding event can be transformed into functional degraders through a PROTAC or hydrophobic tagging [13] campaign and therefore has the potential to expand the druggable proteome. In the future, leveraging those previously identified but overlooked silent binding sites on target proteins for degrader development would be a fruitful direction to expand the degradome.

One limitation of leveraging covalent chemistry for protein degrader development is that mutation on the liganded amino acid may diminish or abolish drug action, as the covalent bond formation is the main driving force for target engagement and degradation. Expanding chemical and E3 toolbox that support TPD could overcome the limitation when certain mutation inactivates E3 ubiquitin ligase's capability for TPD. Identifying additional binding sites on the same substrate or E3 ubiquitin ligase may also overcome mutation-mediated drug resistance. Another limitation of covalent protein degrader is that for substrate/E3 ubiquitin ligase that has fast turnover rate, covalent interaction may hinder the overall degradation efficiency, as covalently targeting those substrates/E3 ubiquitin ligases may make the degraders lose the catalytic feature. Nevertheless, as some fast turnover "undruggable" proteins (for example, Myc) have been targeted using covalent chemistry [35], pursuing covalent degraders for those proteins can still be a promising direction. It should be noted that there are significant interests and applications in both covalent and non-covalent space. In certain cases, we could even consider combining both approaches to achieve maximum target degradation. As we move forward, investigating both covalent and non-covalent POI degraders and choosing the more effective one should be the right practice.

Acknowledgment

Xiaoyu Zhang was supported by the National Cancer Institute of the National Institutes of Health under Award Number R00CA248715 and the Damon-Runyon Cancer Research Foundation (DFS-53-22).

References

1 Samarasinghe, K.T.G. and Crews, C.M. (2021). Targeted protein degradation: a promise for undruggable proteins. *Cell Chem. Biol.* 28 (7): 934–951.
2 De, S., Karim, F., Kiessu, E. et al. (2018). Mechanism of dysfunction of human variants of the IRAK4 kinase and a role for its kinase activity in interleukin-1 receptor signaling. *J. Biol. Chem.* 293 (39): 15208–15220.
3 Nalawansha, D.A. and Crews, C.M. (2020). PROTACs: an emerging therapeutic modality in precision medicine. *Cell Chem. Biol.* 27 (8): 998–1014.
4 Kozicka, Z. and Thoma, N.H. (2021). Haven't got a glue: protein surface variation for the design of molecular glue degraders. *Cell Chem. Biol.* 28 (7): 1032–1047.
5 Kronke, J., Fink, E.C., Hollenbach, P.W. et al. (2015). Lenalidomide induces ubiquitination and degradation of CK1alpha in del(5q) MDS. *Nature* 523 (7559): 183–188.
6 Kronke, J., Udeshi, N.D., Narla, A. et al. (2014). Lenalidomide causes selective degradation of IKZF1 and IKZF3 in multiple myeloma cells. *Science* 343 (6168): 301–305.
7 Lu, G., Middleton, R.E., Sun, H. et al. (2014). The myeloma drug lenalidomide promotes the cereblon-dependent destruction of Ikaros proteins. *Science* 343 (6168): 305–309.
8 Mullard, A. (2021). Targeted protein degraders crowd into the clinic. *Nat. Rev. Drug Discov.* 20 (4): 247–250.
9 Weng, G., Shen, C., Cao, D. et al. (2021). PROTAC-DB: an online database of PROTACs. *Nucleic Acids Res.* 49 (D1): D1381–D1387.
10 Sakamoto, K.M., Kim, K.B., Kumagai, A. et al. (2001). Protacs: chimeric molecules that target proteins to the Skp1-Cullin-F box complex for ubiquitination and degradation. *Proc. Natl. Acad. Sci. U.S.A.* 98 (15): 8554–8559.
11 Ohoka, N., Okuhira, K., Ito, M. et al. (2017). *in vivo* knockdown of pathogenic proteins via specific and nongenetic inhibitor of apoptosis protein (IAP)-dependent protein erasers (SNIPERs). *J. Biol. Chem.* 292 (11): 4556–4570.
12 Clift, D., McEwan, W.A., Labzin, L.I. et al. (2017). A method for the acute and rapid degradation of endogenous proteins. *Cell* 171 (7): 1692–1706.e18.

13 Neklesa, T.K., Tae, H.S., Schneekloth, A.R. et al. (2011). Small-molecule hydrophobic tagging-induced degradation of HaloTag fusion proteins. *Nat. Chem. Biol.* 7 (8): 538–543.

14 Chamberlain, P.P. and Cathers, B.E. (2019). Cereblon modulators: low molecular weight inducers of protein degradation. *Drug Discov. Today Technol.* 31: 29–34.

15 Samarasinghe, K.T.G., Jaime-Figueroa, S., Burgess, M. et al. (2021). Targeted degradation of transcription factors by TRAFTACs: transcription factor targeting chimeras. *Cell Chem. Biol.* 28 (5): 648–661.e5.

16 Takahashi, D., Moriyama, J., Nakamura, T. et al. (2019). AUTACs: cargo-specific degraders using selective autophagy. *Mol. Cell* 76 (5): 797–810.e10.

17 Banik, S.M., Pedram, K., Wisnovsky, S. et al. (2020). Lysosome-targeting chimaeras for degradation of extracellular proteins. *Nature* 584 (7820): 291–297.

18 Li, Z., Wang, C., Wang, Z. et al. (2019). Allele-selective lowering of mutant HTT protein by HTT-LC3 linker compounds. *Nature* 575 (7781): 203–209.

19 Cotton, A.D., Nguyen, D.P., Gramespacher, J.A. et al. (2021). Development of antibody-based PROTACs for the degradation of the cell-surface immune checkpoint protein PD-L1. *J. Am. Chem. Soc.* 143 (2): 593–598.

20 Caianiello, D.F., Zhang, M.W., Ray, J.D. et al. (2021). Bifunctional small molecules that mediate the degradation of extracellular proteins. *Nat. Chem. Biol.* 17 (9): 947–953.

21 Zhang, H., Han, Y., Yang, Y. et al. (2021). Covalently engineered nanobody chimeras for targeted membrane protein degradation. *J. Am. Chem. Soc.* 143 (40): 16377–16382.

22 Edmondson, S.D., Yang, B., and Fallan, C. (2019). Proteolysis targeting chimeras (PROTACs) in 'beyond rule-of-five' chemical space: recent progress and future challenges. *Bioorg. Med. Chem. Lett.* 29 (13): 1555–1564.

23 Schapira, M., Calabrese, M.F., Bullock, A.N., and Crews, C.M. (2019). Targeted protein degradation: expanding the toolbox. *Nat. Rev. Drug Discov.* 18 (12): 949–963.

24 Nowak, R.P., DeAngelo, S.L., Buckley, D. et al. (2018). Plasticity in binding confers selectivity in ligand-induced protein degradation. *Nat. Chem. Biol.* 14 (7): 706–714.

25 Schreiber, S.L. (2021). The rise of molecular glues. *Cell* 184 (1): 3–9.

26 Gerry, C.J. and Schreiber, S.L. (2020). Unifying principles of bifunctional, proximity-inducing small molecules. *Nat. Chem. Biol.* 16 (4): 369–378.

27 Bussiere, D.E., Xie, L., Srinivas, H. et al. (2020). Structural basis of indisulam-mediated RBM39 recruitment to DCAF15 E3 ligase complex. *Nat. Chem. Biol.* 16 (1): 15–23.

28 Faust, T.B., Yoon, H., Nowak, R.P. et al. (2020). Structural complementarity facilitates E7820-mediated degradation of RBM39 by DCAF15. *Nat. Chem. Biol.* 16 (1): 7–14.

29 Alabi, S.B. and Crews, C.M. (2021). Major advances in targeted protein degradation: PROTACs, LYTACs, and MADTACs. *J. Biol. Chem.* 296: 100647.

30 Neklesa, T., Snyder, L.B., Willard, R.R. et al. (2019). ARV-110: an oral androgen receptor PROTAC degrader for prostate cancer. *J. Clin. Oncol.* 37 (7).

31 Winter, G.E., Buckley, D.L., Paulk, J. et al. (2015). Phthalimide conjugation as a strategy for *in vivo* target protein degradation. *Science* 348 (6241): 1376–1381.
32 Bai, L.C., Zhou, H.B., Xu, R.Q. et al. (2019). A potent and selective small-molecule degrader of STAT3 achieves complete tumor regression *in vivo*. *Cancer Cell* 36 (5): 498–511.e17.
33 Singh, J., Petter, R.C., Baillie, T.A., and Whitty, A. (2011). The resurgence of covalent drugs. *Nat. Rev. Drug Discov.* 10 (4): 307–317.
34 Canon, J., Rex, K., Saiki, A.Y. et al. (2019). The clinical KRAS(G12C) inhibitor AMG 510 drives anti-tumour immunity. *Nature* 575 (7781): 217–223.
35 Boike, L., Cioffi, A.G., Majewski, F.C. et al. (2021). Discovery of a functional covalent ligand targeting an intrinsically disordered cysteine within MYC. *Cell Chem. Biol.* 28 (1): 4–13.e17.
36 Ward, C.C., Kleinman, J.I., Brittain, S.M. et al. (2019). Covalent ligand screening uncovers a RNF4 E3 ligase recruiter for targeted protein degradation applications. *ACS Chem. Biol.* 14 (11): 2430–2440.
37 Zhang, X., Luukkonen, L.M., Eissler, C.L. et al. (2021). DCAF11 supports targeted protein degradation by electrophilic proteolysis-targeting chimeras. *J. Am. Chem. Soc.* 143 (13): 5141–5149.
38 Spradlin, J.N., Hu, X., Ward, C.C. et al. (2019). Harnessing the anti-cancer natural product nimbolide for targeted protein degradation. *Nat. Chem. Biol.* 15 (7): 747–755.
39 Zhang, X., Crowley, V.M., Wucherpfennig, T.G. et al. (2019). Electrophilic PROTACs that degrade nuclear proteins by engaging DCAF16. *Nat. Chem. Biol.* 15 (7): 737–746.
40 Sutanto, F., Konstantinidou, M., and Domling, A. (2020). Covalent inhibitors: a rational approach to drug discovery. *RSC Med. Chem.* 11 (8): 876–884.
41 Buckley, D.L., Raina, K., Darricarrere, N. et al. (2015). HaloPROTACS: use of small molecule PROTACs to induce degradation of HaloTag fusion proteins. *ACS Chem. Biol.* 10 (8): 1831–1837.
42 Los, G.V., Encell, L.P., McDougall, M.G. et al. (2008). HaloTag: a novel protein labeling technology for cell imaging and protein analysis. *ACS Chem. Biol.* 3 (6): 373–382.
43 Tovell, H., Testa, A., Maniaci, C. et al. (2019). Rapid and reversible knockdown of endogenously tagged endosomal proteins via an optimized HaloPROTAC degrader. *ACS Chem. Biol.* 14 (5): 882–892.
44 Nabet, B., Roberts, J.M., Buckley, D.L. et al. (2018). The dTAG system for immediate and target-specific protein degradation. *Nat. Chem. Biol.* 14 (5): 431–441.
45 Bond, A.G., Craigon, C., Chan, K.H. et al. (2021). Development of BromoTag: a "bump-and-hole"-PROTAC system to induce potent, rapid, and selective degradation of tagged target proteins. *J. Med. Chem.* 64 (20): 15477–15502.
46 Griffith, E.C., Su, Z., Niwayama, S. et al. (1998). Molecular recognition of angiogenesis inhibitors fumagillin and ovalicin by methionine aminopeptidase 2. *Proc. Natl. Acad. Sci. U.S.A.* 95 (26): 15183–15188.

47 Byrd, J.C., Furman, R.R., Coutre, S.E. et al. (2013). Targeting BTK with Ibrutinib in relapsed chronic lymphocytic leukemia. *New Engl. J. Med.* 369 (1): 32–42.

48 Tinworth, C.P., Lithgow, H., Dittus, L. et al. (2019). PROTAC-mediated degradation of Bruton's tyrosine kinase is inhibited by covalent binding. *ACS Chem. Biol.* 14 (3): 342–347.

49 Dittus, L., Werner, T., Muelbaier, M., and Bantscheff, M. (2017). Differential kinobeads profiling for target identification of irreversible kinase inhibitors. *ACS Chem. Biol.* 12 (10): 2515–2521.

50 Xue, G., Chen, J., Liu, L. et al. (2020). Protein degradation through covalent inhibitor-based PROTACs. *Chem. Commun. (Camb.)* 56 (10): 1521–1524.

51 Guo, W.H., Qi, X., Yu, X. et al. (2020). Enhancing intracellular accumulation and target engagement of PROTACs with reversible covalent chemistry. *Nat. Commun.* 11 (1): 4268.

52 Gabizon, R., Shraga, A., Gehrtz, P. et al. (2020). Efficient targeted degradation via reversible and irreversible covalent PROTACs. *J. Am. Chem. Soc.* 142 (27): 11734–11742.

53 Kim, D., Xue, J.Y., and Lito, P. (2020). Targeting KRAS(G12C): from inhibitory mechanism to modulation of antitumor effects in patients. *Cell* 183 (4): 850–859.

54 Hallin, J., Engstrom, L.D., Hargis, L. et al. (2020). The KRAS(G12C) inhibitor MRTX849 provides insight toward therapeutic susceptibility of KRAS-mutant cancers in mouse models and patients. *Cancer Discov.* 10 (1): 54–71.

55 Fell, J.B., Fischer, J.P., Baer, B.R. et al. (2020). Identification of the clinical development candidate MRTX849, a covalent KRAS(G12C) inhibitor for the treatment of cancer. *J. Med. Chem.* 63 (13): 6679–6693.

56 Janes, M.R., Zhang, J., Li, L.S. et al. (2018). Targeting KRAS mutant cancers with a covalent G12C-specific inhibitor. *Cell* 172 (3): 578–589.e17.

57 Ostrem, J.M., Peters, U., Sos, M.L. et al. (2013). K-Ras(G12C) inhibitors allosterically control GTP affinity and effector interactions. *Nature* 503 (7477): 548–551.

58 Bond, M.J., Chu, L., Nalawansha, D.A. et al. (2020). Targeted degradation of oncogenic KRAS(G12C) by VHL-recruiting PROTACs. *ACS Cent. Sci.* 6 (8): 1367–1375.

59 Zeng, M., Xiong, Y., Safaee, N. et al. (2020). Exploring targeted degradation strategy for oncogenic KRAS(G12C). *Cell Chem. Biol.* 27 (1): 19–31.e6.

60 Burslem, G.M., Smith, B.E., Lai, A.C. et al. (2018). The advantages of targeted protein degradation over inhibition: an RTK case study. *Cell Chem. Biol.* 25 (1): 67–77.e3.

61 Gazdar, A.F. (2009). Activating and resistance mutations of EGFR in non-small-cell lung cancer: role in clinical response to EGFR tyrosine kinase inhibitors. *Oncogene* 28 (Suppl. 1): S24–S31.

62 Lebraud, H., Wright, D.J., Johnson, C.N., and Heightman, T.D. (2016). Protein degradation by in-cell self-assembly of proteolysis targeting chimeras. *ACS Cent. Sci.* 2 (12): 927–934.

63 Seitchik, J.L., Peeler, J.C., Taylor, M.T. et al. (2012). Genetically encoded tetrazine amino acid directs rapid site-specific *in vivo* bioorthogonal ligation with trans-cyclooctenes. *J. Am. Chem. Soc.* 134 (6): 2898–2901.

64 Peng, L., Zhang, Z., Lei, C. et al. (2019). Identification of new small-molecule inducers of estrogen-related receptor alpha (ERRalpha) degradation. *ACS Med. Chem. Lett.* 10 (5): 767–772.

65 Vinogradova, E.V., Zhang, X., Remillard, D. et al. (2020). An activity-guided map of electrophile-cysteine interactions in primary human T cells. *Cell* 182 (4): 1009–1026.e29.

66 Seixas, J.D., Sousa, B.B., Marques, M.C. et al. (2020). Structural and biophysical insights into the mode of covalent binding of rationally designed potent BMX inhibitors. *RSC Chem. Biol.* 1 (4): 251–262.

67 Lu, J., Qian, Y., Altieri, M. et al. (2015). Hijacking the E3 ubiquitin ligase cereblon to efficiently target BRD4. *Chem. Biol.* 22 (6): 755–763.

68 Winter, G.E., Buckley, D.L., Paulk, J. et al. (2015). Drug development. Phthalimide conjugation as a strategy for *in vivo* target protein degradation. *Science* 348 (6241): 1376–1381.

69 Okuhira, K., Ohoka, N., Sai, K. et al. (2011). Specific degradation of CRABP-II via cIAP1-mediated ubiquitylation induced by hybrid molecules that crosslink cIAP1 and the target protein. *FEBS Lett.* 585 (8): 1147–1152.

70 Schneekloth, J.S. Jr., Fonseca, F.N., Koldobskiy, M. et al. (2004). Chemical genetic control of protein levels: selective *in vivo* targeted degradation. *J. Am. Chem. Soc.* 126 (12): 3748–3754.

71 Schneekloth, A.R., Pucheault, M., Tae, H.S., and Crews, C.M. (2008). Targeted intracellular protein degradation induced by a small molecule: en route to chemical proteomics. *Bioorg. Med. Chem. Lett.* 18 (22): 5904–5908.

72 Bondeson, D.P., Smith, B.E., Burslem, G.M. et al. (2018). Lessons in PROTAC design from selective degradation with a promiscuous warhead. *Cell Chem. Biol.* 25 (1): 78–87.e5.

73 Huang, H.T., Dobrovolsky, D., Paulk, J. et al. (2018). A chemoproteomic approach to query the degradable kinome using a multi-kinase degrader. *Cell Chem. Biol.* 25 (1): 88–99.e6.

74 Hay, R.T. (2013). Decoding the SUMO signal. *Biochem. Soc. Trans.* 41 (2): 463–473.

75 Tatham, M.H., Geoffroy, M.C., Shen, L. et al. (2008). RNF4 is a poly-SUMO-specific E3 ubiquitin ligase required for arsenic-induced PML degradation. *Nat. Cell Biol.* 10 (5): 538–546.

76 Filippakopoulos, P., Qi, J., Picaud, S. et al. (2010). Selective inhibition of BET bromodomains. *Nature* 468 (7327): 1067–1073.

77 Elumalai, P., Gunadharini, D.N., Senthilkumar, K. et al. (2012). Induction of apoptosis in human breast cancer cells by nimbolide through extrinsic and intrinsic pathway. *Toxicol. Lett.* 215 (2): 131–142.

78 Bodduluru, L.N., Kasala, E.R., Thota, N. et al. (2014). Chemopreventive and therapeutic effects of nimbolide in cancer: the underlying mechanisms. *Toxicol. in vitro* 28 (5): 1026–1035.

79 Abbas, T. and Dutta, A. (2009). p21 in cancer: intricate networks and multiple activities. *Nat. Rev. Cancer* 9 (6): 400–414.

80 Luo, M., Spradlin, J.N., Boike, L. et al. (2021). Chemoproteomics-enabled discovery of covalent RNF114-based degraders that mimic natural product function. *Cell Chem. Biol.* 28 (4): 559–566.e15.

81 Zhang, D.D., Lo, S.C., Cross, J.V. et al. (2004). Keap1 is a redox-regulated substrate adaptor protein for a Cul3-dependent ubiquitin ligase complex. *Mol. Cell. Biol.* 24 (24): 10941–10953.

82 Cullinan, S.B., Gordan, J.D., Jin, J. et al. (2004). The Keap1-BTB protein is an adaptor that bridges Nrf2 to a Cul3-based E3 ligase: oxidative stress sensing by a Cul3-Keap1 ligase. *Mol. Cell. Biol.* 24 (19): 8477–8486.

83 Kobayashi, A., Kang, M.I., Okawa, H. et al. (2004). Oxidative stress sensor Keap1 functions as an adaptor for Cul3-based E3 ligase to regulate proteasomal degradation of Nrf2. *Mol. Cell. Biol.* 24 (16): 7130–7139.

84 Yamamoto, M., Kensler, T.W., and Motohashi, H. (2018). The KEAP1-NRF2 system: a thiol-based sensor-effector apparatus for maintaining redox homeostasis. *Physiol. Rev.* 98 (3): 1169–1203.

85 Lu, M., Liu, T., Jiao, Q. et al. (2018). Discovery of a Keap1-dependent peptide PROTAC to knockdown Tau by ubiquitination-proteasome degradation pathway. *Eur. J. Med. Chem.* 146: 251–259.

86 Wei, J., Meng, F., Park, K.S. et al. (2021). Harnessing the E3 Ligase KEAP1 for targeted protein degradation. *J. Am. Chem. Soc.* 143 (37): 15073–15083.

87 Wang, Y.Y., Yang, Y.X., Zhe, H. et al. (2014). Bardoxolone methyl (CDDO-Me) as a therapeutic agent: an update on its pharmacokinetic and pharmacodynamic properties. *Drug Des. Devel. Ther.* 8: 2075–2088.

88 Tong, B., Luo, M., Xie, Y. et al. (2020). Bardoxolone conjugation enables targeted protein degradation of BRD4. *Sci. Rep.* 10 (1): 15543.

89 Manford, A.G., Rodriguez-Perez, F., Shih, K.Y. et al. (2020). A cellular mechanism to detect and alleviate reductive stress. *Cell* 183 (1): 46–61.e21.

90 Henning, N.J., Manford, A.G., Spradlin, J.N. et al. (2022). Discovery of a covalent FEM1B recruiter for targeted protein degradation applications. *J. Am. Chem. Soc.* 144 (2): 701–708.

91 Pinch, B.J., Buckley, D.L., Gleim, S. et al. (2021). A strategy to assess the cellular activity of E3 ligase components against neo-substrates using electrophilic probes. *Cell Chem. Biol.* 29 (1): 57–66 e6.

92 Backus, K.M., Correia, B.E., Lum, K.M. et al. (2016). Proteome-wide covalent ligand discovery in native biological systems. *Nature* 534 (7608): 570–574.

93 Soucy, T.A., Smith, P.G., Milhollen, M.A. et al. (2009). An inhibitor of NEDD8-activating enzyme as a new approach to treat cancer. *Nature* 458 (7239): 732–736.

94 Weerapana, E., Wang, C., Simon, G.M. et al. (2010). Quantitative reactivity profiling predicts functional cysteines in proteomes. *Nature* 468 (7325): 790–795.

95 Han, X., Wang, C., Qin, C. et al. (2019). Discovery of ARD-69 as a highly potent proteolysis targeting chimera (PROTAC) degrader of androgen receptor (AR) for the treatment of prostate cancer. *J. Med. Chem.* 62 (2): 941–964.

96 Han, X., Zhao, L., Xiang, W. et al. (2019). Discovery of highly potent and efficient PROTAC degraders of androgen receptor (AR) by employing weak binding affinity VHL E3 ligase ligands. *J. Med. Chem.* 62 (24): 11218–11231.

97 Nusinow, D.P., Szpyt, J., Ghandi, M. et al. (2020). Quantitative proteomics of the cancer cell line encyclopedia. *Cell* 180 (2): 387–402.e16.

98 Wang, C., Weerapana, E., Blewett, M.M., and Cravatt, B.F. (2014). A chemoproteomic platform to quantitatively map targets of lipid-derived electrophiles. *Nat. Methods* 11 (1): 79–85.

99 Rostovtsev, V.V., Green, L.G., Fokin, V.V., and Sharpless, K.B. (2002). A stepwise huisgen cycloaddition process: copper(I)-catalyzed regioselective "ligation" of azides and terminal alkynes. *Angew. Chem. Int. Ed.* 41 (14): 2596–2599.

100 Pappireddi, N., Martin, L., and Wuhr, M. (2019). A review on quantitative multiplexed proteomics. *ChemBioChem* 20 (10): 1210–1224.

101 Li, J., Cai, Z., Bomgarden, R.D. et al. (2021). TMTpro-18plex: the expanded and complete set of TMTpro reagents for sample multiplexing. *J. Proteome Res.* 20 (5): 2964–2972.

102 Resnick, E., Bradley, A., Gan, J. et al. (2019). Rapid covalent-probe discovery by electrophile-fragment screening. *J. Am. Chem. Soc.* 141 (22): 8951–8968.

103 Marino, S.M. and Gladyshev, V.N. (2010). Cysteine function governs its conservation and degeneration and restricts its utilization on protein surfaces. *J. Mol. Biol.* 404 (5): 902–916.

104 Gehringer, M. and Laufer, S.A. (2019). Emerging and re-emerging warheads for targeted covalent inhibitors: applications in medicinal chemistry and chemical biology. *J. Med. Chem.* 62 (12): 5673–5724.

105 Hacker, S.M., Backus, K.M., Lazear, M.R. et al. (2017). Global profiling of lysine reactivity and ligandability in the human proteome. *Nat. Chem.* 9 (12): 1181–1190.

106 Abbasov, M.E., Kavanagh, M.E., Ichu, T.A. et al. (2021). A proteome wide atlas of lysine-reactive chemistry. *Nat. Chem.* 13 (11): 1081–1092.

107 Fadeyi, O.O., Hoth, L.R., Choi, C. et al. (2017). Covalent enzyme inhibition through fluorosulfate modification of a noncatalytic serine residue. *ACS Chem. Biol.* 12 (8): 2015–2020.

108 Hahm, H.S., Toroitich, E.K., Borne, A.L. et al. (2020). Global targeting of functional tyrosines using sulfur-triazole exchange chemistry. *Nat. Chem. Biol.* 16 (2): 150–159.

109 Jia, S., He, D., and Chang, C.J. (2019). Bioinspired thiophosphorodichloridate reagents for chemoselective histidine bioconjugation. *J. Am. Chem. Soc.* 141 (18): 7294–7301.

110 Bach, K., Beerkens, B.L.H., Zanon, P.R.A., and Hacker, S.M. (2020). Light-activatable, 2,5-disubstituted tetrazoles for the proteome-wide profiling of aspartates and glutamates in living bacteria. *ACS Cent. Sci.* 6 (4): 546–554.

9

Extending the Degradation Toolkit – mRNA Targeting as an Alternative Means to Affect Protein Levels

Andrei Ursu, Barbara Herdy and Hendrik Osadnik

Bayer AG, Research & Development, Pharmaceuticals, Life Science Technologies, Building 0520, 42096 Wuppertal, Germany

9.1 Introduction

Drug discovery efforts have been mainly focused on privileged "druggable" protein targets such as enzymes (e.g. kinases and proteases), G protein-coupled receptors (GPCRs), and others [1]. Although applied successfully, the protein-centric approaches can cover only a limited number of human diseases and modes of action (MoA). To expand the druggable space, protein–protein interactions (PPIs) and hard-to-drug targets such as membrane proteins, transcription factors, etc., have been considered [2]. Hence, there is a pressing need to widen the biological space for which safe and effective medicines exhibiting novel MoA can be developed.

RNA-centric therapeutics target upstream events in the life cycle of a protein (Figure 9.1) and therefore represent valuable alternatives to drugging proteins [3]. Indeed, RNA-centric mechanisms that impact an mRNA encoding a diseases-relevant protein [4] have recently gained momentum because of significant advances in next-generation sequencing (NGS), improved capability in analyzing NGS datasets, RNA structural determination, and others. These contributed to a better understanding of endogenous cellular machineries regulating the various stages of RNA maturation [5]. Through splicing and 5′- and 3′-end processing of precursor (pre) messenger (m) RNA (pre-mRNA), a mature mRNA transcript is generated. In many cases, more than one mRNA isoform can be expressed from a pre-mRNA, with frequencies determined by a fine balance at competing splice sites. Mature mRNAs are then transported to the cytoplasm for protein production. Additionally, mRNAs are decorated on both ends with untranslated regions (5′- and 3′-UTRs [untranslated region]), which add an additional layer of regulation and quality control for maintaining cellular homeostasis. For example, RNA interference (RNAi) pathways

Inducing Targeted Protein Degradation: From Chemical Biology to Drug Discovery and Clinical Applications, First Edition. Edited by Philipp Cromm.

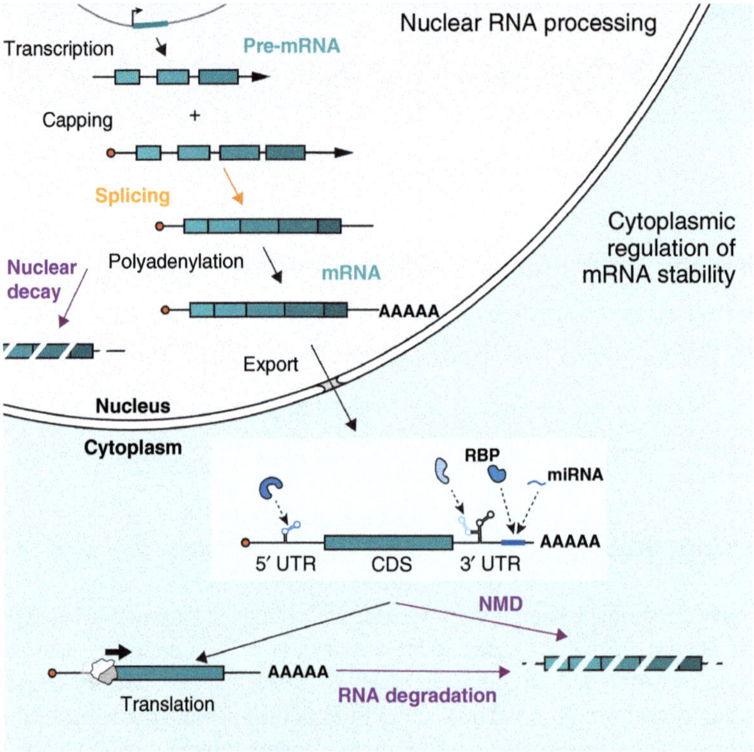

Figure 9.1 Overview of the mRNA's life cycle. During transcription, processing steps in the nucleus (top) convert the pre-mRNA into a mature mRNA, which is exported into the cytoplasm (bottom). Here, interactions of regulatory sequences with RNA binding proteins (RBPs) and small regulatory RNAs (miRNAs) occur. The 5′- as well as the 3′-untranslated regions (UTRs) surrounding the coding sequence (CDS) regulate the mRNA transcript stability. Degradation pathways (purple) occur both in the nucleus and in the cytoplasm to remove incompletely processed RNAs (nuclear decay), RNA transcripts with error-containing CDS (nonsense-mediated decay, NMD), and mRNAs that underwent translation.

operating via microRNAs (miRNAs) bind to 3′-UTRs to induce gene silencing or inhibit translation. Therefore, rational modalities targeting the intricacies of mRNA generation and regulation could yield mechanistically novel RNA-centric entry routes for drug development. However, a deeper understanding of disease-specific mRNA isoform maturation in the disease-relevant transcriptome is required.

Targeting the mRNA of a disease-causing protein for degradation is especially relevant for proteins with unknown function, as well as secreted and disordered proteins. In these cases, deployment of traditional protein-centric targeting modalities is challenging, which further complicates the subsequent drug discovery and development process. mRNA degradation-based approaches have, among others, the following potential advantages: First, preventing the production of a functional protein before or during translation at the mRNA level can be more efficient than targeting the protein itself. On the one hand, the protein's interactome is directly affected because the protein is absent from the cellular environment. On the other hand, the protein is not (immediately) regenerated because the corresponding mRNA is not available for translation. Therefore, a long-lasting therapeutic effect is expected in the case of RNA-centric drugging approaches as compared to transient non-covalent occupancy-driven inhibition of protein function. Second, selective degradation of mRNAs within a highly conserved protein family can be achieved, as their corresponding RNA sequences may differ more substantially among each other, especially in the UTR regions, when compared to amino acid conservation. Lastly, targeting single mRNA isoforms of disease-relevant proteins can afford tissue selectivity if tissue-specific mRNA isoforms are produced.

Chapter 9 provides a focused introduction into post-transcriptional control of mRNA degradation, which directly impacts the protein levels. Adding to the proteolyis targeting chimera (PROTAC) approaches discussed in this book, we explore the possibility of harnessing endogenous RNA processing machineries to downregulate the mRNAs of proteins involved in various human diseases. Firstly, we describe the key protein/macromolecular complexes and various degradation-related regulatory mechanisms responsible for cellular mRNA quality control, occurring both in the nucleus and the cytoplasm. Secondly, we highlight the recurring principles of disturbing or hijacking RNA processing to decrease mRNA and consequently lower protein abundance and will give examples of recent strategies that exploited them. For example, aside from well-known siRNA targeting approaches, we collected a broad set of modalities including small molecules (SMOLs), antisense oligonucleotides (ASOs), SMOL–ASO conjugates, and SMOL chimeric probes that we will introduce and touch upon. Therefore, Chapter 9 provides the state-of-the-art toolbox that harnesses endogenous cellular RNA quality control pathways for targeted degradation of mRNAs. The field of mRNA degradation is vast and challenging but promises to uncover mechanistically novel routes for therapeutic benefit. Therefore, we hope to kindle the interest of the reader to further explore the potential of mRNA degradation in future drug discovery and development campaigns [6, 7].

9.2 Life Cycle of Eukaryotic mRNAs

A typical mRNA is transcribed in the nucleus by RNA polymerase II (Pol II) (Figure 9.1). Immediately after its transcription, the cap structure (m^7GpppN, m = methyl, G = guanosine, p = phosphate, and N = any nucleotide) is added to the 5′-end of the transcript to protect it from degradation [8, 9]. The cap is bound by the nuclear cap binding protein (CBP) complex consisting of nuclear cap binding protein subunit 1 (NCBP1) and 2 (NCBP2), respectively. This event is pivotal to initiate splicing, polyadenylation (poly(A) tail addition), and export of the mRNA into the cytoplasm (Figure 9.1) [10]. The pre-mRNA is further processed by the splicing machinery, which removes non-coding intragenic RNA regions (introns), yielding the mature mRNA (Figure 9.1). Alternative splicing (AS) is of key importance as it defines the identity of the translated coding sequence, shapes the fate of an mRNA, and consequently the expression pattern of the encoded protein. In addition, splicing increases the diversity of the transcriptome as it can generate multiple mRNA isoforms from a single gene by including or excluding different exons.

After nuclear processing and export into the cytoplasm, the 5′-UTR section of the mRNA is scanned by the translation initiation machinery until the first start codon, usually the AUG triplet, of the protein coding sequence (CDS), i.e. the open reading frame (ORF), is found. At the AUG site, the ribosome assembles, and translation is initiated until the stop codon of the ORF is identified (Figure 9.1). Immediately after the stop codon, the 3′-UTR region is encountered, which is followed by the poly(A) tail (Figure 9.1). This part harbors numerous RNA sequences and structures involved in various regulatory functions, such as RNAi pathway, binding of RNA binding proteins (RBPs), etc., which directly impact the mRNA transcript stability and rate of degradation.

In Sections 9.3–9.4, we will describe these maturation stages in more detail, emphasizing the key players and mechanisms involved in the regulation of mRNA degradation, as well as recent modalities modulating mRNA degradation mechanisms for therapeutic benefit.

9.3 Splicing Shapes the Cell's Transcriptome

Alternative splicing is a complex process catalyzed by the spliceosome, a ribonucleoprotein (RNP) complex that recognizes the exon–intron boundaries through conserved sequence motifs and promotes the removal of introns. The spliceosome consists of five small nuclear RNAs (snRNAs) and ~150 proteins that form multiple intermediate complexes along a tightly controlled process. For further information, the reader is directed to excellent comprehensive reviews on splicing and the spliceosome assembly [11–13]. Herein, we focus on key aspects of splice sites recognition and tuning, as they pertain to lowering protein output at the mRNA level.

There are three main sequence determinants of pre-mRNAs: the 5′ splice site (5′SS) at the end of the upstream exon, the 3′ splice site (3′SS) at the start of the downstream exon, and the branch point (BP), featuring an adenine (A) nucleotide residue in the intron preceding the 3′SS (Figure 9.2a). Both the 5′SS and the BP sequence are recognized through Watson–Crick base-pairing interactions by U1 and U2 snRNAs, respectively, and are brought closely together for the first catalytic step of splicing ("branching"). This cleaves the 5′SS to liberate the end of the upstream exon for ligation while attaching the 5′-end of the intron to the 2′OH group of the BP's A residue, resulting in an intron lariat intermediate (Figure 9.2b). The 3′SS is then brought in for the second catalytic step ("exon ligation"). This results in an exon–exon junction by releasing the intron as a lariat, which is degraded. While this concludes the splicing event, parts of the spliceosome remain bound to the exon–exon junctions, also known as the exon junction complex (EJC). The cap and EJCs play a critical role in regulating nuclear export and guide an mRNA toward translation or degradation by nonsense-mediated decay (NMD), which will be discussed in detail in Section 9.4.

In Chapter 9, we are considering two layers of complexity governing AS events. On the one hand, the reliance on base-pairing interactions to recognize splice sites opens the door to rationally manipulate the endogenous AS machinery to alter splicing events related to the gene of interest. Indeed, the vast majority of human pre-mRNAs are alternatively spliced (~92–94%), with ~86% of them having a minor isoform frequency of at least 15% [14]. In addition, variations in the pre-mRNA sequence consensus have been studied on a quantitative [15] as well as a kinetic level [16]. As a result, significant differences in splice site strength have been observed, which could be exploited to induce alternative splicing events for therapeutic benefit. On the other hand, a second layer of splice site activity regulation is conferred by the interplay of cell- or tissue-specific expressed RBP network and/or structured RNA motifs at and in the vicinity of the splice sites. Among the best understood families of splicing, regulating RBPs are the serine and arginine-rich (SR) proteins [17] and heterogeneous nuclear ribonucleoproteins (hnRNPs) [18]. For example, members of these protein families can bind both intronic and exonic regions and act as positive as well as negative splicing regulators via cooperative and competitive interactions [19] with the assembling spliceosome [20] to strengthen or weaken exon inclusion [21]. Much progress has been made in elucidating the secondary layer of splicing regulation in recent years, for example, through mapping the binding sites for a large number of RBPs [22] and by using gene knockdown libraries to identify genes involved in AS networks [23].

In conclusion, an in depth understanding of the various layers of AS regulation in healthy as well as disease tissues is required. This is of key importance to better understand tissue-specific AS regulation and harness this knowledge for drug development and therapeutic targeting.

9.3.1 Aberrant Splicing Impacts the Transcriptome

Aberrant splicing is the cause of a broad spectrum of human diseases. Faulty processing of pre-mRNAs occurs when a bona fide pair of 5′SS and 3′SS splice sites is not properly detected by the spliceosome machinery or if a stretch of pre-mRNA is mistakenly recognized as a splice site (creating a cryptic splice site), thus generating a novel exon (Figure 9.2c). Consequently, aberrant splicing can lead to outcomes such as intron retention, which is the lack of removal of an intron; activation of cryptic splice sites, leading to extended exons or the creation of new ones (cryptic exons); and exon skipping, which is the result of the spliceosome not recognizing particular splice sites and skipping to the downstream ones. Therefore, aberrant splicing of pre-mRNAs results in inclusion of untranslated intronic regions and/or frame shifts in the mRNA's ORF. Some of these events lead to premature

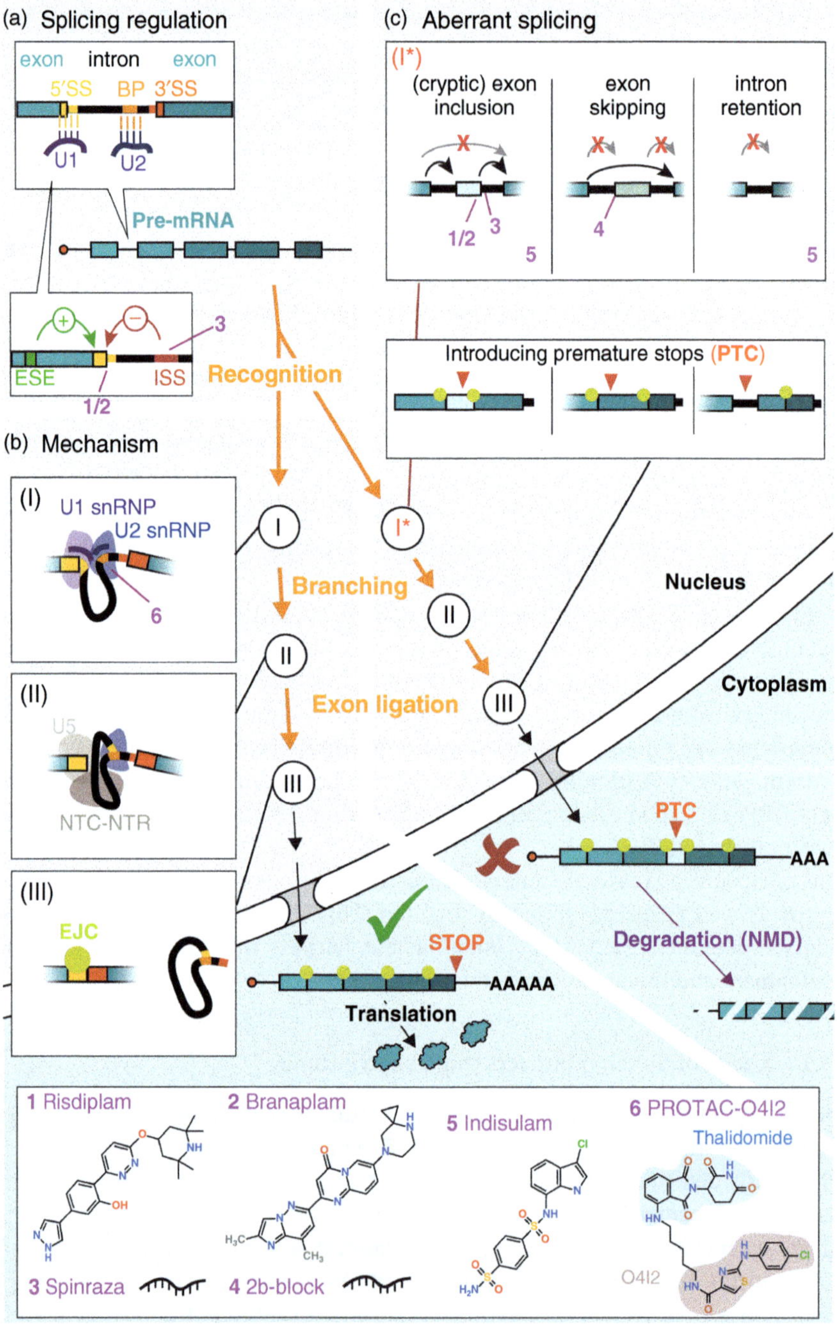
(a) Splicing regulation
exon intron exon
5′SS BP 3′SS
U1
U2
Pre-mRNA
ESE
ISS
1/2
3
Recognition
(b) Mechanism
(I) U1 snRNP
U2 snRNP
6
(II)
U5
NTC-NTR
(III)
EJC
(c) Aberrant splicing
(I*)
(cryptic) exon inclusion
exon skipping
intron retention
1/2
3
4
5
5
Introducing premature stops (PTC)
I
I*
Branching
II
II
Exon ligation
III
III
Nucleus
Cytoplasm
PTC
AAA
STOP
AAAAA
Degradation (NMD)
Translation
1 Risdiplam
2 Branaplam
5 Indisulam
6 PROTAC-O4I2
Thalidomide
O4I2
3 Spinraza
4 2b-block

termination codons (PTCs), which trigger mRNA quality control mechanisms in the cytoplasm, followed by mRNA transcript degradation and therefore lack of protein production.

Here, we distinguish two levels of aberrant splicing. On the one hand, *local* alterations of splicing triggered by mutations in the pre-mRNA sequence change the reactivity of splice sites. These can lead to both the creation of new splice sites, as encountered in cancer [24], and the loss of splice sites, as identified in a variety of genetic disorders [25]. On the other hand, we distinguish *global* alterations of splicing, such as mutations or changes in the expression levels of the spliceosome's constitutive parts. These events profoundly affect transcriptome-wide gene splicing, as seen in some cancers [26, 27]. For example, mutations in the U1 snRNA, which base-pairs with the 5′SS, shift the binding preference of pre-mRNA 5′SS motifs. Consequently, this leads to aberrant splicing changes of multiple cancer-related genes through defective recognition of splice site motifs in chronic lymphocytic leukemia (CLL) and other types of cancers [28].

In conclusion, an in-depth knowledge about disease-specific aberrant splicing events is necessary to therapeutically harness it for targeted degradation of mRNAs.

9.3.2 Therapeutic Strategies to Change Protein Levels Through Splicing Regulation

Splicing can be altered at *local* (i.e. at individual splice site(s)) and *global* (affecting transcriptome-wide splicing regulation) levels. Literature examples covering the two levels will be highlighted in Sections 9.3.2.1–9.4.2.1, with a special emphasis on

Figure 9.2 Principles of splicing regulation and possible therapeutic entry points (pink). (a) Splicing is regulated through motifs on the pre-mRNA that mark the 5′ and 3′ splice sites (SS), as well as the intronic branch point (BP). 5′SS and BP are recognized by base-pairing with small nuclear riboproteins snRNPs (snRNP) U1 and U2, respectively. Regulatory elements such as exonic splicing enhancer (ESE) and intronic splicing silencer (ISS) form an additional layer of regulation that influences splice site recognition by the spliceosome; (b) Mechanism of splicing. (I) At the beginning of the splicing reaction, the U1 and U2 snRNPs harboring the base-pairing bring the bound 5′SS and BP into proximity. (II) After complex remodeling, the branching reaction liberates the exonic part of the 5′SS, while tethering the intronic part to the BP, forming an intron lariat intermediate. (III) During exon ligation, 3′SS is brought into the active site and is ligated to the free 5′SS, producing the spliced mRNA and an intron lariat. Importantly, an exon junction complex (EJC) remains at the splice site and plays a central role in mRNA quality control in the cytoplasm; (c) Downstream effects of aberrant splicing. The improper recognition of splice sites can cause the aberrant inclusion or exclusion of pre-mRNA regions (I*), which can manifest after exon ligation (III) in the production of mRNAs with premature termination codons (PTC), which are degraded in the cytoplasm via NMD.

local gene-specific mRNA degradation. For example, two of the most prominent examples of splicing regulation by a SMOL are the modulation of the survival of motor neuron 2 (SMN2) and huntingtin (HTT) proteins. Both examples highlight the potential of regulating splicing as a novel therapeutic approach, harnessed either to increase (SMN2) or reduce (HTT) protein production in spinal muscular atrophy (SMA) and Huntington's disease (HD), respectively. Although only the reduction of HTT protein levels is relevant for Chapter 9, we added a brief description of SMOL SMN2 modulator **risdiplam (Evrysdi®)** (**1**; Figure 9.2, bottom panel) as the prime example of orally Food and Drug Administration (FDA)-approved drug modulating splicing. Additionally, **branaplam** (**2**; Figure 9.2, bottom panel) was recently reported to reduce HTT protein levels in HD models. Interestingly, **branaplam** also recapitulated **risdiplam**'s MoA, alleviating SMA phenotypic defects *in vitro* and *in vivo* [29].

9.3.2.1 Activating a Weak Splice Site in SMN2 to Increase Protein Production

SMA is a recessive neuromuscular disorder caused by inactivation of the essential gene survival of motor neuron 1 (SMN1) through deletion or mutation. While mapping SMN1, it was discovered that a second copy of the SMN gene exists in a duplicated stretch of the chromosome, termed SMN2 [30]. Although exhibiting high sequence similarity, the SMN2 transcript features a crucial, translationally silent $C \rightarrow T$ (*C280T*) point mutation, which inactivates an exonic splicing enhancer (ESE) site to favor skipping of exon 7. This leads to the translation of a non-functional SMN2 protein, causing SMN2 loss of function. Consequently, rescue of exon 7 splicing represents a promising therapeutic entry point to alleviate SMA phenotypic defects [31].

Indeed, sequence-based design and optimization of ASO blockers yielded **nusinersen** (**Spinraza®**) (**3**; Figure 9.2, bottom panel) as the first SMA RNA therapeutic drug targeting this splicing mechanism to reach the market in 2016 [32]. It acts through inactivating an intronic splicing silencer sequence (ISS-N1) downstream of the splice site, which leads to increased splicing efficiency of the SMN2 transcript and therefore enhanced production of functional SMN2 protein. In parallel, research efforts toward identification of SMOL activators of SMN2 splicing culminated in the approval of **risdiplam** in 2020 [33], as the first orally available SMOL drug to treat SMA [34]. The exact MoA of SMN2-modifiers such as **risdiplam** and **branaplam** is still a matter of debate [35] and includes either SMOL binding to an exonic sequence and stabilizing RBP interactions and/or direct engagement of the 5′SS motif [36–38].

9.3.2.2 mRNA Degradation of HTT by Inducing Aberrant Splicing in HD

HD is a neurodegenerative disease caused by CAG repeat expansions in exon 1 of the HTT transcript. Upon translation, a toxic polyglutamine (polyQ)-containing mutant HTT protein is produced, which leads to various HTT loss of function phenotypes. Although a variety of HTT-lowering approaches have been discussed [39], the SMOL **branaplam** has recently been fast-tracked by the FDA for the treatment of HD and is currently undergoing phase IIb clinical trial (NCT05111249). Originally discovered as an SMN2-splicing activator [29], the recently published results highlighted that **branaplam** treatment triggers the inclusion of a cryptic exon located in intron 49 of the HTT gene [40]. As a result, a PTC is generated within HTT's ORF, which induces HTT mRNA transcript degradation via NMD, thus lowering HTT protein levels. Interestingly, lower HTT protein production upon **branaplam** treatment was recently invoked via (pseudo)exon 50a inclusion, which carries along in-frame stop codons [41].

9.3.2.3 Modulating the MKNK2 Isoform Balance with Splice Switching Oligonucleotides (SSOs)

The identification of genes, whose AS is key for tumorigenesis and tumor progression, is of great therapeutic interest [42]. For example, the MKNK2 gene encodes for the MKNK2 kinase, which upon AS yields two isoforms with dissimilar C-termini. Whereas the MKNK2a isoform exhibits kinase activity because of the ATP binding site, the shorter MKNK2b protein lacks the enzymatic function [43]. The cellular levels of MKNK2a and MKNK2b splice products are governed by the oncogenic splicing factor SRSF1. For example, overexpression of SRSF1 leads to increased MKNK2b protein levels, while the tumor suppressor activity of MKNK2a is mitigated [44]. Indeed, MKNK2a, but not MKNK2b, inhibits Ras-induced transformation *in vitro* and *in vivo* by targeting the Ras/Raf/Mitogen-activated protein kinase (MAPK) signaling pathway [43]. Therefore, shifting MKNK2's AS balance toward MKNK2a over MKNK2b might reduce cancer cell survival by blocking oncogenic transformation and tumorigenesis.

Mogilevsky et al. [45] reported the identification of a single-stranded SSO, which favored production of MKNK2a over MKNK2b in U87MG glioma, HuH7 hepatocellular carcinoma, and MDA-MB-231 triple negative breast cancer (TNBCs) cell lines. Screening various SSOs directed at the 3′SS of MKNK2's exon 14, featuring 2′-*O*-methyl (2′OMe) modification of the sugar moieties and phosphothioate (PS) backbone modifications, yielded **2b-block** (**4**; Figure 9.2, bottom panel). As a result of restoring MKNK2a protein levels, **2b-block** treatment activated p38 mitogen-activated protein (MAP) kinase stress response; triggered apoptosis of U87MG, U251MG, MCF-10A, and MDA-MB-231 cells; and inhibited anchorage-independent growth and tumor formation. Intracranial administration of mCherry-labeled U87MG cells treated with **2b-block** into the murine striatum inhibited glioblastoma tumor development *in vivo*, when analyzed two weeks post-injection.

9.3.2.4 Targeting Global AS with a Molecular "Glue" that Degrades RBM39

Genomic analyses of tumors unveiled protein components of the splicing machinery that can selectively be targeted in patient populations for therapeutic benefit [46]. However, many of the proteins that are involved in the regulation of pre-mRNA splicing fulfill a structural role and lack enzymatic function. Because targeting such proteins can be challenging, a more cost-effective strategy is to uncover the MoA of clinical candidates that failed to show sufficient therapeutic efficacy. On the one hand, such efforts will validate the biological target(s) and the cellular mechanism(s) triggered by the clinical candidate. On the other hand, it will provide insights into the proper selection of the patient population and therefore rationally repurpose the clinical candidate to novel indications.

Han et al. [47] revealed the MoA of **indisulam** (**5**; Figure 9.2, bottom panel), annotated as a carbonic anhydrase inhibitor, which showed modest clinical response in advanced-stage patients with solid tumors in various phase I and II clinical trials. Exome sequencing of **indisulam**-resistant HCT116 clones revealed numerous missense mutations clustered around the RNA recognition motif 2 (RRM2) domain of RNA binding protein 39 (RBM39). Additional experimental evidence highlighted that **indisulam** "glued" the interaction of RBM39, but not of mutated RBM39, with the DDB1- and CUL4-associated factor 15 (DCAF15) of the Cullin-4A (CUL4A) – DNA damage binding protein 1 (DDB1) – DET1- and DDB1-associated protein 1 (DDA1) E3 ubiquitin ligase complex. RNA-seq experiments revealed that **indisulam** treatment triggered global aberrant splicing events such as exon skipping and intron retention, which explained the observed cytotoxicity triggered upon RBM39 degradation. In conclusion, uncovering **indisulam's** MoA aided its repurposing to diseases addicted to RBM39 and/or DCAF15, such as leukemias and lymphomas. For a detailed discussion on "molecular glues" as well as characterization of their mode of binding via X-ray crystallography, we recommend the contributions of Morgan Gadd and Cristina Mayor-Ruiz in Chapters 4 and 6, respectively.

9.3.2.5 PROTAC-Mediated Degradation of Splicing Factor 3B1 (SF3B1)

The spliceosome complex is composed of a multitude of proteins [12], of which the structural protein SF3B1 coordinates the recognition of the 3′SS region at intron–exon junctions as part of the U2 snRNP [48]. As SF3B1 is frequently mutated in myelodysplastic [49] and CLL tumors [50], developing tools that selectively inhibit or ablate mutated SF3B1 protein function will allow the deconvolution of SF3B1's structural role within the spliceosome and its impact on regulating RNA and tumor biology.

Gama-Brambila et al. [51] reported the targeted degradation of the SF3B1 protein via a PROTAC approach. This was generated via the covalent attachment of **thalidomide**, an established SMOL that interacts with the E3 ligase cereblon (CRBN), to a previously reported SF3B1 binder termed **O4I2**. As CRBN is part of the Cullin-4-containing E3 ubiquitin ligase complex CUL4–RBX1–DDB1 (known as CRL4), **PROTAC-O4I2** (**6**; Figure 9.2, bottom panel) triggers proximity-induced degradation via targeted recruitment of the ubiquitin-proteasome cellular machinery to SF3B1. Consequently, the proteome-wide SF3B1-selective degradation triggers apoptosis in K562, HEK293, HepG2, and HeLa cells. Expectedly, splicing of DnaJ homolog subfamily B member 1 (DNAJB1) was affected upon **PROTAC-O4I2** treatment at concentrations ~100-fold less compared to those of pladienolide B, an established small-molecule binder of SF3B1. In addition, the authors showed that the **PROTAC-O4I2** probe improved the survival of a Notch-defective intestinal stem cell (ISC) *in vivo Drosophila* model in an SF3B1-centric manner. In conclusion, the study highlights the straightforward reprogramming of an established targeted binding into a targeted degradation event, which ablates SF3B1 function *in vitro* and *in vivo*.

9.3.3 Nuclear RNA Decay

Immediately after transcription, RNA transcripts are stepwise bound by various sets of protein complexes for further processing and subsequent nuclear export steps. Although it has been assumed that mRNA decay occurs exclusively in the cytoplasm, nuclear mRNA degradation has been recently reported to be an essential quality control mechanism for cellular homeostasis [52, 53]. For example, nuclear decay removes transcriptional by-products, for example, when RNA Pol II stalls or terminates before reaching completion or when mRNAs are improperly processed (Figure 9.3a). In addition, nuclear surveillance mechanisms via nuclear exosome complexes also degrade unspliced mRNA [54] and transcripts that were prematurely cleaved and polyadenylated at cryptic polyadenylation sites [52, 55]. For example, mRNA transcripts lacking nuclear cap binding complex (CBC) undergo decapping by exoribonuclease protein 1 (DXO1) and are degraded by XRN2 [56]. Expectedly, there are various nuclear RNA exosome complexes that consist of, among others, exosome complex exonucleases RRP6 and RRP44. In conclusion, such endogenous RNA degradation mechanisms represent a promising source of possible therapeutic entry points for targeted degradation of disease-causing mRNAs.

9.3.3.1 Small-Molecule-Mediated Nuclear Decay of CUG Repeat Expansions

RNA repeat expansions are responsible for more than 40 diseases, covering various neurological and muscular atrophies, and others [57]. CUG trinucleotide repeat expansions (r(CUG)^{exp}) are the main cause for myotonic dystrophy type 1 (DM1) and fuchs endothelial corneal dystrophy (FECD). Whereas the former is observed in patients harboring r(CUG)^{exp} in the 3′-UTR of dystrophia myotonica protein kinase (DMPK), the latter is localized within intron 3 of transcription factor 4 (TCF4). Both disease etiologies emerge from an RNA gain-of-function mechanism, whereby r(CUG)^{exp} sequesters the splicing regulator muscleblind-like 1 protein (MBNL1) in nuclear foci. Consequently, the availability of MBNL1 is reduced, leading to global aberrant splicing defects. Attractive therapeutic approaches are either to compete with the MBNL1 sequestration via addition of a SMOL or trigger degradation of toxic r(CUG)^{exp}.

Angelbello et al. [58] reported the SMOL **compound 2b** (**7**; Figure 9.3, bottom panel) that binds and engages r(CUG)^{exp} and potently inhibits the r(CUG)^{exp} MBNL1 interaction *in vitro* and in cells. For example, in patient-derived DM1 fibroblasts and myotubes, **compound 2b** corrected DM1 phenotypes, such as the number of MBNL1-positive nuclear foci and inclusion of MBNL1 exon 5. As expected, **compound 2b**'s bioactivity was recapitulated in FECD patient-derived cells.

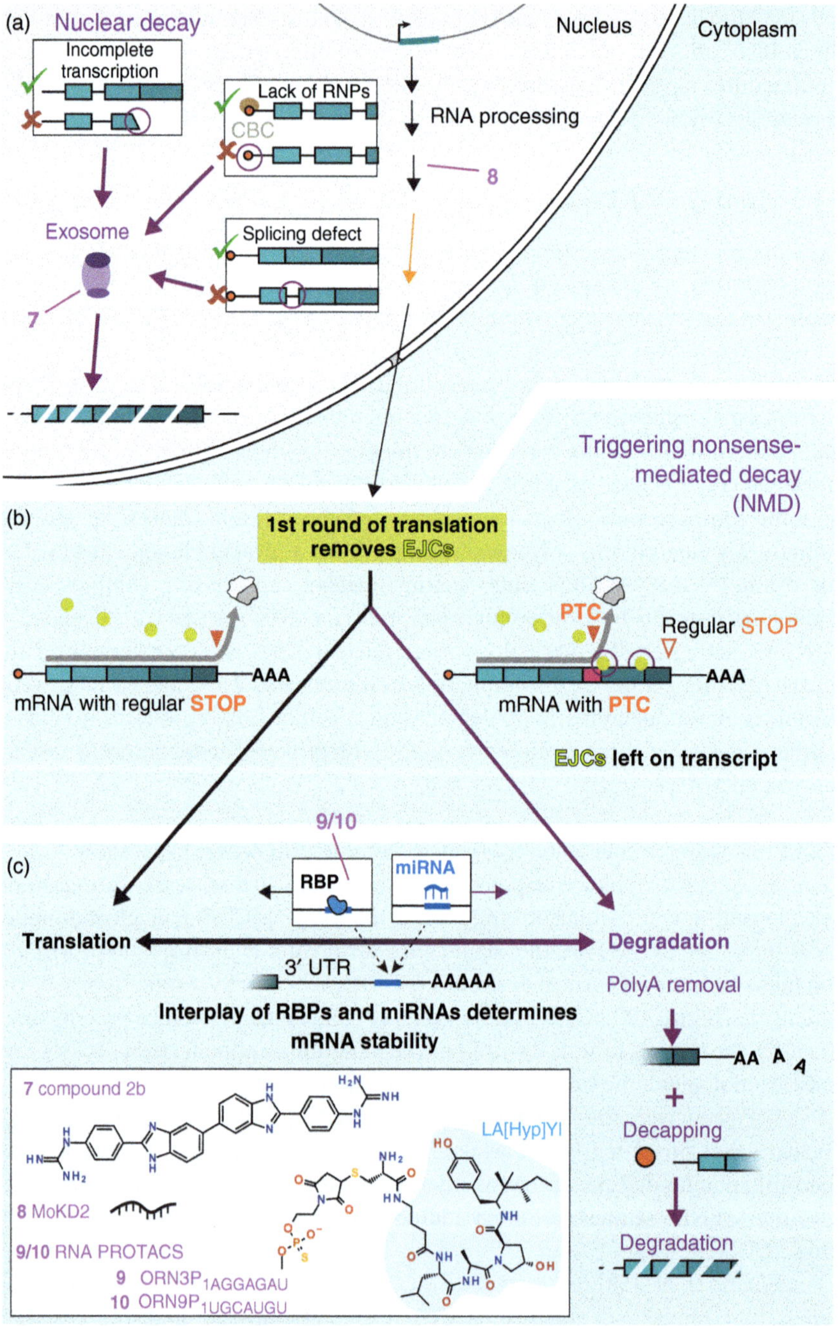
(a) Nuclear decay
Nucleus
Cytoplasm
Incomplete transcription
Lack of RNPs
CBC
RNA processing
8
Exosome
Splicing defect
7
Triggering nonsense-mediated decay (NMD)
(b)
1st round of translation removes EJCs
PTC
Regular STOP
AAA
mRNA with regular STOP
mRNA with PTC
EJCs left on transcript
9/10
(c)
RBP
miRNA
Translation
Degradation
3′ UTR
AAAAA
PolyA removal
Interplay of RBPs and miRNAs determines mRNA stability
AA A A
Decapping
7 compound 2b
LA[Hyp]YI
8 MoKD2
9/10 RNA PROTACS
9 ORN3P1AGGAGAU
10 ORN9P1UGCAUGU

However, targeted real-time quantitative PCR (RT-qPCR) analysis revealed that **compound 2b** treatment did not affect the intron 3-excised, i.e. intronless, TCF4 mature mRNA levels, but lowered the intron 3-retained TCF4 mRNA transcript levels harboring r(CUG)^{exp}. Further mechanistic studies revealed that this biological effect is mediated by RRP6 and RRP44, but not XRN1. Although further investigations are needed to completely elucidate **compound 2b**'s MoA, it highlights the possibility of harnessing intrinsic RNA decay pathways to promote targeted degradation of other disease-causing RNAs, as recently reported by the same group [59, 60].

9.4 Cytoplasmatic RNA Quality Control Mechanisms

Multiple quality control pathways target defective mRNA transcripts for degradation both in the nucleus and in the cytoplasm, thereby shaping the transcriptome to maintain cellular homeostasis, prevent emergence of disease, and swiftly adapt to extra- and intracellular stimuli. For instance, under different conditions, the half-lives of selected mRNA transcripts can be extended or reduced over the range of ~1000-fold. Therefore, key cytoplasmic mRNA quality surveillance mechanisms have evolved to safeguard mRNA transcripts along their life cycle. Section 9.4 will briefly highlight the protein complexes and the corresponding cellular processes involved in these steps.

9.4.1 Incorrect Splicing Triggers NMD in the Cytoplasm

One of the best characterized and evolutionary-conserved mRNA quality control mechanism occurs during the first round of translation via NMD in the cytoplasm (Figure 9.3b) [61]. For example, it was found that NMD targets one-third of mutated,

Figure 9.3 Major principles of RNA degradation pathways and possible therapeutic entry points (pink). (a) Incompletely processed mRNAs or unprotected intermediates of mRNA processing are guided to the nuclear RNA degradation machinery (exosome) for removal; (b) Nonsense-mediated decay (NMD) is triggered when exon junction complexes (EJCs) remain bound to the mRNA after the first round of translation. This is caused by PTCs that lead to premature dissociation of the ribosome and signal erroneous splicing. If no EJCs remain, mRNA is stabilized and further translated; (c) The interplay of stabilizing and destabilizing interactions regulates the fate of mRNAs in the cytoplasm. RBPs and miRNAs can compete for overlapping binding regions and cause the recruitment of the degradation machinery or prevent it. RNA degradation is initiated through decapping of the 5′-end, which then leads to shortening of the poly(A) tail and degradation.

disease-causing mRNAs. However, it recently has been revealed that NMD also targets ~10% of non-disease-related mRNAs to control the appropriate cellular responses to environmental changes [62].

In the nucleus, large messenger ribonucleoprotein particles (mRNPs) are processing pre-mRNAs by directing them toward capping, splicing, and polyadenylation. These events result in tagging of mRNAs with distinct EJC complexes ~20–24 nucleotides (nt) upstream of exon–exon junctions [63]. Interestingly, EJCs remain bound to the mRNAs during their export from the nucleus and throughout the "pioneer round" of translation, where the EJCs are removed by the processing ribosomes (Figure 9.3b, left branch). An mRNA efficiently marked for degradation via NMD features a PTC located at ≥50–55 nt upstream of an exon–exon junction. As a result, the downstream EJC remains attached to the mRNA as the ribosome falls off before the PTC (Figure 9.3b, right branch) [64]. The mRNA decay via NMD is mostly centered around the regulator of nonsense transcripts 1 (UPF1), which also hubs the recruitment of decapping and deadenylation complexes (Figure 9.3c) [65, 66].

Cytoplasmic mRNA degradation is also highly dependent on the removal of the poly(A) tail, as it protects mRNAs from 3′-end degradation (Figure 9.3c). A key player in stabilizing the poly(A) tail is the cytoplasmic polyadenylate binding protein (PABPC), which binds to ~25–30 adenine units. When intra- or extracellular cues signal the degradation of a particular mRNA or mRNA subsets, two main exonuclease (deadenylase) complexes, the CCR4–negative on TATA-less (NOT) and the PAN2–PAN3 complex, can be recruited by RBPs to shorten the poly(A) tail. Upon shortening it by ~10–12 nt, canonical mRNA decay is initiated by removing the 5′-cap, i.e. decapping, and degradation in a 5′–3′ direction by XRN1 or in a 3′–5′ direction by the cytoplasmic exosome complexes [62, 67]. The sheer abundance of different decapping enzymes, as well as exonucleases, points toward a highly regulated and more complex mRNA surveillance system, which remains yet to be explored for targeted degradation of disease-causing mRNAs as possible entry routes for therapeutic benefit.

9.4.1.1 Harnessing Intronic Poly(A) Activation with ASOs

At least 50% of human genes feature alternative polyA sites (PAS) within their corresponding RNA transcripts. As a result of alternative intronic polyadenylation (IPA), truncated protein isoforms with altered biological functions can be generated at the expense of native full-length counterparts. IPA has been shown to be relevant in receptor tyrosine kinase (RTK) isoform generation, where PAS usage generates protein isoforms termed soluble decoy RTKs (sdRTKs), which lack the transmembrane (TM) domain and the intracellularly located ATP binding kinase domain. As RTKs biological function is regulated via lateral dimerization at the surface of the plasma membrane, such "decoy" RTK products interfere with signal transduction to the cytoplasm via non-functional dimerization. Therefore, rational manipulation of the RTK isoform composition via IPA represents a potential therapeutic modality in human malignancies triggered by aberrant activation of RTK signaling pathways.

Vorlová et al. [68] used ASOs to target 5′SS in RTK mRNA that feature a PAS in the downstream intron. The ASOs were designed to mask the 5′SS so that the intronic sequence containing the PAS is retained, and IPA is triggered instead. Indeed, targeting vascular endothelial growth factor 2 (VEGFR2)'s intron 13 with **MoKD2** (**8**; Figure 9.3, bottom panel) led to the production, at both the RNA and protein levels, of a soluble decoy isoform of VEGFR2 at the expense of the full length. Consequently, the number of endothelial tubes and nodes were decreased, which ultimately inhibited the endothelial tube formation. In conclusion, induction of sdRTK highlights exciting novel therapeutic modalities in human diseases, where the RTK pathway is aberrantly upregulated.

9.4.2 RNA Binding Proteins Recruit the mRNA Degradation Machinery

The basic ingredient of RNA–protein complexes are the RBPs that bind (un)structured RNA sequences. Not only do they directly interact with a multitude of RNA targets in a cellular contextual manner but they also provide the scaffolding capacity to assemble highly complex macromolecular assemblies. Over 1500 evolutionary-conserved RBPs have been identified in humans [22] that regulate every aspect of RNA processing and maturation. The integrated result of RBP binding is complex, as RBPs can significantly impact mRNA biology depending on the localization of the binding site within the mRNA transcript, the cellular context, and others. Prominent examples are RBPs regulating 5′- and 3′-UTRs, such as tristetraprolin (TTP) and human antigen R (HuR). In addition, members of the embryonic lethal abnormal vision (ELAV) protein family recognize AU-rich elements (AREs) [69, 70] and the Pumilio RBPs recognize Pumilio-rich elements (PRE) in 3′-UTRs [71–73]. The literature of RBPs is vast [74], and because of space limitations, we cannot comprehensively cover this topic in Chapter 9. We are of the opinion that better understanding mRNA RBP interactions could provide another path forward for selective degradation of disease-causing mRNAs. Indeed, progress has been made in modulating RBPs with SMOLs and we direct the reader to an excellent review published recently [75].

9.4.2.1 RNA-PROTAC-Mediated Degradation of LIN28A and RBFOX1

As RBPs are essential players that regulate the stability of mRNA transcripts, targeted removal of a disease-specific RBP, such as Lin-28 homolog A (LIN28A) and RNA binding Fox-1 homolog 1 (RBFOX1), can affect the life cycle of a selected or a subset of disease-relevant mRNAs simultaneously. Ghidini et al. [76] reported the proteasome-mediated degradation of LIN28A and RBFOX1 via peptide–ASO conjugates termed RNA PROTACs. The RNA PROTACs comprise of two covalently linked modules: (i) a short ASO oligonucleotide that matches the preferred consensus binding sequence of LIN28A or RBFOX1, respectively, and (ii) a peptide sequence that binds components of the ubiquitin E3-ligase complex(es). Therefore, RNA PROTAC brings the RBP in the vicinity of the canonical ubiquitin-proteasome machinery, inducing targeted RBP degradation. As a proof of concept, a conserved

5′-AGGAGAU-3′ motif reported to bind the zinc knuckle domain (ZKD) of LIN28A was selected. The ASO's cellular permeability and stability were increased via introduction of diastereomeric PS backbone and 2′-OMe or 2′-methoxyethyl (2′-MOE) modifications. The RNA PROTAC **ORN3P$_1$** (**9**; Figure 9.3, bottom panel) was generated via covalently linking the ASO with the **LA[Hyp]YI** peptide, which is derived from the **ALAPYI**P amino acid sequence of the transcription factor hypoxia-inducible factor 1-alpha (HIF1α). The hydroxylation of the central proline residue is recognized by the von Hippel–Lindau disease tumor suppressor (VHL) ubiquitination complex, leading to the proteasomal degradation of LIN28A. Indeed, **ORN3P$_1$** efficiently degraded LIN28A in K562 and human testicular embryonal carcinoma NT2/D1 cells. To further strengthen the proof of concept, the authors designed an additional RNA PROTAC directed toward targeted degradation of RBFOX1, termed **ORN9P$_1$** (**10**; Figure 9.3, bottom panel). Although the proteome and transcriptome-wide effects of degrading LIN28A and RBFOX1 were not investigated, the study highlights RNA PROTAC as a promising modality to targeted proteasomal degradation of RBPs.

9.4.3 RNA Interference (RNAi) – microRNA, siRNA, and ASO Gapmers

RNAi was first discovered in *Caenorhabditis elegans* [77], where this double-stranded RNA (dsRNA)-based regulatory mechanism triggered post-transcriptional gene silencing (Figure 9.4). In general, RNA Pol II-mediated transcription generates primary transcripts, termed pri-miRNAs. Pri-miRNAs are then processed into precursor miRNAs (pre-miRNAs) by the microprocessor complex Drosha ribonuclease III (Drosha)-Microprocessor complex subunit DGCR8 (DGCR8) and exported into the cytoplasm. Here, they are further processed by endoribonuclease Dicer (Dicer) and RISC-loading complex subunit TARBP2 (TRBP2). Dicer cleaves the terminal loop of the pre-miRNA, leading to a dsRNA intermediate. Finally, the sense strand of the miRNA duplex is degraded, while the guide strand (antisense; mature miRNA) remains in the RNA-induced silencing complex (RISC)–loading complex (RLC) containing Argonaute proteins (Ago1–Ago4). As soon as the mature miRNA is loaded into the RISC complex, it hybridizes with its cognate target mRNA sequence in the 3′-UTR (Figure 9.4).

Synthetic short double-stranded RNAs as in short interfering (siRNAs) or shRNAs are therapeutically attractive [78] because they exploit the maturation pathways of endogenous miRNAs to modulate gene silencing (Figure 9.4) [78]. On the one hand, shRNA sequences are encoded in a DNA vector that requires intracellular delivery via plasmid transfection or viral transduction. Upon transcription, a hairpin RNA construct is produced, which is then cleaved by Dicer to yield a dsRNA that is subsequently integrated into the RISC complex. On the other hand, siRNAs are synthetic dsRNAs, typically in the range of 20–24 base pairs, which are recognized by the RISC complex. Similar to shRNAs, siRNAs require intracellular delivery via transient transfection or viral vectors.

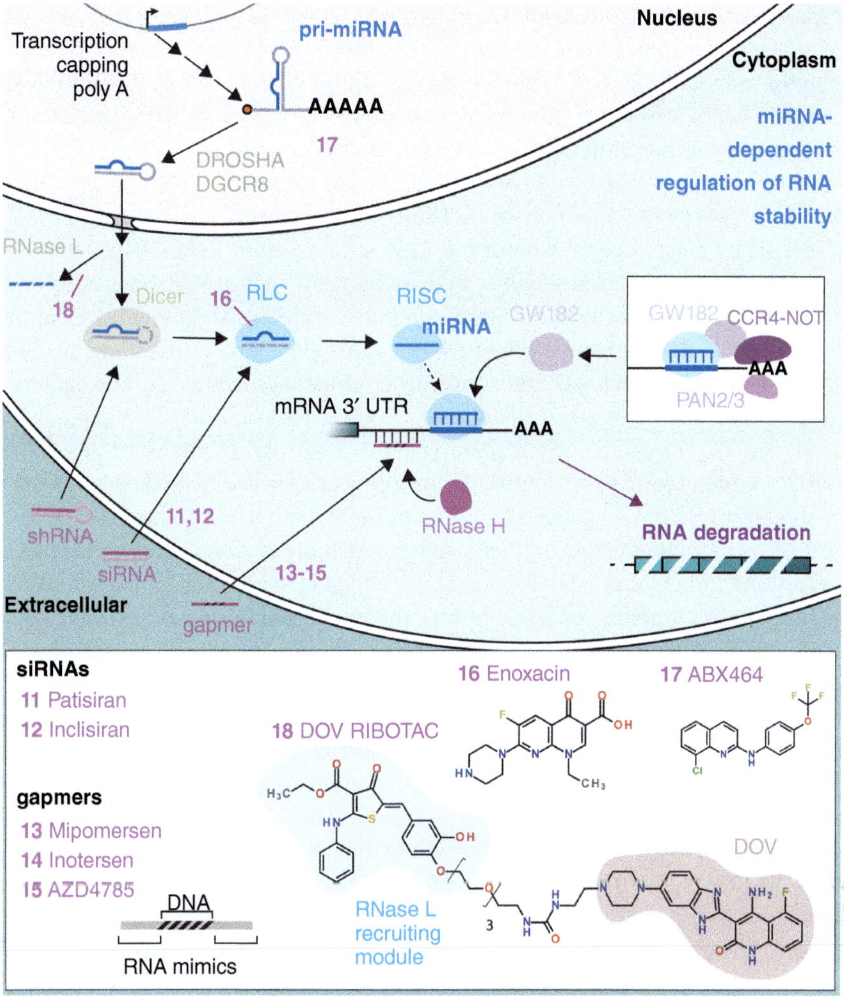

Figure 9.4 Description of the miRNA/siRNA and RNase H-mediated degradation pathways and their involvement in the regulation of mRNA stability. After transcription and early processing (top), pri-miRNAs are processed through several steps in the nucleus and cytoplasm (bottom), before being bound by the RISC. The interaction of the miRNA-loaded RISC with complementary regions in 3′-UTRs recruits proteins responsible for decapping and poly(A) removal, thus triggering mRNA decay. Using the later processing steps of miRNA maturation, therapeutic small-hairpin RNAs (shRNA), synthetic small-interfering RNAs (siRNAs, bottom left), and ASO gapmers can be used to perform targeted degradation of mRNAs.

siRNAs and shRNAs are widely considered robust tools for targeted modulation of gene expression and can be designed based on sequence complementarity. Transferring their potential into RNA therapeutic drugs has been challenging because of, for example, effective and organ-specific delivery, off-target effects leading to non-specific activation of the innate immune system, and others [79, 80].

Despite these hurdles, **Patisiran** (**Onpattro**®; **11**, Figure 9.4, bottom panel) was the first siRNA drug approved by the FDA in 2018 for the treatment of hereditary transthyretin amyloidosis (hATTR) with polyneuropathy [78], while **inclisiran** (**Leqvio**®; **12**, Figure 9.4, bottom panel) got marketed in 2021 for patients suffering from atherosclerotic cardiovascular disease (ASCVD).

Among the sequence-based ASO tools, single-stranded ASO gapmers have received considerable attention [81]. Their MoA capitalizes on ribonuclease H (RNase H)-mediated degradation of the RNA strand within RNA–DNA heteroduplexes. Whereas ASO blockers highlighted in Chapter 9, such as **Spinraza**, **2b-block**, and **MoKB2**, are single-stranded RNA oligonucleotides, ASO gapmers are single-stranded DNA–RNA mixmers (Figure 9.4) featuring a central DNA sequence that triggers RNase H-mediated degradation. Structural and functional studies centered around RNase H1 highlighted the optimal DNA sequence of an ASO gapmer for effective RNA transcript degradation (Figure 9.4). For example, at least five (8–10 have been found to be optimal) central consecutive deoxynucleotide residues are necessary for an ASO gapmer to be an optimal substrate for RNase H1. The central deoxynucleotide-containing region is flanked at the 5′ and 3′-ends with various 2′-substituted nucleotides, i.e. RNA mimics, which contribute to higher affinity to the target RNA sequence and help improve the physicochemical and pharmacological properties of ASO gapmers [81]. Exploiting RNase H1-mediated degradation of disease-causing RNAs lead to the approval of **mipomersen** (**Kynamro**®; **13**, Figure 9.4, bottom panel) by the FDA in 2013 for the treatment of homozygous familial hypercholesterolemia (HoFH), whereas **inotersen** (**Tegsedi**®; **14**, Figure 9.4, bottom panel) got marketed in 2018 for the treatment of hATTR. Whereas **mipomersen** cleaves apolipoprotein B-100 (APOB), **inotersen** degrades transthyretin (TTR) mRNA. In addition, a recent study reports the preclinical results of **AZD4785** (**15**; Figure 9.4, bottom panel), an ASO gapmer targeting the 3′-UTR of Kirsten rat sarcoma virus (KRAS) mRNA. **AZD4785** potently and selectively degraded KRAS mRNA. As a result of depleting KRAS protein, downstream signaling pathways were inhibited, triggering antiproliferative effects in KRAS mutant cells. The same phenotypic effects were recapitulated *in vivo*, where KRAS mRNA and protein degradation was measured in a broad set of tissues without any observable adverse effects. Furthermore, **AZD4785**'s safety was demonstrated in mice and monkeys, highlighting **AZD4785** as an attractive RNA therapeutic for the treatment of KRAS-driven cancer in humans. As a result of a staggering number of antisense therapies already undergoing various stages of (pre)clinical development, we expect the number of approved antisense therapies for a broad range of human conditions to increase.

9.4.3.1 Small-Molecule Enhancement of microRNA Processing

While siRNAs drugs have been approved by the FDA, lowering their therapeutically effective dose might mitigate off-target effects, leading to safer clinical candidates. Using a phenotypic screening on ~2000 SMOL library, Shan et al. [82] identified **enoxacin** (**Penetrex**®; **16**, Figure 9.4, bottom panel) that increased the siRNA-mediated degradation of a stable enhanced green fluorescent protein (EGFP) in a human embryonic kidney (HEK293) cell line (termed 293-EGFP) by an order of magnitude. In other words, the siRNA dosage required to degrade EGPF mRNA was considerably reduced upon **enoxacin** treatment. Further experimental evidence highlighted that **enoxacin** promotes loading of siRNA/miRNA duplexes onto the RISC complex by "glueing" transactivation response element RNA-binding protein (TRBP) to selected RNAs [83]. Indeed, **enoxacin**'s MoA is dependent on TRBP, as the knockdown of this protein abolished the bioactivity of the SMOL. This study highlights the identification of a SMOL modulator of the siRNA/miRNA processing machinery, thereby uncovering a promising avenue of selectively manipulating siRNA/miRNA pathways for therapeutic benefit.

9.4.3.2 SMOL-Mediated Upregulation of miR-124 in Inflammatory Diseases

Aberrant inflammatory signaling of immune cells is often associated with disease pathogenesis, such as autoimmune diseases. Among many layers of regulation, non-coding miRNAs have shown to safeguard the immune system by impacting intracellular signaling pathways. For example, miR-124 has emerged as a promising RNA target in patients suffering of rheumatoid arthritis (RA) [84] or pediatric intestinal failure [85], where miR-124 is downregulated. Consequently, elevation of miR-124 levels increases the miRNA-mediated degradation of endogenous mRNA targets.

Tazi et al. [86] have reported the identification of a selective SMOL upregulator of miR-124 expression, **ABX464** (**17**; Figure 9.4, bottom panel). Studies have demonstrated that miR-124 is transcribed from three genomic loci. A single locus generates long non-coding RNA (lncRNA 0599-205), which is subsequently spliced to produce miR-124. Mechanistically, **ABX464** might inhibit degradation of lncRNA 0599-205 by targeting the CBC–nuclear exosome targeting (NEXT) complex. Administration of **ABX464** offered long-term protection against dextran sulfate (DSS)-induced intestinal inflammation and inhibited colitis in an miR-124-centric manner. Because of the favorable safety profile *in vivo*, **ABX464** advanced to phase IIb trials in ulcerative colitis (UC) and phase IIa in RA. In conclusion, **ABX464**'s MoA led to upregulation of miR-124 levels, which is therapeutically viable in clinical indications, where an miR-124-centric attenuation of inflammation is required.

9.4.3.3 RIBOTAC-Mediated Degradation of Pre-miR-21 via Targeted Recruitment of RNase L

Ribonuclease targeting chimeras (RIBOTAC) have recently been reported as a novel proximity-induced modality for targeted degradation of RNAs [87]. In general, proximity-inducing chimera strategies [88] use SMOLs (molecular glues and bifunctional molecules) and hybrids (SMOL-antibody and SMOL-ASO conjugates) to rewire endogenous cellular processes toward targeted protein/RNA cleavage, degradation, or post-transcriptional editing [88]. Consequently, such technologies can extend beyond the traditional target occupancy agonism or inhibition to a new therapeutic avenue described as event-driven pharmacology. For example, proximity-induced modalities often exhibit catalytic behavior; in other words, sub-stoichiometric amounts of the targeting chimeras (TACs) are needed to affect the cellular fate of a biological target. Because of the catalytic MoA, TACs often feature increased potency and selectivity compared to traditional target binders/inhibitors [89]. Therefore, the application of TACs is highly suited to challenging biological targets, where traditional intervention modalities failed to provide robust solutions toward successful drug discovery and development campaigns.

RIBOTACs degrade disease-causing RNAs via proximal recruitment of ribonucleases [87]. This is achieved via a modular probe featuring two covalently linked components: First, a SMOL that binds and engages a specific RNA motif within a disease-causing RNA of interest; Second, a second SMOL that binds and/or activates a suitable ribonuclease. By covalently linking the two modules, the RIBOTAC probe recruits the ribonuclease in the vicinity of the RNA motif and subsequently initiates nuclease-mediated degradation in a targeted manner. The current generation of RIBOTACs exploits the ribonuclease function of 2′-5′ oligoadenylate synthetase-dependent ribonuclease or RNase L. RNase L is a key member of the cell's antiviral program and under steady-state conditions only present in minute amounts in the cytosol in an inactive form. The ribonuclease activity of RNase L is only activated upon dimerization via endogenous ligands such as 2′,5′-phosphodiester-linked oligoadenylates (2′–5′A_ns), which are often produced as a response of the innate immune system to viral infections. At least three 2′,5′-As (2′,5′-A_3) and a single 5′-phosphoryl group are necessary for RNase's moderate degradation ability of single-stranded RNAs. Consequently, the first RIBOTAC report in 2018 by the Disney lab used a SMOL-2′-5′A_4 chimeric probe for RNase L-mediated degradation of pri-miRNA-96 [90]. The same group reported in 2020 the replacement of RNase L's activation/dimerization 2′-5′A_4 module with a SMOL [91]. The newly generated bifunctional RIBOTAC successfully degraded pre-miRNA-21 *in vitro* and *in vivo* and featured superior potency and selectivity, when compared to the pre-miRNA-21 SMOL binder lacking the RNase L-recruiting module. Since 2020, the successful application of RIBOTAC-mediated degradation has been reported for severe acute respiratory syndrome (SARS)-CoV-2 frame-shifting element [92], hexanucleotide repeat expansions, r$(G_4C_2)^{exp}$ [93], and miRNAs [94]. This is no surprise as dysregulation of miRNA biogenesis is a hallmark of various diseases [95, 96]. miRNA-21 is among the best studied miRNAs, and its upregulation is associated with several of human disorders [97]. Consequently, modalities that restore the native levels of this miRNA represent promising therapeutic interventions.

Zhang et al. [94] reported the conversion of the established, clinically used RTK inhibitor **dovitinib (DOV)** into a potent and selective degrader of precursor miRNA-21 (pre-miRNA-21) *in vitro* and *in vivo*. Functional studies revealed that **DOV** inhibited miRNA-21 biogenesis in MDA-MB-231 cells by selectively affecting pre-miRNA-21 processing. As a result of lower levels of mature miRNA-21, expression of direct targets of mature miRNA-21 such as programmed cell death protein 4 (PDCD4) and phosphatidylinositol 3,4,5-trisphosphate 3-phosphatase and dual-specificity protein phosphatase PTEN (phosphatase and tensin homolog [PTEN]) was restored.

DOV was then converted into a RIBOTAC degrader of pre-miRNA-21, termed **DOV RIBOTAC** (**18**; Figure 9.4, bottom panel). Conversion to **DOV RIBOTAC** led to ~25-fold improved potency and selectivity compared to **DOV**. In addition, an ~100-fold decrease in RTK phosphorylation was observed, suggesting a dramatic decrease in RTK protein occupancy in cells treated with **DOV RIBOTAC**. Finally, the **DOV RIBOTAC** degrader mitigated tumor burden in a lung xenograft mouse model and improved kidney function in an Alport syndrome *in vivo* model.

9.5 Conclusions

In recent years, new modalities have been explored to tackle disease-relevant targets. This trend has been fueled by the need to identify novel approaches of drugging disease-relevant biological targets, other than kinases, proteases, GPCRs, etc. As highlighted in this chapter, targeting, or exploiting RNA biology, particularly mRNA degradation mechanisms, extends beyond the traditional protein-centric approaches, tapping into a multitude of post-transcriptional regulatory mechanisms. Consequently, novel and potentially biologically relevant protein targets, RNA sequences, and structures, or RNA–protein interactions, could foster the development of next-generation therapeutics towards "undruggable" targets, as well as new avenues of yet underexplored disease indications. Indeed, the recent approval of **risdiplam**, as the first SMOL oral medication for SMA, spurred the interest into exploring pre-mRNA splicing for a multitude of human conditions.

To make mRNA degradation amenable to therapeutic targeting with novel modalities in a rational manner, a better understanding of the context-dependent interactions between the protein and RNA single-stranded regions/structures involved in regulating RNA biology is needed. The examples comprised in Chapter 9 are highlighting the current status of this very promising research direction. First, deploy the already-established targeting chimera technologies, such as (RNA) PROTAC and RIBOTAC, toward validated RBP and RNA structures, respectively. Secondly, a major contribution in exploiting endogenous cellular mechanisms for targeted mRNA degradation will arise from integrating (RNA) chemical biology tools, especially when combined with genomic analyses of patient cohorts and/or readily available *in vivo* models. On the one hand, **indisulam** is a prime example of the importance of MoA elucidation to explore more effective or novel indications for already existing chemical matter. Indeed, recent studies proposed **indisulam** as a highly efficacious treatment against neuroblastoma [98, 99]. On the other hand, **compound 2b** and **DOV** in **DOV RIBOTAC** highlighted the potential of targeting RNA structures and validating RNA-centric target occupancy MoAs. Such findings facilitated the emergence of novel modalities such as RIBOTACs that endows target occupancy SMOLs with RNA degradation-driven pharmacology, featuring the catalytic activity and drastically improved potency and selectivity at lower doses [89].

Third, compared to a single orally administered and marketed SMOL drug, there are numerous antisense therapies currently in use [78, 81]. In addition, many such RNA therapeutics are undergoing various stages of (pre)clinical investigations for a plethora of human disease indications, which (yet) lack a SMOL oral drug. This is not surprising considering the unparalleled sequence-based programmability of ASOs to target designated regions of the disease-causing (pre)-mRNA of interest. Indeed, the ASO-based RNA therapeutic modalities covered in this book chapter highlight their straightforward design from sequence, for robust hypothesis and/or target validation *in vitro* and *in vivo* by various regulatory processes.

Lastly, many of the biological targets and processes covered in Chapter 9 have not (yet) been harnessed toward targeted mRNA degradation by either modality. Therefore, it is our hope that the SMOL modulators of splicing, RNA therapeutics (ASO blockers and gapmers, siRNAs, and shRNAs), (RNA) PROTAC, and RIBOTAC examples highlighted herein will soon be part of the pharmaceutical companies' portfolios. In addition, key to drugging these mRNA degradation mechanisms will be the selection of the therapeutically most relevant entry point for any disease-causing mRNA via the safest modality that will bring therapeutic benefit to patients.

Acknowledgments

We acknowledge Dr. Razvan Nutiu, Dr. Nicole Biber, Dr. Nathalie Legrand, and Dr. Andreas Timmermann for critically reviewing the content of the book chapter. In addition, we thank members of the RNA Team at Bayer for helpful discussions and insights provided.

Conflict of Interest

Barbara Herdy, Hendrik Osadnik and Andrei Ursu are employees of Bayer AG.

References

1 Santos, R., Ursu, O., Gaulton, A. et al. (2017). A comprehensive map of molecular drug targets. *Nat. Rev. Drug Discov.* 16 (1): 19–34.

2 Lazo, J.S. and Sharlow, E.R. (2016). Drugging undruggable molecular cancer targets. *Annu. Rev. Pharmacol. Toxicol.* 56: 23–40.

3 Wang, F., Zuroske, T., and Watts, J.K. (2020). RNA therapeutics on the rise. *Nat. Rev. Drug Discov.* 19 (7): 441–442.

4 Harries, L.W. (2019). RNA biology provides new therapeutic targets for human disease. *Front. Genet.* 10 (205): 1–12.

5 Quake, S.R. (2021). The cell as a bag of RNA. *Trends Genet.* 37 (12): 1064–1068.

6 Cheneval, D., Kastelic, T., Fuerst, P., and Parker, C.N. (2010). A review of methods to monitor the modulation of mRNA stability: a novel approach to drug discovery and therapeutic intervention. *J. Biomol. Screen.* 15 (6): 609–622.

7 Ursu, A., Costales, M.G., Childs-Disney, J.L., and Disney, M.D. (2020). Chapter 15 small-molecule targeted degradation of RNA. In: *Protein Degradation with New Chemical Modalities: Successful Strategies in Drug Discovery and Chemical Biology*, 317–336. Cambridge, UK: The Royal Society of Chemistry.

8 Shatkin, A.J. (1976). Capping of eucaryotic mRNAs. *Cell* 9 (4, Part 2): 645–653.

9 Pelletier, J., Schmeing, T.M., and Sonenberg, N. (2021). The multifaceted eukaryotic cap structure. *WIREs RNA* 12 (2): e1636.

10 Topisirovic, I., Svitkin, Y.V., Sonenberg, N., and Shatkin, A.J. (2011). Cap and cap-binding proteins in the control of gene expression. *Wiley Interdiscip. Rev. RNA* 2 (2): 277–298.

11 Wilkinson, M.E., Charenton, C., and Nagai, K. (2020). RNA splicing by the spliceosome. *Annu. Rev. Biochem.* 89 (1): 359–388.

12 Yan, C., Wan, R., and Shi, Y. (2019). Molecular mechanisms of pre-mRNA splicing through structural biology of the spliceosome. *Cold Spring Harb. Perspect. Biol.* 11 (1): a032409.

13 Kastner, B., Will, C.L., Stark, H., and Lührmann, R. (2019). Structural insights into nuclear pre-mRNA splicing in higher eukaryotes. *Cold Spring Harb. Perspect. Biol.* 11 (11): a032417.

14 Wang, E.T., Sandberg, R., Luo, S. et al. (2008). Alternative isoform regulation in human tissue transcriptomes. *Nature* 456 (7221): 470–476.

15 Wong, M.S., Kinney, J.B., and Krainer, A.R. (2018). Quantitative activity profile and context dependence of all human 5′ splice sites. *Mol. Cell* 71 (6): 1012–1026.e3.

16 Wachutka, L., Caizzi, L., Gagneur, J., and Cramer, P. (2019). Global donor and acceptor splicing site kinetics in human cells. *eLife* 8: e45056.

17 Jeong, S. (2017). SR proteins: binders, regulators, and connectors of RNA. *Mol. Cells* 40 (1): 1–9.

18 Geuens, T., Bouhy, D., and Timmerman, V. (2016). The hnRNP family: insights into their role in health and disease. *Hum. Genet.* 135 (8): 851–867.

19 Pandit, S., Zhou, Y., Shiue, L. et al. (2013). Genome-wide analysis reveals SR protein cooperation and competition in regulated splicing. *Mol. Cell* 50 (2): 223–235.

20 Shen, H. and Green, M.R. (2004). A pathway of sequential arginine-serine-rich domain-splicing signal interactions during mammalian spliceosome assembly. *Mol. Cell* 16 (3): 363–373.

21 Saha, K., Fernandez, M.M., Biswas, T. et al. (2021). Discovery of a pre-mRNA structural scaffold as a contributor to the mammalian splicing code. *Nucleic Acids Res.* 49 (12): 7103–7121.

22 Van Nostrand, E.L., Freese, P., Pratt, G.A. et al. (2020). A large-scale binding and functional map of human RNA-binding proteins. *Nature* 583 (7818): 711–719.

23 Han, H., Braunschweig, U., Gonatopoulos-Pournatzis, T. et al. (2017). Multilayered control of alternative splicing regulatory networks by transcription factors. *Mol. Cell* 65 (3): 539–553.

24 Jayasinghe, R.G., Cao, S., Gao, Q. et al. (2018). Systematic analysis of splice-site-creating mutations in cancer. *Cell Rep.* 23 (1): 270–281.

25 Anna, A. and Monika, G. (2018). Splicing mutations in human genetic disorders: examples, detection, and confirmation. *J. Appl. Genet.* 59 (3): 253–268.

26 Zhang, Y., Qian, J., Gu, C., and Yang, Y. (2021). Alternative splicing and cancer: a systematic review. *Signal Transduct. Target. Ther.* 6 (1): 78.

27 Sveen, A., Kilpinen, S., Ruusulehto, A. et al. (2016). Aberrant RNA splicing in cancer; expression changes and driver mutations of splicing factor genes. *Oncogene* 35 (19): 2413–2427.

28 Shuai, S., Suzuki, H., Diaz-Navarro, A. et al. (2019). The U1 spliceosomal RNA is recurrently mutated in multiple cancers. *Nature* 574 (7780): 712–716.

29 Cheung, A.K., Hurley, B., Kerrigan, R. et al. (2018). Discovery of small molecule splicing modulators of survival motor neuron-2 (SMN2) for the treatment of spinal muscular atrophy (SMA). *J. Med. Chem.* 61 (24): 11021–11036.

30 Lefebvre, S., Bürglen, L., Reboullet, S. et al. (1995). Identification and characterization of a spinal muscular atrophy-determining gene. *Cell* 80 (1): 155–165.

31 Lorson, C.L., Hahnen, E., Androphy, E.J., and Wirth, B. (1999). A single nucleotide in the SMN gene regulates splicing and is responsible for spinal muscular atrophy. *Proc. Natl. Acad. Sci.* 96 (11): 6307–6311.

32 Ottesen, E.W. (2017). ISS-N1 makes the first FDA-approved drug for spinal muscular atrophy. *Transl. Neurosci.* 8 (1): 1–6.

33 Ratni, H., Ebeling, M., Baird, J. et al. (2018). Discovery of risdiplam, a selective survival of motor neuron-2 (SMN2) gene splicing modifier for the treatment of spinal muscular atrophy (SMA). *J. Med. Chem.* 61 (15): 6501–6517.

34 Dhillon, S. (2020). Risdiplam: first approval. *Drugs* 80 (17): 1853–1858.

35 Singh, R.N., Ottesen, E.W., and Singh, N.N. (2020). The first orally deliverable small molecule for the treatment of spinal muscular atrophy. *Neurosci. Insights* 15: 1–11. 2633105520973985.

36 Sivaramakrishnan, M., McCarthy, K.D., Campagne, S. et al. (2017). Binding to SMN2 pre-mRNA-protein complex elicits specificity for small molecule splicing modifiers. *Nat. Commun.* 8 (1): 1476.

37 Wang, J., Schultz, P.G., and Johnson, K.A. (2018). Mechanistic studies of a small-molecule modulator of SMN2 splicing. *Proc. Natl. Acad. Sci.* 115 (20): E4604–E4612.

38 Campagne, S., Boigner, S., Rüdisser, S. et al. (2019). Structural basis of a small molecule targeting RNA for a specific splicing correction. *Nat. Chem. Biol.* 15 (12): 1191–1198.

39 Tabrizi, S.J., Ghosh, R., and Leavitt, B.R. (2019). Huntingtin lowering strategies for disease modification in Huntington's disease. *Neuron* 101 (5): 801–819.

40 Bhattacharyya, A., Trotta, C.R., Narasimhan, J. et al. (2021). Small molecule splicing modifiers with systemic HTT-lowering activity. *Nat. Commun.* 12 (1): 7299.

41 Keller, C.G., Shin, Y., Monteys, A.M. et al. (2022). An orally available, brain penetrant, small molecule lowers huntingtin levels by enhancing pseudoexon inclusion. *Nat. Commun.* 13 (1): 1150.

42 Bonnal, S.C., López-Oreja, I., and Valcárcel, J. (2020). Roles and mechanisms of alternative splicing in cancer — implications for care. *Nat. Rev. Clin. Oncol.* 17 (8): 457–474.

43 Maimon, A., Mogilevsky, M., Shilo, A. et al. (2014). Mnk2 alternative splicing modulates the p38-MAPK pathway and impacts Ras-induced transformation. *Cell Rep.* 7 (2): 501–513.

44 Karni, R., de Stanchina, E., Lowe, S.W. et al. (2007). The gene encoding the splicing factor SF2/ASF is a proto-oncogene. *Nat. Struct. Mol. Biol.* 14 (3): 185–193.

45 Mogilevsky, M., Shimshon, O., Kumar, S. et al. (2018). Modulation of MKNK2 alternative splicing by splice-switching oligonucleotides as a novel approach for glioblastoma treatment. *Nucleic Acids Res.* 46 (21): 11396–11404.

46 Kahles, A., Lehmann, K.-V., Toussaint, N.C. et al. (2018). Comprehensive analysis of alternative splicing across tumors from 8,705 patients. *Cancer Cell* 34 (2): 211–224.e6.

47 Han, T., Goralski, M., Gaskill, N. et al. (2017). Anticancer sulfonamides target splicing by inducing RBM39 degradation via recruitment to DCAF15. *Science* 356 (6336): eaal3755.

48 Golas, M.M., Sander, B., Will, C.L. et al. (2003). Molecular architecture of the multiprotein splicing factor SF3b. *Science* 300 (5621): 980–984.

49 Papaemmanuil, E., Cazzola, M., Boultwood, J. et al. (2011). Somatic SF3B1 mutation in myelodysplasia with ring sideroblasts. *N. Engl. J. Med.* 365 (15): 1384–1395.

50 Wang, L., Lawrence, M.S., Wan, Y. et al. (2011). SF3B1 and other novel cancer genes in chronic lymphocytic leukemia. *N. Engl. J. Med.* 365 (26): 2497–2506.

51 Gama-Brambila, R.A., Chen, J., Zhou, J. et al. (2021). A PROTAC targets splicing factor 3B1. *Cell Chem. Biol.* 28 (11): 1616–1627.e8.

52 Schmid, M. and Jensen, T.H. (2018). Controlling nuclear RNA levels. *Nat. Rev. Genet.* 19 (8): 518–529.

53 Wolin, S.L. and Maquat, L.E. (2019). Cellular RNA surveillance in health and disease. *Science* 366 (6467): 822–827.

54 Bousquet-Antonelli, C., Presutti, C., and Tollervey, D. (2000). Identification of a regulated pathway for nuclear pre-mRNA turnover. *Cell* 102 (6): 765–775.

55 Chiu, A.C., Suzuki, H.I., Wu, X. et al. (2018). Transcriptional pause sites delineate stable nucleosome-associated premature polyadenylation suppressed by U1 snRNP. *Mol. Cell* 69 (4): 648–663.

56 Chang, J.H., Jiao, X., Chiba, K. et al. (2012). Dxo1 is a new type of eukaryotic enzyme with both decapping and 5'-3' exoribonuclease activity. *Nat. Struct. Mol. Biol.* 19 (10): 1011–1017.

57 Depienne, C. and Mandel, J.-L. (2021). 30 years of repeat expansion disorders: what have we learned and what are the remaining challenges? *Am. J. Hum. Genet.* 108 (5): 764–785.

58 Angelbello, A.J., Benhamou, R.I., Rzuczek, S.G. et al. (2021). A small molecule that binds an RNA repeat expansion stimulates its decay via the exosome complex. *Cell Chem. Biol.* 28 (1): 34–45.

59 Wagner-Griffin, S., Abe, M., Benhamou, R.I. et al. (2021). A druglike small molecule that targets r(CCUG) repeats in myotonic dystrophy type 2 facilitates degradation by RNA quality control pathways. *J. Med. Chem.* 64 (12): 8474–8485.

60 Benhamou, R.I., Angelbello, A.J., Wang, E.T., and Disney, M.D. (2020). A toxic RNA catalyzes the cellular synthesis of its own inhibitor, shunting it to endogenous decay pathways. *Cell Chem. Biol.* 27 (2): 223–231.

61 Nagy, E. and Maquat, L.E. (1998). A rule for termination-codon position within intron-containing genes: when nonsense affects RNA abundance. *Trends Biochem. Sci.* 23 (6): 198–199.

62 Kurosaki, T., Popp, M.W., and Maquat, L.E. (2019). Quality and quantity control of gene expression by nonsense-mediated mRNA decay. *Nat. Rev. Mol. Cell Biol.* 20 (7): 406–420.

63 Le Hir, H., Izaurralde, E., Maquat, L.E., and Moore, M.J. (2000). The spliceosome deposits multiple proteins 20–24 nucleotides upstream of mRNA exon–exon junctions. *EMBO J.* 19 (24): 6860–6869.

64 Thermann, R., Neu-Yilik, G., Deters, A. et al. (1998). Binary specification of nonsense codons by splicing and cytoplasmic translation. *EMBO J.* 17 (12): 3484–3494.

65 Grudzien-Nogalska, E. and Kiledjian, M. (2017). New insights into decapping enzymes and selective mRNA decay. *WIREs RNA* 8 (1): e1379.

66 Kramer, S. and McLennan, A.G. (2019). The complex enzymology of mRNA decapping: enzymes of four classes cleave pyrophosphate bonds. *WIREs RNA* 10 (1): e1511.

67 Garneau, N.L., Wilusz, J., and Wilusz, C.J. (2007). The highways and byways of mRNA decay. *Nat. Rev. Mol. Cell Biol.* 8 (2): 113–126.

68 Vorlová, S., Rocco, G., Lefave, C.V. et al. (2011). Induction of antagonistic soluble decoy receptor tyrosine kinases by intronic polyA activation. *Mol. Cell* 43 (6): 927–939.

69 Lykke-Andersen, J. and Wagner, E. (2005). Recruitment and activation of mRNA decay enzymes by two ARE-mediated decay activation domains in the proteins TTP and BRF-1. *Genes Dev.* 19 (3): 351–361.

70 Brooks, S.A. and Blackshear, P.J. (2013). Tristetraprolin (TTP): interactions with mRNA and proteins, and current thoughts on mechanisms of action. *Biochim. Biophys. Acta* 1829 (6-7): 666–679.

71 Goldstrohm, A.C., Hall, T.M.T., and McKenney, K.M. (2018). Post-transcriptional regulatory functions of mammalian Pumilio proteins. *Trends Genet.* 34 (12): 972–990.

72 Wickens, M., Bernstein, D.S., Kimble, J., and Parker, R. (2002). A PUF family portrait: 3′UTR regulation as a way of life. *Trends Genet.* 18 (3): 150–157.

73 Goldstrohm, A.C., Hook, B.A., Seay, D.J., and Wickens, M. (2006). PUF proteins bind Pop2p to regulate messenger RNAs. *Nat. Struct. Mol. Biol.* 13 (6): 533–539.

74 Gebauer, F., Schwarzl, T., Valcárcel, J., and Hentze, M.W. (2021). RNA-binding proteins in human genetic disease. *Nat. Rev. Genet.* 22 (3): 185–198.

75 Wu, P. (2020). Inhibition of RNA-binding proteins with small molecules. *Nat. Rev. Chem.* 4 (9): 441–458.

76 Ghidini, A., Cléry, A., Halloy, F. et al. (2021). RNA-PROTACs: degraders of RNA-binding proteins. *Angew. Chem. Int. Ed.* 60 (6): 3163–3169.

77 Fire, A., Xu, S., Montgomery, M.K. et al. (1998). Potent and specific genetic interference by double-stranded RNA in *Caenorhabditis elegans*. *Nature* 391 (6669): 806–811.

78 Setten, R.L., Rossi, J.J., and Han, S.-p. (2019). The current state and future directions of RNAi-based therapeutics. *Nat. Rev. Drug Discov.* 18 (6): 421–446.

79 Kleinman, M.E., Yamada, K., Takeda, A. et al. (2008). Sequence- and target-independent angiogenesis suppression by siRNA via TLR3. *Nature* 52 (7187): 591–597.

80 DeVincenzo, J., Lambkin-Williams, R., Wilkinson, T. et al. (2010). A randomized, double-blind, placebo-controlled study of an RNAi-based therapy directed against respiratory syncytial virus. *Proc. Natl. Acad. Sci.* 107 (19): 8800–8805.

81 Crooke, S.T., Baker, B.F., Crooke, R.M., and Liang, X.H. (2021). Antisense technology: an overview and prospectus. *Nat. Rev. Drug Discov.* 20 (6): 427–453.

82 Shan, G., Li, Y., Zhang, J. et al. (2008). A small molecule enhances RNA interference and promotes microRNA processing. *Nat. Biotechnol.* 26 (8): 933–940.

83 Fareh, M., Yeom, K.-H., Haagsma, A.C. et al. (2016). TRBP ensures efficient Dicer processing of precursor microRNA in RNA-crowded environments. *Nat. Commun.* 7 (1): 13694.

84 Nakamachi, Y., Kawano, S., Takenokuchi, M. et al. (2009). MicroRNA-124a is a key regulator of proliferation and monocyte chemoattractant protein 1 secretion in fibroblast-like synoviocytes from patients with rheumatoid arthritis. *Arthritis Rheumatol.* 60 (5): 1294–1304.

85 Xiao, Y.T., Wang, J., Lu, W. et al. (2016). Downregulated expression of microRNA-124 in pediatric intestinal failure patients modulates macrophages activation by inhibiting STAT3 and AChE. *Cell Death Dis.* 7 (12): e2521.

86 Tazi, J., Begon-Pescia, C., Campos, N. et al. (2021). Specific and selective induction of miR-124 in immune cells by the quinoline ABX464: a transformative therapy for inflammatory diseases. *Drug Discov. Today* 26 (4): 1030–1039.

87 Dey, S.K. and Jaffrey, S.R. (2019). RIBOTACs: small molecules target RNA for degradation. *Cell Chem. Biol.* 26 (8): 1047–1049.

88 Ng, C.S.C. and Banik, S.M. (2022). Recent advances in induced proximity modalities. *Curr. Opin. Chem. Biol.* 67: 102107.

89 Ursu, A., Childs-Disney, J.L., Angelbello, A.J. et al. (2020). Gini coefficients as a single value metric to define chemical probe selectivity. *ACS Chem. Biol.* 15 (8): 2031–2040.

90 Costales, M.G., Matsumoto, Y., Velagapudi, S.P., and Disney, M.D. (2018). Small molecule targeted recruitment of a nuclease to RNA. *J. Am. Chem. Soc.* 140 (22): 6741–6744.

91 Costales, M.G., Aikawa, H., Li, Y. et al. (2020). Small-molecule targeted recruitment of a nuclease to cleave an oncogenic RNA in a mouse model of metastatic cancer. *Proc. Natl. Acad. Sci.* 117 (5): 2406–2411.

92 Haniff, H.S., Tong, Y., Liu, X. et al. (2020). Targeting the SARS-CoV-2 RNA genome with small molecule binders and ribonuclease targeting chimera (RIBOTAC) degraders. *ACS Cent. Sci.* 6 (10): 1713–1721.

93 Bush, J.A., Aikawa, H., Fuerst, R. et al. (2021). Ribonuclease recruitment using a small molecule reduced c9ALS/FTD r(G_4C_2) repeat expansion *in vitro* and *in vivo* ALS models. *Sci. Transl. Med.* 13 (617): eabd5991.

94 Zhang, P., Liu, X., Abegg, D. et al. (2021). Reprogramming of protein-targeted small-molecule medicines to RNA by ribonuclease recruitment. *J. Am. Chem. Soc.* 143 (33): 13044–13055.

95 Ha, M. and Kim, V.N. (2014). Regulation of microRNA biogenesis. *Nat. Rev. Mol. Cell Biol.* 15 (8): 509–524.

96 Ardekani, A.M. and Naeini, M.M. (2010). The role of microRNAs in human diseases. *Avicenna J. Med. Biotechnol.* 2 (4): 161–179.

97 Kumarswamy, R., Volkmann, I., and Thum, T. (2011). Regulation and function of miRNA-21 in health and disease. *RNA Biol.* 8 (5): 706–713.

98 Singh, S., Quarni, W., Goralski, M. et al. (2021). Targeting the spliceosome through RBM39 degradation results in exceptional responses in high-risk neuroblastoma models. *Sci. Adv.* 7 (47): eabj5405.

99 Nijhuis, A., Sikka, A., Yogev, O. et al. (2022). Indisulam targets RNA splicing and metabolism to serve as a therapeutic strategy for high-risk neuroblastoma. *Nat. Commun.* 13 (1): 1380.

10

The Future of Heterobifunctional Compounds: PROTACs and Beyond

George M. Burslem

University of Pennsylvania, Department of Biochemistry and Biophysics, Department of Cancer Biology and Penn Epigenetics Institute, Perelman School of Medicine, Philadelphia, PA, 19104, USA

10.1 Introduction

Over the past 20 years, the use of heterobifunctional compounds to induce targeted protein degradation has gained traction and progressed from proof-of-concept chemical biology experiments to a burgeoning industry, with a multitude of companies working in this space and multiple compounds in clinical trials [1–3]. As with any new technology, there has been an initial skepticism surrounding the approach, followed by excitement as we enter the peak of inflated expectations as we progress along the Gartner hype cycle (Figure 10.1). At some point, we will inevitably enter the trough of disillusionment, perhaps we already have, but as we progress further as a community, I think it is fair to say targeted protein degradation as a modality is here to stay. Perhaps not as the cure-all, drug the undruggable, magic bullet that we might hope [4] for but certainly as a component of medicinal chemistry and drug discovery campaigns and definitely as a tool for biological discovery [5]. In this chapter, I will speculate about the future of heterobifunctional compounds for targeted protein degradation, discuss recent technological advances, and highlight the emerging possibilities for editing post-translational modifications beyond ubiquitin that the heterobifunctional revolution has inspired.

10.2 Protein Degradation Beyond Cancer

Although huge strides have been made in the progression of heterobifunctional compounds into the clinic, there remain some questions, at least in the public domain, about the ideal physicochemical properties required for oral bioavailability, the safety of prolonged use of E3 ligase modulating compounds, blood–brain barrier penetration, and potential resistance mechanisms *in vivo*. Addressing these concerns, among others, will be necessary for the progression of heterobifunctional

Inducing Targeted Protein Degradation: From Chemical Biology to Drug Discovery and Clinical Applications, First Edition. Edited by Philipp Cromm.

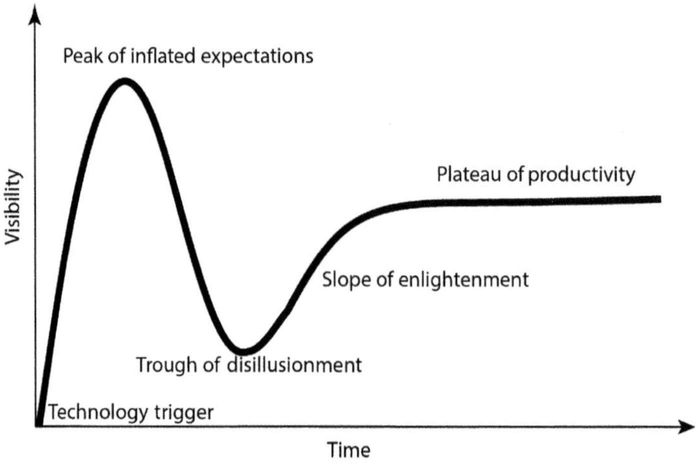

Figure 10.1 The Gartner hype curve.

compounds into the clinic for non-oncology targets as the safety requirements are more rigorous for treatments given to patients with chronic disease rather than to patients fighting for additional months of life [6]. For example, phase 1 trials for oncology drugs are generally performed in cancer patients as the risk–benefit analysis makes it unethical to use healthy human volunteers, but this will not be the case for other indications [7]. Additionally, investigational new drugs for oncology are often given only after other treatments have failed and are therefore not placebo or standard of care controlled. The bar for safety and indeed efficacy for heterobifunctional protein degraders to enter trials for non-oncology indications is clearly higher, but there are several classes of protein targets where protein degradation approaches are appealing.

For example, proteins with defined scaffolding roles are promising targets for protein degradation approaches, even if they also have enzymatic function. The furthest progressed example of this in the heterobifunctional field, outside of oncology, is interleukin-1 receptor-associated kinase 4 (IRAK4). IRAK4 is a kinase with an essential role in innate immunity [8], including the scaffolding of the Myddosome [9]. Several groups have developed IRAK4 degraders for the treatment of autoimmune diseases [10–12], and while some groups have reported no differential biology between inhibition and degradation, thus bringing into question the validity of this approach [10, 11], Kymera have progressed a IRAK4 degrader into clinical trials as the first example of a non-oncology heterobifunctional protein degrader (http://ClinicalTrials.gov Identifier: NCT04772885) [12].

Another application of heterobifunctional induced protein degradation that has garnered a lot of attention is their use against tau. The hyperphosphorylation of tau results in filament formation, which is implicated in Alzheimer's disease, frontotemporal dementia, and other tauopathies [13]. Several groups have developed heterobifunctional compounds that result in the degradation of tau by the proteasome [14–16]. These compounds are able to reduce the tau burden in cell culture [15] and have some effect on cognitive performance *in vivo*, albeit via intracerebroventricular infusion [16]. However, despite tantalizing hints of blood–brain barrier penetration in press releases, there have yet to be any peer-reviewed reports on blood–brain barrier-penetrant heterobifunctional compounds, leading to some healthy skepticism about their use for central nervous system drug discovery [17].

10.3 Emerging Heterobifunctional Modalities for Protein Degradation

10.3.1 PROTAC Variations

The predominant heterobifunctional approach for protein degradation is, of course, the proteolysis targeting chimera (PROTAC) technology that started it all. This has already been discussed extensively elsewhere in the literature [5, 18, 19], and within this volume, this will not be covered in detail. However, there are tricks in the PROTAC space left to uncover and adaptations that may prove advantageous, including but not limited to the discovery of ligands for additional E3 ligases [20–24]. For example, the Ciulli lab continues to innovate in the PROTAC space, developing PROTAC variants such as the macrocyclic PROTACs (Figure 10.2) [25], which constrain the heterobifunctional compound into the bioactive conformation, thus reducing entropic costs for ternary complex formation, in a similar manner to stapled peptides [26]. This approach relies on structure-guided design as the bioactive conformation must be known from an X-ray crystal structure to be effectively constrained. To date, macrocyclic PROTACs have only been demonstrated for the BET proteins, but they nevertheless provide an interesting proof of principle that may be used further in future, albeit only for systems with a previously solved ternary complex structure.

Similarly, the Ciulli group has also reported trivalent PROTACs [27], expanding the bifunctional paradigm with the addition of an extra recruiting element (Figure 10.2). Again, the BET family proteins were used as a proof of principle for this concept, demonstrating concurrent binding of two bromodomains and a single E3 ligase, as well as decreased DC_{50} values for BRD2/3/4 with these triskelion-inspired compounds. Beyond the ability to leverage the multivalent effect for increased target occupancy, multivalent PROTACs open up a wealth of intriguing possibilities. For example, it may well be possible to develop trivalent PROTACs with differential recruiting elements on each of the three arms opening up the possibility of degrading protein complexes by simultaneously binding both proteins in the complex. This may provide a mechanism for context-dependent degradation such that only complexed proteins are degraded while monomers are spared. Additionally, it will be interesting to explore the effect of recruiting multiple E3 ligases to the same protein via the use of 1 : 2 ratios of target ligand to E3 ligand or by recruiting two different ligases simultaneously. One could imagine that this could have drastic effects on the rate of degradation or even provide a tool to rapidly screen potential E3 ligase/protein pairs.

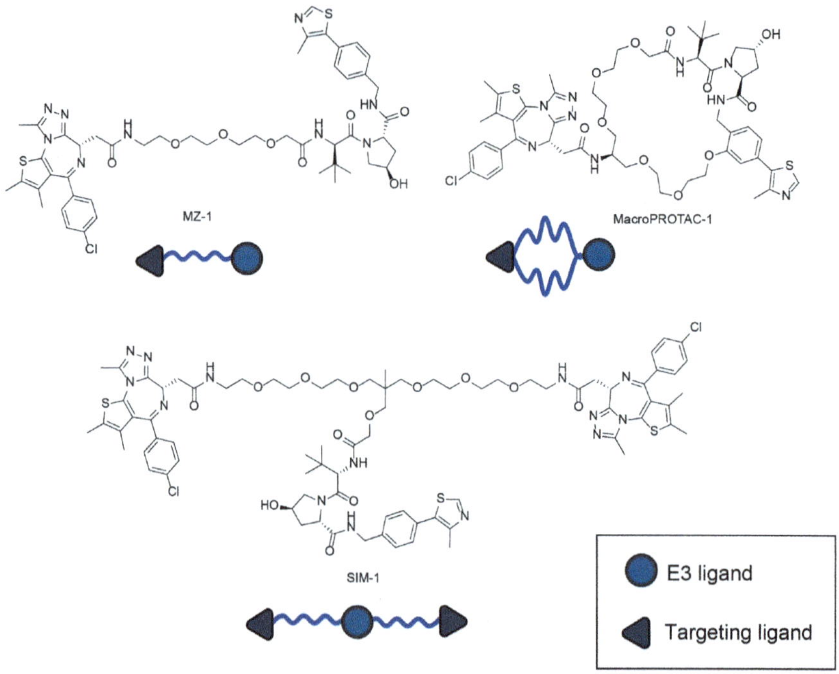

Figure 10.2 Structures of PROTAC variants.

Another recent expansion of the PROTAC concept is the use of oligonucleotides as recruiting elements [28–33], which again provides enticing possibilities for modular approaches to the degradation of RNA binding proteins [29], DNA binding proteins [30], or transcription factors [31–33] but simultaneously incurring new issues with compound stability, cell permeability, and *in vivo* delivery.

Various approaches have been employed to impart additional temporal or spatial control over PROTAC action. The earliest of which was the phosphoPROTACs that only enact degradation in response to specific growth factors [34]. More recently, there has been a slew of photo-controlled PROTACs that employ either photoswitches [35–37] or photocages [38–41] to control the action of a PROTAC. In the case of photo-switchable PROTACs (or PHOTACs) [35–37], this photocontrol is reversible, arising from diazobenzene photoisomerization, enabling transient PROTAC activity and therefore precise control of when and where degradation occurs. Similar, although irreversible, approaches have been reported using photocages for both CRBN [38, 39, 41] and VHL ligands [39, 40]. Finally, there have been reports on making PROTACs specific to certain cell types, either by antibody-mediated delivery to only cells expressing certain cell surfaces proteins [42] or by caged PROTACs that are only released in cells expressing certain hydrolase enzymes [43].

As the applications of heterobifunctional compounds for protein degradation continue to expand, I anticipate additional technical variations and extensions such as those discussed above will continue to emerge and indeed may be necessary to cross the so-called trough of disillusionment into widespread use.

10.4 PROTAC-Inspired Technologies

Beyond the canonical heterobifunctional approaches for protein degradation, additional PROTAC-inspired technologies have arisen over the past few years. These chiefly employ the concept of induced proximity but utilize alternative biological protein degradation machinery in place of the ubiquitin proteasome system. Intriguingly, a recent publication introduced the concept of deubiquitinase targeting chimera (DUBTAC) [44], which modulates the ubiquitin proteasome system, but for protein stabilization rather than protein degradation. Heterobifunctional recruitment of OTUB1 can remove ubiquitin and subsequently prevent proteasomal degradation.

10.5 Highjacking Autophagy

After the ubiquitin proteasome system, the most frequently used approach for targeted protein degradation is to highjack autophagy, in which materials are sequestered into autophagosomes. These autophagosomes then fuse with lysosomes, and the contents are degraded via the hydrolytic enzymes contained within. In place of the E3 ligase ligand employed in PROTACs, a ligand resulting in autophagosome encapsulation can be used for targeted protein degradation. This approach has been referred to as autophagy-targeting chimeras (AUTACs) [45] or autophagosome-tethering compounds (ATTECs) [46] but are fundamentally the same approach (Figure 10.3).

AUTACs use guanine derivatives to trigger autophagosome formation, mimicking the xenophagic response to certain bacteria [45]. This triggers polyubiquitination of the targeted protein but with K63-linked chains resulting in autophagosome formation, rather than K48-linked chains that signal for proteasomal degradation (Figure 10.3). AUTAC effects are limited to the cytosol but have the advantage of being able to induce the degradation of not just proteins but entire organelles (e.g. mitochondria). The full mechanism of how AUTACs function has yet to be elucidated, and the applications for targeted protein degradation are yet to be truly realized, but this approach holds promise.

ATTECs function via a similar mechanism, but rather than actively inducing autophagosome formation, they tag cargo along with already forming autophagosomes via heterobifunctional recruitment to LC-3 [47], a component of the phagophore precursor of the autophagosome (Figure 10.3). Various LC-3 ligands have been used to induce the degradation of mutant huntingtin, polyQ proteins, lipid droplets [48], and BRD4 [49].

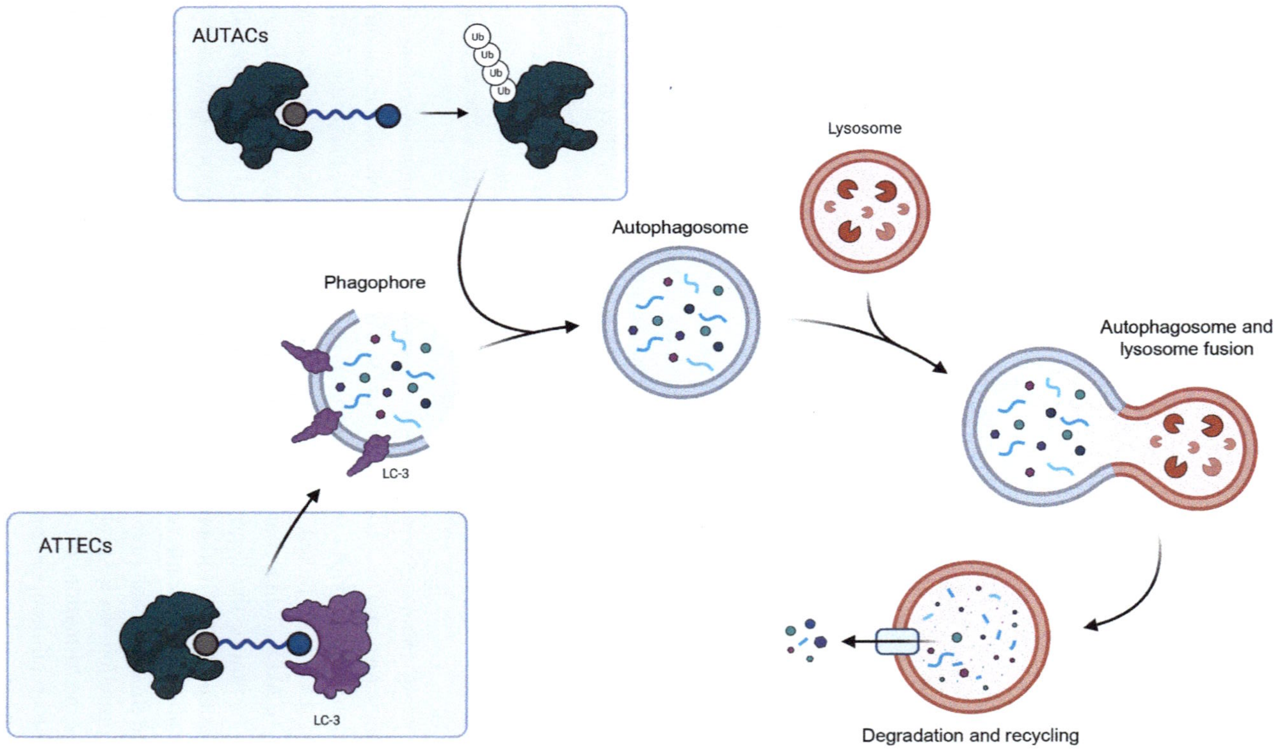

Figure 10.3 High jacking autophagy by AUTACs and ATTECs. Cellular debris, proteins, and damaged organelles are enclosed in phagophores resulting in autophagosomes. Autophagosomes subsequently fused with lysosomes resulting in the degradation of contents by lysosomal proteases. AUTACs and ATTECs can recruit proteins to this cascade.

Extensive additional characterization of these compound classes is still required, and it remains to be seen if the increased autophagic flux induced by AUTACs is problematic or if ATTEC-mediated degradation is limited by the rate of autophagosome formation. Nevertheless, together AUTACs and ATTECs may provide an orthogonal mechanism for targeted protein degradation as compared to PROTACs and provide proof-of-concept demonstrations for additional development of targeted autophagy. Additionally, as the entire ternary complex appears to be included in the autophagosome, targeted autophagy may lack the duration of effect or catalytic nature of PROTACs.

10.6 Degradation of Extracellular Proteins

Relatedly, lysosome targeting chimeras (LyTACs) [50] have emerged as a technology, derived from PROTACs, but for the degradation of extracellular and cell surface proteins via the lysosome (Figure 10.4). LyTACs rely on lysosome targeting receptors on the cell surface, which shuttle glycosylated proteins from the extracellular space to lysosome, where they are degraded. The first-generation LyTACs use antibodies to target the protein to be degraded and serine-*O*-mannose-6-phosphonate (M6Pn)-derived glycopolypeptides as ligands for the cation-independent mannose-6-phosphate receptor (CI-M6PR) as the lysosome targeting receptor [50]. These compounds are capable of inducing internalization and degradation of endogenous extracellular proteins as well as cell surface proteins such as EGFR, transferrin receptor 1, and PD-L1. Because of the unique mechanism of LyTACs, cell permeability of the heterobifunctional protein–glycopeptide conjugates is not a concern, and they hold promise for the addition of the ability to degrade substrates to the already powerful therapeutic antibody toolbox. However, it is important to note the fact that the antibody is degraded along with the target and therefore LYTACs are not catalytic.

A subsequent generation of LyTACs employs the same approach but crucially uses a different lysosome targeting receptor, the asialoglycoprotein receptor (ASGPR) that is only expressed in the liver [51]. ASGPR recognizes *N*-acetylgalactosamine (GalNAc) glycoproteins and has been used for liver-specific delivery of RNAi. Trivalent GalNAc ligands are sufficient for ASGPR mediated internalization and lysosomal degradation and can readily be conjugated to antibodies or peptide ligands for cell surface receptors. Ahn et al. demonstrate liver cell-specific degradation of HER family proteins and integrins using GalNAc LyTACs [51]. The concept of lysosome targeting receptors specific to certain cell types could conceivably be extended to other lysosome targeting receptors with restricted expression patterns, thus providing a tissue-specific degradation mechanism. Simultaneously, Zhou et al. also reported similar studies using GalNAc LyTACs [52]. An all-small molecule class of compounds, molecular degraders of extracellular proteins through the ASGPR (MoDE-As), which work by the same mechanism, have also been reported [53]. Several companies are exploring the LYTAC strategy, but it remains to be seen if they will provide advantageous over other antibody therapeutics that can often induce target internalization and degradation without LYTAC conversion or if target degradation is more effective than antibody blockade.

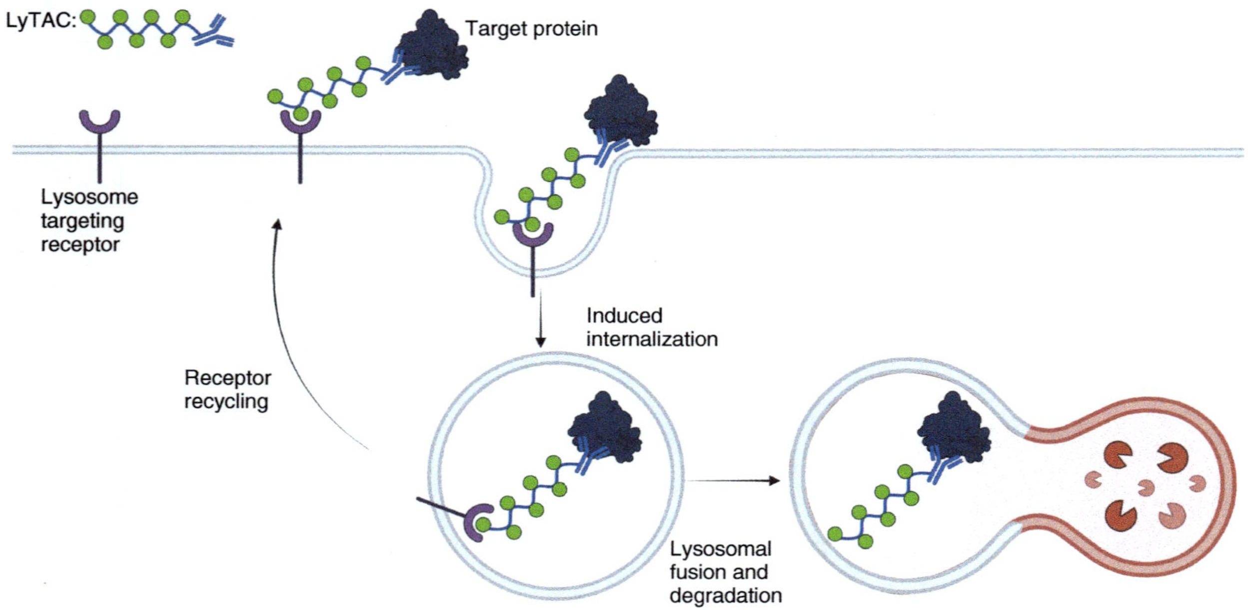

Figure 10.4 Degradation of extracellular proteins via LyTAC.

10.7 Heterobifunctional Compounds Beyond Protein Degradation

Perhaps, some of the most exciting applications of heterobifunctional compounds lie outside the realms of targeted protein degradation but draw on the learnings from PROTACs and other heterobifunctionals to enact alternative outcomes.

10.8 Degradation of RNA

One of the first examples of heterobifunctionals beyond protein degradation was the use of heterobifunctional compounds for the targeted degradation of RNA rather than protein. The Disney lab employed heterobifunctional small molecules, ribonuclease targeting chimeras (RIBOTACs), to recruit RNase L to specific transcripts, resulting in their degradation [54]. This approach has been employed to target RNAs involved in cancers [54, 55], viruses [56], and neurodegenerative diseases [57], highlighting again the applications of heterobifunctional compounds beyond oncology and has delivered *in vivo* proof of principle as a therapeutic strategy [57]. It could essentially function as small-molecule RNA interference but is only capable of degrading RNA transcripts with defined secondary structures and has the normal caveats surround RNA targeting small molecules [58].

10.9 Modulating Phosphorylation

Another recent technological advance is the application of heterobifunctional approaches to modulate the phosphorylation status of proteins. Of course, kinase inhibitors have been able to inhibit phosphorylation downstream of specific kinases to great effects for therapeutic benefits for many years [59], but phosphatases have proven challenging targets for drug discovery [60]. Additionally, the use of heterobifunctional compounds imparts catalytic qualities by invoking an event-driven, rather than occupancy-driven, pharmacology [61]. Finally, and most importantly, the use of heterobifunctional compounds for induced proximity enables the substrate reprogramming of effector proteins, thus inducing the phosphorylation or dephosphorylation of non-native targets (Figure 10.5).

The Choudhary lab pioneered the use of heterobifunctional compounds, called phosphorylation inducing chimera (PHICS) [62], for the targeted phosphorylation of BRD4 and BTK by linking ligands for these proteins to allosteric activators of AMP-activated protein kinase (AMPK) and protein kinase C (PKC) (Figure 10.5). Using these model systems, they validated targeted phosphorylation *in vitro* and in a cellular context. To date, no functional data for PHIC application has been reported, but with such compelling proof of principle, the applications of targeted phosphorylation to modulate signaling pathways is enticing and likely to deliver interesting results in the coming years.

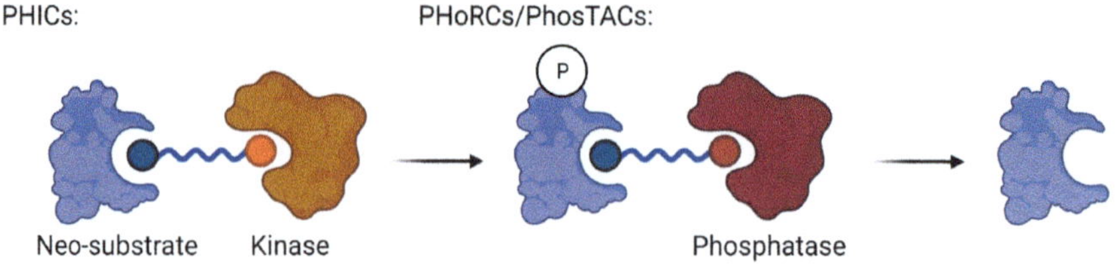

Figure 10.5 Heterobifunctional editing of phosphorylation.

Crucially, phosphorylation, along with many other PTMs, is a reversible process, and therefore, the removal of the phosphate can also be induced by proximity. The recruitment of phosphatases to phosphorylated substrates has been reported by both Yamazoe et al. and Chen et al. under the titles of phosphatase recruiting chimeras (PhoRCs) [63] or phosphorylation targeting chimeras (PhosTACs) [64], respectively. Crucially, these studies demonstrated for the first time that PTMs can be removed by heterobifunctional compounds (Figure 10.5).

PhoRCs utilize heterobifunctional compounds to recruit protein–phosphatase 1 (PP1) to neosubstrates, initially via a halotag fusion protein but latterly with PP1 activating peptides [63]. Yamazoe et al. demonstrate proof of concept by reducing the phosphorylation of both Akt and EGFR, albeit only at high concentrations and without any demonstrated phenotypic outcome. Clearly, higher affinity, more cell-penetrant ligands for PP1 will be required for the progression of this approach, but the ability of heterobifunctional approaches to remove PTMs is clearly established.

The Crews lab took a chemical biology approach, using fusion proteins and generic ligands for them, to probe the possibility of recruiting a subunit of protein phosphatase 2 (PP2A) and hence the rest of the catalytically active complex to neosubstrates via the heterobifunctional approach [64]. FKBP-fused PP2A can be directly recruited to Halo-tagged programmed cell death protein 4 (PDCD4) or the FOXO3a transcription factor. Reduced phosphorylation of FOXO3a results in enhanced transcriptional activity, read out via luciferase activity, demonstrating for the first-time biological consequences of heterobifunctional targeted dephosphorylation. Although this chemical biology approach cannot be directly translated into a therapeutic strategy, it validates another phosphatase for recruitment and demonstrates that this approach can have functional consequences.

10.10 Targeted Acetylation

Recently, a similar chemical biology approach has been employed to induce targeted acetylation via heterobifunctional compounds referred to as Ace-TAGs [65]. These compounds use ligands for the bromodomain of the p300/CBP acetyltransferases linked to FKBP ligands to induce the acetylation of FKBP fusion proteins. So far, this approach has been demonstrated for fusion proteins of histone H3.3, p53, and RelA, which are all known substrates of p300, therefore posing the question as to whether true enzyme reprogramming is possible in the case of acetylation or if it will remain a tool to increase the level of endogenous acetylation. Nevertheless, this is an intriguing and potentially powerful approach and adds to the toolbox of heterobifunctional induced post-translational modifications.

10.11 Potential Applications of Heterobifunctional Compounds to Modulate PTMS

The examples provided above, alongside the success of the PROTAC approach, reveal the power and breadth of modulations that can be induced by heterobifunctional compounds. This makes it tempting to speculate that eventually it will be possible to edit any post-translational modification and/or alter levels of any biomolecule using induced proximity. For example, one can envision the use of targeted methylation/demethylation of chromatin to induce epigenetic reprogramming or targeted glycosylation of cell surface proteins to alter immunoreactivity.

Despite this promise, each heterobifunctional approach will need to be individually developed, validated, and applied, likely first by chemical biology approaches, followed by careful bespoke ligand development efforts and eventual progression toward therapeutic use. Importantly, it remains to be seen how portable concepts such as linker optimization and ternary complex formation are between different recruited proteins and how amenable each class of effector protein is to substrate reprogramming by heterobifunctional compounds.

10.12 Conclusions and Outlook

Only time can tell how things will play out as the burgeoning world of heterobifunctional compounds continues to expand. However, one thing is for certain, there will be a lot of trials and tribulations as we, as a community, continue to explore the possibilities, solve the problems, and push the boundaries of using induced proximity modalities. Nevertheless, I am sure we are all excited to see what the future holds in this intriguing area of biomedical research.

References

1 Sakamoto, K.M., Kim, K.B., Kumagai, A. et al. (2001). Protacs: chimeric molecules that target proteins to the Skp1–Cullin–F box complex for ubiquitination and degradation. *Proc. Natl. Acad. Sci.* 98 (15): 8554–8559.
2 Neklesa, T., Snyder, L.B., Willard, R.R. et al. (2019). ARV-110: an oral androgen receptor PROTAC degrader for prostate cancer. *J. Clin. Oncol.* 37 (7_suppl): 259–259.

3 Flanagan, J., Qian, Y., Gough, S. et al. (2019). Abstract P5-04-18: ARV-471, an oral estrogen receptor PROTAC degrader for breast cancer. *Cancer Res.* 79 (4 Supplement): P5-04-18–P5-04-18.
4 Crews, C.M. (2010). Targeting the undruggable proteome: the small molecules of my dreams. *Chem. Biol.* 17 (6): 551–555.
5 Burslem, G.M. and Crews, C.M. (2020). Proteolysis-targeting chimeras as therapeutics and tools for biological discovery. *Cell* 181 (1): 102–114.
6 Moreau, K., Coen, M., Zhang, A.X. et al. (2020). Proteolysis-targeting chimeras in drug development: a safety perspective. *Br. J. Pharmacol.* 177 (8): 1709–1718.
7 Karakunnel, J.J., Palaniappan, L., Schmidt, K.T. et al. (2018). Reviewing the role of healthy volunteer studies in drug development. *J. Transl. Med.* 16 (1): 336.
8 Suzuki, N., Suzuki, S., Duncan, G.S. et al. (2002). Severe impairment of interleukin-1 and toll-like receptor signalling in mice lacking IRAK-4. *Nature* 416 (6882): 750–754.
9 Gay, N.J., Gangloff, M., and O'Neill, L.A.J. (2011). What the myddosome structure tells us about the initiation of innate immunity. *Trends Immunol.* 32 (3): 104–109.
10 Nunes, J., McGonagle, G.A., Eden, J. et al. (2019). Targeting IRAK4 for degradation with PROTACs. *ACS Med. Chem. Lett.* 10 (7): 1081–1085.
11 Zhang, J., Fu, L., Shen, B. et al. (2020). Assessing IRAK4 functions in ABC DLBCL by IRAK4 kinase inhibition and protein degradation. *Cell Chem. Biol.* 27 (12): 1500–1509.e13.
12 Mullard, A. (2020). IRAK4 degrader to take on innate immunity. *Nat. Biotechnol.* 38 (11): 1221–1223.
13 Alonso, A.d.C., Zaidi, T., Novak, M. et al. (2001). Hyperphosphorylation induces self-assembly of τ into tangles of paired helical filaments/straight filaments. *Proc. Natl. Acad. Sci.* 98 (12): 6923–6928.
14 Chu, T.-T., Gao, N., Li, Q.-Q. et al. (2016). Specific knockdown of endogenous tau protein by peptide-directed ubiquitin-proteasome degradation. *Cell Chem. Biol.* 23 (4): 453–461.
15 Silva, M.C., Ferguson, F.M., Cai, Q. et al. (2019). Targeted degradation of aberrant tau in frontotemporal dementia patient-derived neuronal cell models. *eLife* 8: e45457.
16 Wang, W., Zhou, Q., Jiang, T. et al. (2021). A novel small-molecule PROTAC selectively promotes tau clearance to improve cognitive functions in Alzheimer-like models. *Theranostics* 11 (11): 5279–5295.
17 Farrell, K. and Jarome, T.J. (2021). Is PROTAC technology really a game changer for central nervous system drug discovery? *Expert Opin. Drug Discov.* 16 (8): 833–840.
18 Luh, L.M., Scheib, U., Juenemann, K. et al. (2020). Prey for the proteasome: targeted protein degradation—a medicinal chemist's perspective. *Angew. Chem. Int. Ed.* 59 (36): 15448–15466.
19 Bond, M.J. and Crews, C.M. (2021). Proteolysis targeting chimeras (PROTACs) come of age: entering the third decade of targeted protein degradation. *RSC Chem. Biol.* 2 (3): 725–742.
20 Spradlin, J.N., Hu, X., Ward, C.C. et al. (2019). Harnessing the anti-cancer natural product nimbolide for targeted protein degradation. *Nat. Chem. Biol.* 15: 747–755.

21 Ward, C.C., Kleinman, J.I., Brittain, S.M. et al. (2019). Covalent ligand screening uncovers a RNF4 E3 ligase recruiter for targeted protein degradation applications. *ACS Chem. Biol.* 14 (11): 2430–2440.

22 Zhang, X., Crowley, V.M., Wucherpfennig, T.G. et al. (2019). Electrophilic PROTACs that degrade nuclear proteins by engaging DCAF16. *Nat. Chem. Biol.* 15 (7): 737–746.

23 Henning, N.J., Manford, A.G., Spradlin, J.N. et al. (2022). Discovery of a covalent FEM1B recruiter for targeted protein degradation applications. *J. Am. Chem. Soc.* 144 (2): 701–708.

24 Belcher, B.P., Ward, C.C., and Nomura, D.K. (2021). Ligandability of E3 ligases for targeted protein degradation applications. *Biochemistry* .

25 Testa, A., Hughes, S.J., Lucas, X. et al. (2020). Structure-based design of a macrocyclic PROTAC. *Angew. Chem. Int. Ed.* 59 (4): 1727–1734.

26 Cromm, P.M., Spiegel, J., and Grossmann, T.N. (2015). Hydrocarbon stapled peptides as modulators of biological function. *ACS Chem. Biol.* 10 (6): 1362–1375.

27 Imaide, S., Riching, K.M., Makukhin, N. et al. (2021). Trivalent PROTACs enhance protein degradation via combined avidity and cooperativity. *Nat. Chem. Biol.* 17 (11): 1157–1167.

28 Patil, K.M., Chin, D., Seah, H.L. et al. (2021). G4-PROTAC: targeted degradation of a G-quadruplex binding protein. *Chem. Commun.* 57 (95): 12816–12819.

29 Ghidini, A., Cléry, A., Halloy, F. et al. (2021). RNA-PROTACs: degraders of RNA-binding proteins. *Angew. Chem. Int. Ed.* 60 (6): 3163–3169.

30 Shao, J., Yan, Y., Ding, D. et al. (2021). Destruction of DNA-binding proteins by programmable oligonucleotide PROTAC (O'PROTAC): effective targeting of LEF1 and ERG. *Adv. Sci.* 8 (20): 2102555.

31 Samarasinghe, K.T.G.; An, E.; Genuth, M. A.; et al. (2021) OligoTRAFTACs: A Generalizable Method for Transcription Factor Degradation. bioRxiv: p. 2021.12.20.473482.

32 Samarasinghe, K.T.G., Jaime-Figueroa, S., Burgess, M. et al. (2021). Targeted degradation of transcription factors by TRAFTACs: transcription factor targeting chimeras. *Cell Chem. Biol.* 28 (5): 648–661.e5.

33 Liu, J., Chen, H., Kaniskan, H.Ü. et al. (2021). TF-PROTACs enable targeted degradation of transcription factors. *J. Am. Chem. Soc.* 143 (23): 8902–8910.

34 Hines, J., Gough, J.D., Corson, T.W., and Crews, C.M. (2013). Posttranslational protein knockdown coupled to receptor tyrosine kinase activation with phosphoPROTACs. *Proc. Natl. Acad. Sci.* 110 (22): 8942–8947.

35 Reynders, M., Matsuura, B.S., Bérouti, M. et al. (2020). PHOTACs enable optical control of protein degradation. *Sci. Adv.* 6 (8): eaay5064.

36 Pfaff, P., Samarasinghe, K.T.G., Crews, C.M., and Carreira, E.M. (2019). Reversible spatiotemporal control of induced protein degradation by bistable PhotoPROTACs. *ACS Central Sci.* 5 (10): 1682–1690.

37 Jin, Y.-H., Lu, M.-C., Wang, Y. et al. (2020). Azo-PROTAC: novel light-controlled small-molecule tool for protein knockdown. *J. Med. Chem.* 63 (9): 4644–4654.

38 Xue, G., Wang, K., Zhou, D. et al. (2019). Light-induced protein degradation with photocaged PROTACs. *J. Am. Chem. Soc.* 141 (46): 18370–18374.

39 Naro, Y., Darrah, K., and Deiters, A. (2020). Optical control of small molecule-induced protein degradation. *J. Am. Chem. Soc.* 142 (5): 2193–2197.

40 Kounde, C.S., Shchepinova, M.M., Saunders, C.N. et al. (2020). A caged E3 ligase ligand for PROTAC-mediated protein degradation with light. *Chem. Commun.* 56 (41): 5532–5535.

41 Liu, J., Chen, H., Ma, L. et al. (2020). Light-induced control of protein destruction by opto-PROTAC. *Sci. Adv.* 6 (8): eaay5154.

42 Maneiro, M.a., Forte, N., Shchepinova, M.M. et al. (2020). Antibody–PROTAC conjugates enable HER2-dependent targeted protein degradation of BRD4. *ACS Chem. Biol.* 15 (6): 1306–1312.

43 Liu, J., Chen, H., Liu, Y. et al. (2021). Cancer selective target degradation by folate-caged PROTACs. *J. Am. Chem. Soc.* 143 (19): 7380–7387.

44 Henning, N.J.; Boike, L.; Spradlin, J. N.; et al., Deubiquitinase-Targeting Chimeras for Targeted Protein Stabilization. bioRxiv, 2021: p. 2021.04.30.441959.

45 Takahashi, D., Moriyama, J., Nakamura, T. et al. (2019). AUTACs: cargo-specific degraders using selective autophagy. *Mol. Cell* 76 (5): 797–810.e10.

46 Li, Z., Zhu, C., Ding, Y. et al. (2020). ATTEC: a potential new approach to target proteinopathies. *Autophagy* 16 (1): 185–187.

47 Li, Z., Wang, C., Wang, Z. et al. (2019). Allele-selective lowering of mutant HTT protein by HTT–LC3 linker compounds. *Nature* 575 (7781): 203–209.

48 Fu, Y., Chen, N., Wang, Z. et al. (2021). Degradation of lipid droplets by chimeric autophagy-tethering compounds. *Cell Res.* 31 (9): 965–979.

49 Pei, J., Pan, X., Wang, A. et al. (2021). Developing potent LC3-targeting AUTAC tools for protein degradation with selective autophagy. *Chem. Commun.* 57 (97): 13194–13197.

50 Banik, S.M., Pedram, K., Wisnovsky, S. et al. (2020). Lysosome-targeting chimaeras for degradation of extracellular proteins. *Nature* 584 (7820): 291–297.

51 Ahn, G., Banik, S.M., Miller, C.L. et al. (2021). LYTACs that engage the asialoglycoprotein receptor for targeted protein degradation. *Nat. Chem. Biol.* 17 (9): 937–946.

52 Zhou, Y., Teng, P., Montgomery, N.T. et al. (2021). Development of triantennary *N*-acetylgalactosamine conjugates as degraders for extracellular proteins. *ACS Central Sci.* 7 (3): 499–506.

53 Caianiello, D.F., Zhang, M., Ray, J.D. et al. (2021). Bifunctional small molecules that mediate the degradation of extracellular proteins. *Nat. Chem. Biol.* 17 (9): 947–953.

54 Costales, M.G., Matsumoto, Y., Velagapudi, S.P., and Disney, M.D. (2018). Small molecule targeted recruitment of a nuclease to RNA. *J. Am. Chem. Soc.* 140 (22): 6741–6744.

55 Costales, M.G., Suresh, B., Vishnu, K., and Disney, M.D. (2019). Targeted degradation of a hypoxia-associated non-coding RNA enhances the selectivity of a small molecule interacting with RNA. *Cell Chem. Biol.* 26 (8): 1180–1186.e5.

56 Haniff, H.S., Tong, Y., Liu, X. et al. (2020). Targeting the SARS-CoV-2 RNA genome with small molecule binders and ribonuclease targeting chimera (RIBOTAC) degraders. *ACS Central Sci.* 6 (10): 1713–1721.

57 Bush, J.A., Aikawa, H., Fuerst, R. et al. (2021). Ribonuclease recruitment using a small molecule reduced c9ALS/FTD r(G_4C_2) repeat expansion *in vitro* and *in vivo* ALS models. *Sci. Transl. Med.* 13 (617): eabd5991.

58 Falese, J.P., Donlic, A., and Hargrove, A.E. (2021). Targeting RNA with small molecules: from fundamental principles towards the clinic. *Chem. Soc. Rev.* 50 (4): 2224–2243.

59 Ferguson, F.M. and Gray, N.S. (2018). Kinase inhibitors: the road ahead. *Nat. Rev. Drug Discov.* 17 (5): 353–377.

60 Barr, A.J. (2010). Protein tyrosine phosphatases as drug targets: strategies and challenges of inhibitor development. *Future Med. Chem.* 2 (10): 1563–1576.

61 Lai, A.C. and Crews, C.M. (2016). Induced protein degradation: an emerging drug discovery paradigm. *Nat. Rev. Drug Discov.* 16: 101.

62 Siriwardena, S.U., Munkanatta Godage, D.N.P., Shoba, V.M. et al. (2020). Phosphorylation-inducing chimeric small molecules. *J. Am. Chem. Soc.* 142 (33): 14052–14057.

63 Yamazoe, S., Tom, J., Fu, Y. et al. (2020). Heterobifunctional molecules induce dephosphorylation of kinases–a proof of concept study. *J. Med. Chem.* 63 (6): 2807–2813.

64 Chen, P.-H., Hu, Z., An, E. et al. (2021). Modulation of phosphoprotein activity by phosphorylation targeting chimeras (PhosTACs). *ACS Chem. Biol.* 16 (12): 2808–2815.

65 Wang, W.W., Chen, L.-Y., Wozniak, J.M. et al. (2021). Targeted protein acetylation in cells using heterobifunctional molecules. *J. Am. Chem. Soc.* 143 (40): 16700–16708.

11

Destruction with a Purpose: Targeted Protein Degradation in Drug Discovery

Paola Martinelli, Christiane Kofink, Georg Boeck, Harald Weinstabl and Manfred Koegl

Boehringer Ingelheim RCV GmbH & Co KG, Dr. Boehringer Gasse 5-11, A-1121, Vienna, Austria

11.1 PROTACs in Drug Discovery: Why?

Man-made drugs are typically small, in the range of 500 Da, which is beneficial for their pharmacokinetic properties: on average, smaller compounds are more soluble, more easily absorbed, and more stable, leading to more efficacious drugs. Proteolysis-targeting chimeras (PROTACs), on the other hand, are built from two such molecules, plus a linker, which makes them on average roughly at least twice in size. In addition to having to optimize a small molecule that binds your target of interest, you have to optimize the way the two binders (target and E3) are linked together as this has been shown to have profound effects on degradation efficacy.

In other words, from a medicinal chemistry perspective, it is harder to optimize PROTACs than classical drugs. Therefore, what are the reasons that justify trying it anyway?

In this chapter, we will first look at the four main reasons to engage in PROTAC drug discovery, discuss the challenges of PROTAC optimization, touch briefly upon other routes of administration than oral, and finally take a look at molecular glues as alternatives to PROTACs.

11.1.1 Targeting Proteins that Do Not Respond to Inhibition

Not all potential drug targets that have nice druggable pockets respond to filling up these pockets with small molecules. This can be exemplified by the chromatin modulating protein SMARCA2. Its loss halts cell proliferation in cells that have lost SMARCA4 [1–3]. As loss of SMARCA4 occurs in a sizable fraction of lung cancers, this makes SMARCA2 an interesting potential drug target. The acetyl-lysine pocket of SMARCA2's bromodomain provides medicinal chemists with a convenient point of attack as it can be successfully targeted by small molecules. However, this does not

Inducing Targeted Protein Degradation: From Chemical Biology to Drug Discovery and Clinical Applications, First Edition. Edited by Philipp Cromm.

stop SMARCA2-dependent cells from growing. As it turns out, this bromodomain is simply not necessary for keeping the cells alive [4]. Mutational disruption of the bromodomain is also without consequence for cell proliferation, confirming the above conclusion. For this reason, SMARCA2 bromodomain binders have been used to generate PROTACs, which efficiently induced SMARCA2 degradation followed by a profound antiproliferative and apoptotic response in SMARCA2-dependent cells [5].

A similar case can be made for BRD9, which is part of a chromatin remodeling complex termed the noncanonical BAF (ncBAF) or GLTSCR-containing BAF complex (GBAF) [6, 7]. The activity of this complex is indispensable for synovial sarcomas and malignant rhabdoid tumors. As in the case of SMARCA2, the inhibition of the bromodomain of BRD9 is not sufficient to elicit strong antiproliferative responses. Removing the whole BRD9 protein from the cells, however, destabilizes the ncBAF complex. Consequently, in malignant rhabdoid tumors and synovial sarcomas, degradation of BRD9 has stronger antiproliferative effects than inhibition of its bromodomain [8–10]. Two BRD9 degrading compounds are presently in early stages of preclinical and clinical development by C4 Therapeutics and Foghorn Therapeutics, respectively (Table 11.1).

Another and possibly even more compelling example can be found in PROTACs targeting the estrogen or androgen receptors (ER and AR). Selective ER modulators such as tamoxifen are successfully applied to treat ER-positive breast cancer [11] but can eventually lose their effectiveness in blocking the receptor's activity [12]. In this case, the ER-degrading drug fulvestrant can be successfully applied. Despite its clinical success, PROTACs built to degrade ER surpass fulvestrant in efficacy and potency (reviewed in Ref. [13]). Arvinas' ARV-417 is the clinically most advanced ER PROTAC [14]. It is currently in phase II of clinical development.

In the case of castration-resistant prostate cancers, response to AR-inhibiting drugs such as enzalutamide can be lost by genetic changes that turn these drugs into AR-stimulating drugs: their binding to AR is not lost, but their inhibition of AR is circumvented [15]. As they still bind AR, they can be used as target binders to generate AR degrading PROTACs. Degradation of AR will negate any activating activity that the binders have on AR and thus tumor growth. Arvinas' AR-based PROTAC ARV-110 has been shown to be bioavailable and tolerated upon oral dosing and has shown promising signs of efficacy in phase I [16]. It is currently in clinical phase II (see Table 11.1 for a list of PROTACs used in clinical development).

Another target that may be worth the extra resources required for PROTAC development is the kinase IRAK4. This protein is part of an inflammatory signal cascade downstream of interleukin-1 and Toll-like receptor activation. Following receptor activation, the formation of a multiprotein complex, the myddosome, is triggered, which is nucleated by multimerization of the protein MYD88 and which drives pathway signaling [17]. IRAK4 is part of this structure. Thus, in addition to its function as a kinase, IRAK4 has a scaffolding function, which cannot be inhibited by kinase inhibitors, but can be efficiently disrupted by degradation of IRAK4. The expectation is that degradation of IRAK4, removing both the kinase and the scaffolding function of IRAK4, will be more efficacious in blocking signaling via the myddosome than merely blocking its kinase activity. Blocking signal transduction at that level can be

Table 11.1 PROTACs currently in clinical development.

Compound	Target	E3 ligase	RoA	Indication	Sponsor	Phase	Expected primary completion date	Trial id
ARV-110	AR	CRBN	Oral	Prostate cancer	Arvinas Inc.	I/II	2022-10-31	NCT-03888612
ARV-471	ER	CRBN	Oral	Breast cancer	Arvinas Inc.	I/II	2022-03-30	NCT-04072952
ARV-471 + Palbociclib	ER	CRBN	Oral	Breast cancer	Arvinas Inc.	Ib	2022-03-30	NCT-04072952
ARV-766	AR	n.a.	Oral	Prostate cancer	Arvinas Inc.	I	2024-12-06	NCT-05067140
AR-LDD (CC-94676)	AR	n.a.	Oral	Prostate cancer	Bristol Myers Squibb	I	2022-06-28	NCT-04428788
DT2216	Bcl-xL	VHL	iv	Liquid and solid cancers	Dialectic Therapeutics	I	2022-10-31	NCT-04886622
FHD-609	BRD9	n.a.	iv	Synovial sarcoma	Foghorn Therapeutics	I	2024-12-21	NCT-04965753
GT20029	AR	n.a.	topical	Androgenic alopecia, acne	Kintor Pharmaceutical	I	–	n.a.
KT-474	IRAK4	n.a.	Oral	Immune-mediated inflammatory diseases	Kymera Therapeutics/Sanofi	I	2022-02-01	NCT-04772885
NX-2127	BTK	CRBN	Oral	B-cell malignancies	Nurix Therapeutics	I	Nov. 23	NCT-04830137
HSK29116	BTK	n.a.	Oral	B-cell malignancies	Sichuan Haisco Pharmaceutical	I	Aug. 23	NCT-04861779
GB-16673	BTK	n.a.	Oral	B-cell malignancies	BeiGene	I	2023-12-17	NCT-05006716

RoA, route of administration.

beneficial in tumors that are driven by activating mutations in MYD88, which allows for constitutive signaling [18]. In inflammatory diseases driven by signaling from Toll-like receptors and from IL-1 family cytokines via the myddosome, such as atopic dermatitis and hidradenitis suppurativa, taking out IRAK4 is expected to block signaling [19]. An IRAK4 degrading PROTAC, KT-474, is currently in phase I of clinical development [20].

The ability to target proteins outside of their active centers leads to a significant increase in the number of proteins that can be targeted by small molecules. Schneider et al. [21] have recently systematically approached the question of the size of the "PROTACable genome," i.e. how many proteins can be modulated by PROTACs based on several criteria, including the availability of a binding pocket, their localization, and their natural half-life. Based on their criteria, they arrive at the number of 1336 PROTAC targets. The authors state that this is likely an underestimation as their selection results in inclusion of only 166 of the already 269 PROTAC targets that can be found in the literature.

11.1.2 Selective Inhibition of Isoforms

When the number of proteins bound by a given small molecule (a "binder") is compared to the number of proteins degraded by a PROTAC built using that binder, it has been consistently observed that the PROTAC is more selective than the binder. This has been seen for kinases [22–24] as well as for BET proteins [25]. The phenomenon is likely explained by additional requirements for the ternary interaction of the target protein, the PROTAC, and the E3 ligase to be effective: not every protein bound by the PROTAC can form into a trimeric complex that is sufficiently stable and adequately positioned to allow efficient ubiquitination. For drug discovery, this poses the extra challenge that only a fraction of the possible PROTACs will be effective in protein degradation, and optimization of PROTACs has a lot to do with getting the attachment sites, geometry, and length of the linker right [25]. A benefit of this observation is that with PROTACs, selectivity values can be attained that are unattainable with traditional inhibitors, as exemplified best in the selective degradation of p38 isoforms p38α and p38δ using a nonselective kinase inhibitor as the PROTAC handle [26]. This isoform selectivity was linked to differences in ternary complex affinities. It has to be noted, however, that PROTACs can also result in the unexpected degradation of proteins that are only weakly bound by the used binder: e.g. a PROTAC based on dabrafenib unexpectedly leads to degradation of CDK17 [27].

It is worth noting here that every PROTAC is still an inhibitor. Although selectivities for the degrading activity are typically higher, the less selective inhibiting activity can contribute to any effects measured during drug optimization programs. This complicates the picture unless the increased potency of the PROTAC cause by its catalytic mode of action sufficiently separates the IC_{50} values of the degrading and inhibiting activities.

11.1.3 Increase in Potency Because of Catalytic Activity

PROTACs are nonstoichiometric agents: one PROTAC can drive the degradation of many copies of its substrate, which is frequently referred to as event-driven pharmacology. This is different from inhibitors, where at least one inhibitor is required for every instance of the target inhibited (occupancy-driven pharmacology). For this reason, PROTACs can be a lot more potent than their respective binders, leading to exquisite potencies as can be seen, e.g. for BRD4 [28], AR [29], or RIPK2 PROTACs [30]. In practical work, this gain in potency is very often counterbalanced by a loss in cellular uptake *in vitro* and even more so by poor pharmacokinetic (PK) properties. To put it more positively, PROTACs may be able to compensate challenging PK properties by their potency.

11.1.4 Prolonged Duration of Effects

Trivial to say, in occupancy-driven pharmacology, an inhibitor only inhibits the activity of its target as long as it is present. In drug discovery, this means that the pharmacokinetic profile limits the duration of activity of a classical drug. The effects of protein degradation, on the other hand, persist until resynthesis of the protein reaches a level sufficient for the protein's function. For proteins with a slow rate of synthesis, this can lead to a prolonged efficacy of the drug up to time points where drug levels have fallen below the limit of detection, as has been found for degraders of RIPK2 [30].

RIPK2 is a kinase that functions downstream of the pattern recognition receptors NOD1 and NOD2, which recognize bacterial peptidoglycans. Its dysregulation is associated with several immune disorders, such as inflammatory bowel diseases, making it a potential target for drug discovery. RIPK2 has a half-life of 50 hours or longer in immune cells *in vitro* as measured by stable isotope labeling by aminoacids in cell culture (SILAC) labeling and a correspondingly slow resynthesis rate. Mares et al. [30] synthesized RIPK2 degrading PROTACs based on the inhibitor of apoptosis family E3 ligases (IAPs). Their best compounds are exquisitely potent with half-maximal activities in the subnanomolar range and efficacies greater than 90% degradation of RIPK2. When the optimized compound is subcutaneously administered to rats in a single, low dose of 0.3 mg/kg, suppression of inflammatory cytokines persists for an impressive period of 6–10 days, including a period in which the PROTAC levels in the blood have fallen below the lower limit of detection. Such a prolonged pharmacodynamic effect allows a less than once daily dose to be efficacious, which will be of importance when subcutaneous (s.c.) or intravenous (i.v.) routes of administration are pursued for use in human patients. Miah et al. then extended this work by further improving the solubility and metabolic stability of the PROTACs while preserving potency and biological efficacy [31]. Impressively, they show that upon subcutaneous application of a slow-release formulation based on poly(lactic-*co*-glycolic acid) (PLGA), RIPK2 levels can be kept suppressed for up to 60 days [31]. Where such slow-release subcutaneous formulations are possible and efficacious, they may well offer a route of administration that is equivalent to or better than oral administration with respect to patient compliance. In addition, the slow release may help avoid toxicities associated with high maximal concentrations of the drug.

In summary, PROTACs are harder to make compared to classical inhibitors, but the possibilities of an enlarged target space, higher selectivity, potency, and duration of effect can make the endeavor worth the effort.

11.2 Routes of Application for PROTACs

Oral application typically is the preferred route for patients and is the easiest way to self-administer medication. However, achieving oral bioavailability is very challenging for PROTACs (see also Section 11.3) [32]. PROTAC molecules are typically large, lipophilic, poorly soluble, and poorly permeable and often are a good substrate to gastrointestinal efflux transporters, such as *P*-gp. As compounds will be absorbed only in the dissolved state, solubility is a key factor for a reasonable oral bioavailability. The second most important factor is permeability through the gut wall. As both are at the lower end, PROTAC molecules are categorized as BCS IV compounds according to the Biopharmaceutical Classification System (BCS) [33]: low solubility and low permeability, the most challenging compound class for a formulation developer (Figure 11.1). Poor solubility can be addressed with formulations to some extent, but permeability and efflux typically cannot. Therefore, permeability and efflux assays should become the most important tools for the early absorption, distribution, metabolism, excretion (ADME) characterization of oral PROTAC compounds.

If permeability cannot be improved by modifying the molecule and oral bioavailability remains low, the parenteral route could be an alternative as in this case, the permeability boundary of the body is overcome by a needle. One has to bear in mind, however, that for parenteral administration, the solubility of the compound is the most important parameter for a successful formulation development.

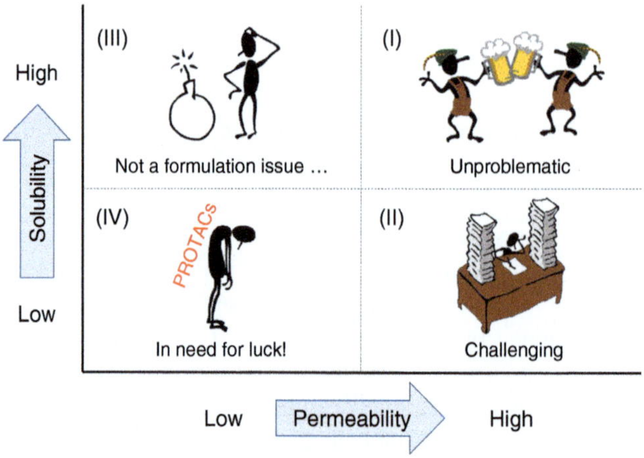

Figure 11.1 Biopharmaceutical Classification System (BCS) for oral compounds.

The parenteral route seems to be a straightforward formulation approach but reveals specific challenges as well:

- The choice of excipients for the pharmaceutical formulation is much more limited than for the oral route.
- The formulation has to comply with a narrow, physiological pH range in order not to create pain upon injection.
- For poorly soluble compounds, there is a high risk of precipitation at the injection site, which can lead to adverse effects.
- Osmolality has to remain in the isotonic range, which limits the concentration range of API and excipients.
- For the most ways of parenteral application other than i.v., (e.g. s.c. or i.m., see also below), the volume of injection is limited to a few milliliters only.
- In a ready-to-use solution, the stability of the API in aqueous formulation is crucial.
- For the sterility of the formulation, a terminal sterilization step (autoclaving) or aseptic manufacturing is needed and adds complexity to the drug product.
- For administration, a device, at least a syringe, is needed, as well as often an assisted administration by a health care professional (HCP), e.g. a nurse.
- Finally, one should not forget about the fear of needles (belonephobia) that might compromise the compliance of the patients.

The parenteral application is not a route of administration itself but summarizes many different routes with i.v. (intravenous), i.m. (intramuscular), and s.c. (subcutaneous) as the most prominent ones. Among these, s.c. is the only way to a self-administered medication by the patient and therefore the most popular one, especially when the frequency of injection is high, e.g. daily. For a frequency of injection of once a week or less, i.v. and i.m. administration can become an alternative, accompanied by the option of more complex formulations if health care providers are involved and can perform the final steps of preparation of the medication, e.g. the reconstitution of a solution for injection out of a powder or lyophilisate. For s.c., self-administered formulations, device and formulation should be as simple and easy to use as possible and ready-to-use solutions are highly preferred. The main determinant for the frequency of injection of a compound is the clearance, which determines the half-life of the compound *in vivo* and should be in focus for optimization from the beginning. Although s.c. and i.m. depot formulations are available for sustained release, it should be kept in mind that this is reasonable for very highly efficacious and low-dosed PROTACs only. Different technologies allow for different drug loadings of the formulation, but as a rule of thumb, the daily dose should be not more than 10 mg, preferably less than 1 mg. The volume of injection is subcutaneously limited to not more than roughly 2 ml, if standard devices (needle safety devices, autoinjector, and pen) are used. For compliance reasons and to lower the pain upon injection, the volume per single injection should not exceed 1 ml preferably. Recently, many new devices have become available for the s.c. delivery of volumes up to 50 ml. These adhesive devices, called as patch pumps, on-body devices, or large-volume injectors, are typically easy to use, automatically inject the needle, and deliver the medication subcutaneously over several minutes to hours. As these highly engineered devices are expensive, they significantly increase the cost of goods for the medication. Moreover, their relatively large size adds complications for the supply chain, both in pharmacies and at home for the patient. For these reasons, patch pumps normally are not considered for daily dosing.

In addition to all technical hurdles for the s.c. delivery of PROTAC molecules, parenteral administration can cause local irritations and adverse events (inflammation, flush, edema, etc.) at the injection site. Given our limited understanding of the subcutaneous immunogenicity [34], unexpected adverse effects can occur and are sometimes hard to explain. To avoid surprises at a late stage of drug optimization, macroscopic as well as histopathological examinations of the injection sites should be thoroughly considered.

11.3 Tackling DMPK Challenges of PROTACs

Most successful small-molecule drugs are administered to patients via the oral route. With very few exceptions, intravenous administration is only acceptable to patients for drugs with long half-lives in human blood, such as antibody-based drugs that can be efficacious when administered less than once weekly. Despite being twice the size of normal small molecules, the half-lives of PROTACs are not significantly different from those of classical small molecules. Thus, i.v. administration is not a valid option in most cases. Subcutaneous administration may be an option (see above), but all things being equal, oral administration will be preferred by patients and health care professionals alike. However, just how hard is it to make PROTACs bioavailable as a swallowed pill?

As we have initially discussed, because of their bifunctional nature, PROTACs are usually large lipophilic molecules with challenging physicochemical properties that fall into the "beyond rule of 5" space. This is often directly reflected in poor oral bioavailability for these molecules. To achieve orally bioavailable degraders, hurdles such as poor solubility and permeability have to be overcome [35]. That PROTAC-specific properties represent a significant challenge for the optimization of drug metabolism and pharmacokinetics (DMPK) becomes clear when compounds from a BRD4 inhibitor program are compared to SMARCA2 PROTACs (Figure 11.2).

While BRD4 inhibitors populate a chemical space between 10 and 45 heavy atoms and cover a large lipophilicity range with cLogP values from −1 to 5.8, PROTACs only start at a heavy atom count of 55 and increases to 100, with cLogPs ranging from 3 to 6. This high lipophilicity generally results in poor solubility of PROTACs at pH = 6.8 in aqueous media, where only around 5% of the PROTACs show measurable solubility. On the contrary, the majority of BRD4 inhibitors shows a good solubility of >50 μg/ml at pH = 6.8. Apart from solubility, permeability is also a critical issue in the optimization of PROTACs toward oral bioavailability. Most small molecules from the BRD4 inhibitor program show a good to excellent apical–basolateral permeability (AB) in Caco-2 cells of at least $>5\times10^{-6}$ cm/s, while for PROTACs, only a small number of compounds reach a permeability of $>5\times10^{-6}$ cm/s

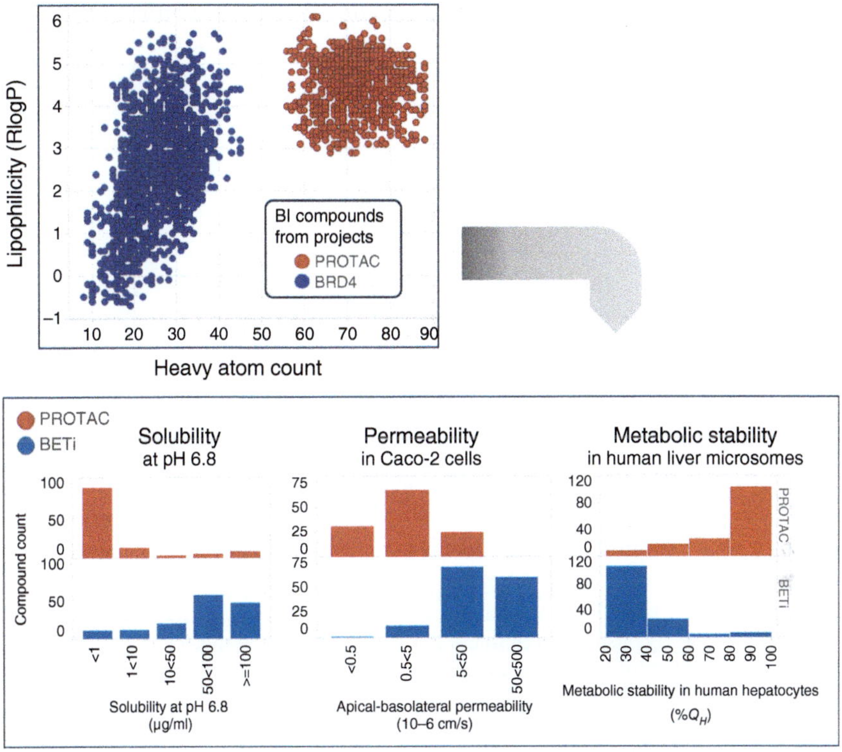

Figure 11.2 The large size and high lipophilicity of PROTACs translate into challenges with respect to solubility, permeability, and metabolic stability. Data are taken from two programs at Boehringer Ingelheim aiming at the optimization of VHL-based SMARCA2 PROTACs and BET protein bromodomain inhibitors.

(Figure 11.2). Furthermore, the metabolic stability in human liver microsomes is heavily influenced by the physicochemical properties of the PROTACs. The majority of PROTACs show a high clearance of >80% of the hepatic blood flow (>80% Q_H; note that high % Q_H values indicate low metabolic stability) in human liver microsomes, whereas most compounds from the BRD4 inhibitor program show a good stability of <40% Q_H in human hepatocytes. The required multiparameter optimization of large lipophilic molecules illustrates the main challenge in achieving orally bioavailable degraders.

One possibility to improve the overall properties of a PROTAC is to design a specific protein of interest (POI) binder that shows already-improved physicochemical properties compared to the published starting points, e.g. by reducing the H-bond donor (HBD)/H-bond acceptor (HBA) counts. Another possibility to tweak the overall compound properties lies in the choice of your E3 ligase. Despite the fact that there are more than 600 known E3 ligases, the most frequently precedented E3 ligases leading to functional degraders in the literature are based on mouse double minute 2 homolog (MDM2), inhibitor of apoptosis proteins (IAP), Von Hippel–Lindau tumor suppressor (VHL), or cereblon (CRBN). Each of the ligase binders

Table 11.2 Comparison of physicochemical parameters of different E3 ligase binders.

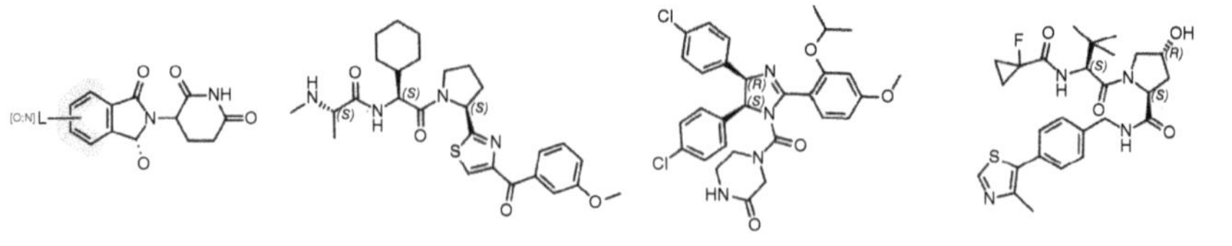

<table>
<tr><th></th><th>Lidomides</th><th>LCL-161</th><th>Nutlin-3</th><th>Ciulli motif</th></tr>
<tr><th>Ligase</th><th>CRBN</th><th>IAP</th><th>MDM2</th><th>VHL</th></tr>
<tr><td>MW</td><td>244–259</td><td>513</td><td>582</td><td>517</td></tr>
<tr><td>K_d/IC50 (nM)</td><td>~600</td><td>~5</td><td>~100</td><td>~50</td></tr>
<tr><td>cLogP</td><td>0.5</td><td>3.5</td><td>8</td><td>2.7</td></tr>
<tr><td>TPSA</td><td>66–93</td><td>101</td><td>84</td><td>112</td></tr>
<tr><td>HBD|HBA</td><td>1–2|3–4</td><td>2|6</td><td>1|5</td><td>3|5</td></tr>
<tr><td>LE|LLE</td><td>0.39|6.6</td><td>0.32|5.1</td><td>0.25|3</td><td>0.28|4.5</td></tr>
</table>

Molecular weight (MW), dissociation constant (K_d), inhibitory concentration of 50% (IC_{50}), calculated logarithmic partition coefficient (cLogP), topological polar surface area (TPSA), hydrogen bond donor (HBD), hydrogen bond acceptor (HBA), ligand efficiency (LE), and lipophilic ligand efficiency (LLE).

has its strength and weaknesses (Table 11.2). MDM2 and VHL binders show a high binding affinity toward their corresponding ligase; however, they already come with a high heavy atom (HA) count, HBD/HBA count, and lipophilicity. The peptidic nature of most known IAP binders limits their suitability for oral PROTAC design. CRBN binders on the other hand display a comparably weak binding affinity toward their target but feature a low molecular weight and lipophilicity resulting in better starting points to achieve orally bioavailable PROTACs [36, 37].

Pike et al. summarized extensively their data on the ADME properties of PROTACs [32]. Based on the analysis of their chemical matter, they outlined that VHL-targeted heterobifunctional degraders failed to achieve any appreciable oral exposure, despite the low total plasma clearance. In contrast, because of their lower molecular weight, HBD/HBA counts, and lipophilicity, CRBN-targeted molecules displayed a more "drug-like" behavior: roughly one-third of the cereblon-based PROTACs tested achieved a good oral bioavailability (>30%). For comparison, this is true for approximately two-thirds of conventional small molecules.

The beneficial physicochemical properties of CRBN binders are directly reflected in the fact that currently most degraders entering the clinic being orally administered [20] use CRBN as the E3 ligase. The most advanced compounds under clinical investigation are the CRBN-based degraders ARV-110 (Arvinas, androgen receptor degrader) and ARV-471 (Arvinas, Estrogen receptor degrader), which recently entered phase II clinical trials (Figure 11.3).

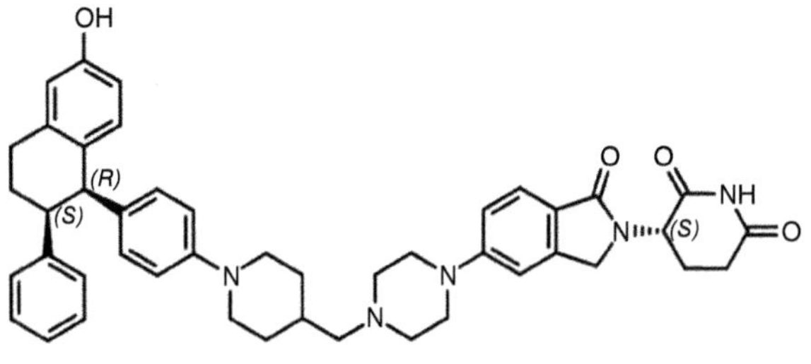

ARV-471

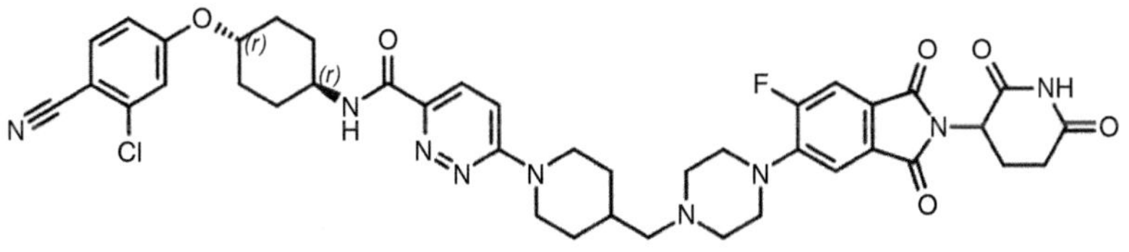

ARV-110

Figure 11.3 Structure of estrogen receptor degrading PROTAC ARV-471 [14] and androgen receptor degrading PROTAC ARV-110. *Source:* Snyder et al. [79]/Arvinas Inc.

Besides the described strategies to improve the physicochemical properties of small-molecule PROTACs, this class of molecules also offer a new angle for optimization: Because of their constructive tri-fold nature (POI binder, linker, and ligase binder), PROTACs possess the ability to adopt different conformations in solution and upon binding [38] often referred to as "chameleonicity" [39]. This ability – although difficult to design – can prove valuable when it comes to the intramolecular compensation of hydrogen bond donors, thus facilitating the cellular uptake of PROTAC molecules or improving their efflux transporter liabilities, ultimately improving oral bioavailability.

Although SBPD (structure-based PROTAC design) has been successfully applied to rationalize the design of potency improvements, for example, improving cooperativity (the ratio between binary and ternary binding affinities) via back-binding, scientists have failed so far to successfully apply this concept for the improvement of ADME properties. However, merging learnings in the field of chameleonicity and SBPD have the potential to generate drug candidates unifying both beneficial ADME properties and potencies.

Although the use of SBPD in the optimization of DMPK properties of PROTACs is limited, it can have great impact in optimizing the proteolytic activity of PROTACs. The approach requires information on the ternary complex, ideally a molecular structure consisting of POI, E3 ligase, and PROTAC. The feasibility to obtain these ternary structures very much depends on the properties of the E3 ligase and the protein of interest. Although several examples of ternary structures are published for the E3 ligase VHL [25], for the other prominent E3 ligases CRBN and IAP, this has only been described in singular studies [40, 41].

Once a ternary complex structure is solved, it provides an efficient way to optimize the degrader based on rational design using cooperativity as an optimization parameter. An example of structure-based drug design for PROTACs was exemplified in the optimization of the linker region of PROTAC1 ending in a PROTAC ACBI1 with significantly improved cooperativity by Farnaby et al. [5]. Furthermore, SBPD can be used to constrain a flexible PROTAC molecule in its bioactive conformation, e.g. by marcocyclization, hence leading to PROTACs targeting the interfacial binding sites between the E3 ligase and target protein, resulting in the formation of a more stable ternary complex with increased cooperativity [42]. Although cooperativity seems to be a predictive optimization parameter for ternary complex structure for VHL, this does not necessarily need to be the case for other E3 ligases, such as CRBN or IAP.

A recent report, describing the first ternary crystal structures between the E3 ligase IAP and the kinase domain of BTK, suggests a much more dynamic complex with no preference for a single conformation [40]. Interestingly, in this case, the optimization toward enhanced protein–protein contacts and more restricted conformational dynamics leads to undesired weaker cellular degradation. Similar observations have been made for complexes of the E3 ligase CRBN and the bromodomain of BRD4 as a protein of interest [41]. The study describes that despite the absence of a tight binding or positive cooperativity, one can achieve highly efficient compound-dependent degradation.

To conclude, the DMPK optimization of PROTACs remains difficult because of their challenging physicochemical parameters. However, despite multiple "rule of 5 violations," PROTACs can be optimized to comply with the criteria required for oral bioavailability, including solubility, permeability, microsomal stability, and potency. For cereblon-based PROTACs, Arvinas' successful phase I trials have shown that oral bioavailability is possible in humans, and it will be interesting to see which other E3 ligase binders will also be able to achieve this.

11.4 Molecular Glue Degraders: Definition, Advantages, and Challenges

Proximity-induced protein degradation is at the basis of the mode of action of Revlimid (lenalidomide), which is approved for multiple myeloma and is one of the best-selling drugs in oncology with a multibillion market size. Therefore, agents inducing targeted protein degradation have the true potential to become drugs. However, lenalidomide is not a large bifunctional PROTAC but a representant of a different family of proteolytic drugs, the much smaller so-called molecular glues.

Molecular glues are generally defined as small molecules that induce new protein–protein interactions (PPI) or stabilize the pre-existing ones. As proximity is a crucial factor in a plethora of different cellular events, the biological and pharmacological effects of molecular glues are highly diverse and depend on the proteins involved [43].

The term "molecular glue" was first introduced in the early 1990s by Stuart Schreiber [44], after his group elucidated the mode of action of the immunosuppressants cyclosporin A (CsA) and FK506, and it became clear that both drugs induce the formation of a complex between calcineurin and a non-natural partner, cyclophilin for CsA and FKBP for FK506 [45, 46]. This discovery, which was confirmed and further clarified when the X-ray structure of the complexes was solved a few years later [47, 48], paved the road toward the discovery of numerous compounds with molecular glue features.

Molecular glue degraders can induce or stabilize PPIs between an E3 ubiquitin ligase and a target protein, thereby inducing ubiquitination and proteasome-dependent degradation of the latter, much like PROTACs. However, unlike PROTACs, molecular glues lack a linker between the ligase-binding and the POI-binding moieties and, most importantly, do not need to have high binary affinity for both proteins involved in the PPI, as they rely on extensive direct interactions between the E3 ligase and the target protein, in addition to the protein–ligand interactions. For this reason, molecular glue degraders are particularly attractive for targeting proteins lacking an obvious binding pocket. Additionally, as molecular glue degraders engage the E3 ligase and the substrate with much higher affinity when they are in the ternary complex than as a binary interaction, they generally have no measurable hook effect (Figure 11.4).

Compared to PROTACs, molecular glue degraders have much more favorable physicochemical properties, including smaller molecular weight, better oral bioavailability, and rather a good PK/PD profile. They are therefore more "drug-like" and generally fall within the "rule of five." On the other hand, however, they have been so far discovered serendipitously, and there is still relatively less knowledge regarding the principles of their discovery and optimization, which makes their rational design hard.

11.4.1 Serendipitously Discovered Molecular Glue Degraders

11.4.1.1 Thalidomide Analogs

Thalidomide was first marketed in the mid-1950s to treat insomnia and morning sickness in pregnant women and was banned from the market less than 10 years later after it was shown to be highly teratogenic [49]. Unfortunately, it had already affected between 8000 and 12 000 patients who gave birth to babies with severe deformities, most often limb defects. In 1965, new pharmacological activities of thalidomide were identified, leading to a resurgence of interest in the drug [49]. Over the years, it was discovered that thalidomide and its analogs lenalidomide and pomalidomide ("IMiDs" for "immunomodulatory imide drugs") have immunomodulatory, anti-inflammatory, and antitumor properties. However, their mode of action remained unknown until CRBN was first identified as the target of thalidomide [50]. Subsequently, IMiD-bound CRBN was shown to interact with several non-natural substrates, or "neosubstrates," and induce their ubiquitination and

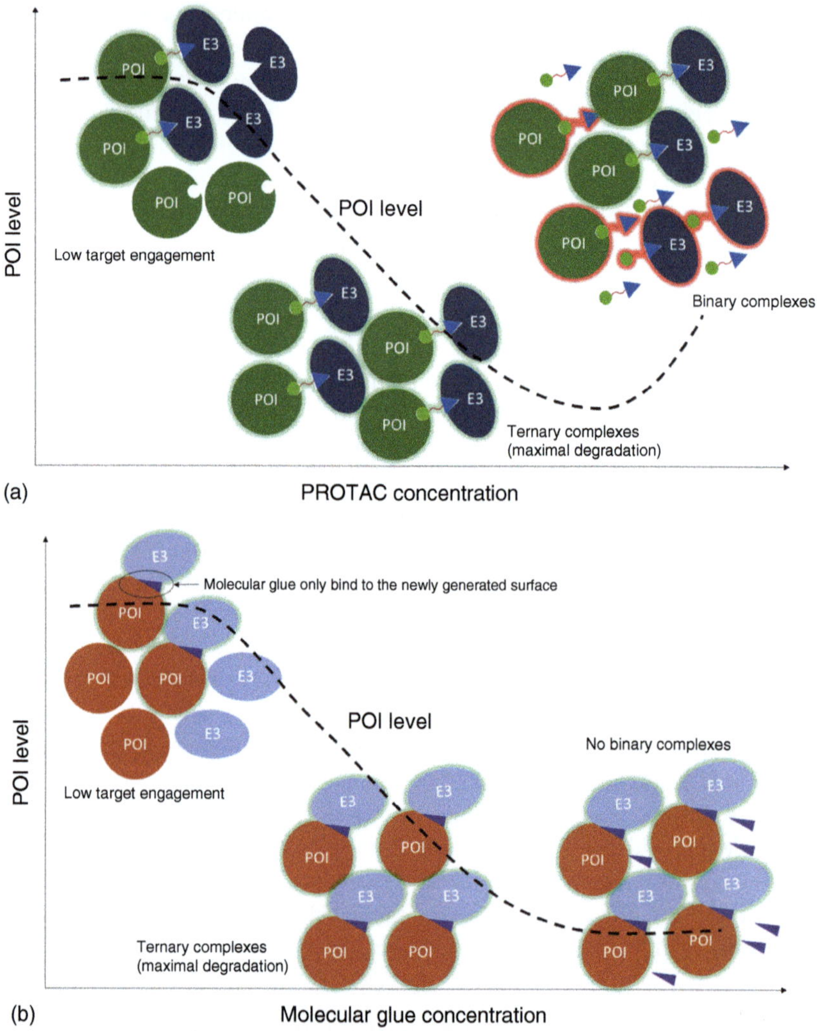

Figure 11.4 PROTACs can suffer from the "hook effect," molecular glue degraders do not. Increasing concentrations of PROTACs (a) initially correspond to increased numbers of productive ternary complexes (green halo) and therefore to higher rates of degradation of the protein of interest (POI). However, as the PROTAC concentration increases, the proportion of nonproductive binary complexes (red halo) where the PROTAC only binds to either E3 or the POI increases and the efficacy of degradation is lower. This is called the "hook effect." In contrast, molecular glue degraders (b) usually do not have a high binary affinity for either the E3 or the POI and only bind efficiently when ternary complexes are formed. Therefore, nonproductive binary complexes do not form, even at high concentrations of the molecular glue.

degradation. Degradation of the transcription factors Ikaros (IKZF1) and Aiolos (IKZF3) was shown to be linked to the immunomodulatory and antitumor effect of IMiDs [51–55] while degradation of casein kinase 1α (CK1α) was shown to be involved in the efficacy of lenalidomide in the 5q-myelodysplastic syndrome [56]. As mentioned, lenalidomide is currently approved for multiple myeloma and is commercialized under the name Revlimid.

Following the clinical success of the early thalidomide analogs, IMiDs have received some attention in the past years, and they have been used to develop PROTACs, including those that are currently in the clinic. However, their rational design to improve selectivity and avoid unexpected polypharmacology is still challenging. In particular, the structure–activity relationship of IMiDs can be confusing, as relatively small changes in the molecules often result in steep transitions in the degradation of specific substrates.

11.4.1.2 Aryl Sulfonamides

Indisulam, an aryl sulfonamide derivative, was first discovered in a phenotypic screening for antitumor drugs [57] and has been tested in clinical trials for advanced solid tumors [58]. However, like for thalidomide analogs, its mode of action was elucidated only several years later, when two studies independently reported that indisulam acts as molecular glue between the CUL4-DCAF15 E3 ligase and the splicing factor RNA binding motif protein 39 (RBM39, also known as CAPERα) [59, 60]. Other aryl sulfonamides, such as E7820, tasisulam, and chloroquinoxaline sulfonamide (CQS), also induce degradation of RMB39 via binding to CRL4-DCAF15 [59–61]. The RBM39 paralog RBM23 was shown to be degraded by aryl sulfonamides through the same mechanism, although it seems that the antitumor effect of indisulam is independent of RBM23 degradation [61].

In contrast to IMiDs, which show a reasonable affinity for CRBN, aryl sulfonamides bind DCAF15 only weakly, with K_d values as high as >50 μM for indisulam and tasisulam [62] demonstrating that molecular glue degraders do not depend on high-affinity binary interactions [63]. With a total area of 1150 Å^2, the DCAF15-RBM39 interaction surface is almost twice as large as the one of CRBN and its neosubstrates, which compensates for the low binary affinity of the aryl sulfonamides for DCAF15. The functionalization of a shallow, nonconserved pocket in DCAF15 and the weak binary affinity of aryl sulfonamide indicate that molecular glue degraders can be obtained for nonligandable E3 ligases. On the other hand, the extensive PPI surface that characterizes the DCAF15-RBM39 complex around aryl sulfonamides, which are buried into the complex, suggest that these compounds only recruit neosubstrates with a very specific geometry and are therefore not easily tunable toward other targets. Nevertheless, a DCAF15-based PROTAC directed toward BRD4 was recently reported, which uses JQ1 and E7820 as target-binding and E3-binding moieties, respectively [64].

11.4.1.3 BCL6 Degrader BI-3802

Although thalidomide analogs and aryl sulfonamides cause degradation by mediating the interaction of the target protein with an E3 ligase, a completely different mechanism for glue-induced degradation was recently reported for BI-3802, a BCL6 degrader discovered by Boehringer Ingelheim [65].

Kerres, Koegl, and colleagues were aiming at finding potent inhibitors of the interaction between the BCL6 transcription factor – a known oncogenic driver in lymphoid malignancies such as diffuse large B cell lymphomas (DLBCL) – and its co-repressors, when they noticed a subset of compounds with an atypical behavior in biophysical assays. They surprisingly but consistently induced protein precipitation in co-crystallization and nuclear magnetic resonance (NMR) experiments. When tested in cells, these compounds were found to induce ubiquitylation and proteasome-dependent degradation of BCL6, which resulted in extensive derepression of several targets and ultimately reduced the proliferation of DLBCL cell lines. Closer analyses revealed that these compounds inhibited the binding of co-repressors to the BTB domain of BCL6, but they did not inhibit dimerization of the BTB domain itself. Interestingly, BI-3802-induced degradation of BCL6 was not rescued by treatment with the neddylase inhibitor MLN4924, thus indicating that no cullin-RING E3 ligase was involved in the ubiquitylation of BCL6.

More recently, the Ebert lab further characterized the molecular basis of BI-3802-induced BCL6 degradation [66]. When treating cells with BI-3802, they observed the rapid formation of BCL6 foci, which subsequently disappeared, consistent with protein degradation. These foci appeared as regular structures with a sinusoidal shape using electron microscopy, and the authors hypothesized that BI-3802 induced the formation of higher order BCL6-containing structures. The structure of BI-3802-induced BCL6 filaments analyzed with cryo-electron microscopy revealed that BI3802 promoted BCL6 polymerization by binding to a groove between dimers, thus facilitating the assembly of supramolecular filaments. Subsequently, SIAH1 was shown to be the responsible E3 ligase for the ubiquitylation of BCL6. Interestingly, SIAH1 showed a weak affinity for BCL6, which was highly enhanced when the transcription factor was in BI-3802-induced polymers. As opposed to other molecular glue degraders, BI-3802 does not directly bind the E3 ligase in the ternary complex but only the target protein. This novel polymerization-driven mode of action opens new potential avenues in the field of molecular glue degraders.

11.4.2 PROTACs that Are also Molecular Glues: NX-2127 and KT-413

Thalidomide analogs are currently the most common E3 ligands used for PROTAC design, mostly because of their more favorable physicochemical properties when compared to VHL ligands [67]. More than 30 different proteins have been successfully degraded with CRBN-based PROTACs, including oncogenic targets, proteins involved in immune disorders, the neurodegenerative disease-associated protein Tau, and even a protein from hepatitis C virus [36]. Given the glue behavior of CRBN ligands, the risk of unwanted degradation of neosubstrates is a common concern when developing PROTACs based on IMiDs, especially within nononcology indications, where the regulations concerning treatment-related adverse effects are stricter. Degradation of neosubstrates is generally monitored and optimized against. However, there are at least two examples of CRBN-based PROTACs that also act as molecular glues, which are being developed toward the clinic.

NX-2127, developed by Nurix Therapeutics, is composed of an inhibitor of BTK, a tyrosine kinase involved in B-cell malignancies, linked to a thalidomide analog binding to CRBN [68]. The resulting molecule induces degradation of BTK as well as the two classical CRBN neosubstrates, IKZF1 (Ikaros) and IKZF3 (Aiolos). Oral administration of NX-2127 was shown to inhibit tumor growth in xenografts more effectively than the BTK inhibitor ibrutinib. The added molecular glue activity on IKZF1 and IKZF3 can increase T-cell activation and antitumor immune response.

KT-413, from Kymera Therapeutics, shows some similarities: it induces degradation of IRAK4, a protein involved in B-cell lymphomas, as well as the two CRBN neosubstrates IKFZ1 and IKFZ2, with a single-digit nanomolar potency [69]. Based on this double activity, this molecule was named "IRAKIMiD."

Such dual PROTAC-molecular glue molecules might be very rare and probably limited to therapeutic indications where degradation of CRBN neosubstrates is beneficial per se, as suggested by the observation that selective degradation of IRAK4 had only a modest effect on the downstream NF-κB and MAPK signaling pathways and did not affect cell proliferation or apoptosis in diffuse large B-cell lymphoma cell lines [70]. However, such molecules highlight the versatility of targeted protein degradation.

11.4.3 Rational Discovery of Molecular Glue Degraders

Although molecular glue degraders present some important advantages over PROTACs, especially their favorable DMPK properties, it is still unclear to what extent they can be rationally discovered. Successful prospective discovery of molecular glue degraders has been achieved both through screening-based and target-based approaches.

11.4.3.1 Screening-Based Discovery: CDK12 Inhibitors Degrade Cyclin K

In the summer of 2020, the groups of Georg Winter, Nicolas Thomä, and Benjamin Ebert described two distinct approaches aimed at discovering new molecular glue degraders. Interestingly, both reports identified CDK12 inhibitors that caused the degradation of cyclin K.

Słabicki et al. started from an in silico analysis correlating large-scale drug sensitivity data covering 4518 clinical and preclinical compounds with the mRNA expression of 499 E3 ligase components over 578 cancer cell lines [71]. The group observed a correlation between sensitivity to the CDK inhibitor CR8 and the expression of the CUL4 adaptor DDB1. Proteomics, genome-wide CRISPR-Cas9 resistance screens, and structural studies revealed that CR8 selectively degrades cyclin K by binding to CDK12 and converting it into a substrate receptor for DDB1, bypassing the requirement for a canonical DCAF substrate receptor. CDK12 was shown to have a basal weak affinity for DDB1, which was greatly enhanced by CR8 binding. As opposed to other molecular glue degraders that engage a ligandable pocket in the E3 ligase, CR8 binds the ATP pocket of CDK12 but does not have an independent binding site on DDB1. This might broaden the spectrum of target proteins and E3 ligases that can be used for targeted protein degradation.

Mayor-Ruiz and colleagues identified compounds with a similar mode of action by screening about 2000 known cytotoxic and cytostatic compounds on wt or hyponeddylated cells carrying a mutation in the UBE2M E2 ligase and comparing the results [72]. Neddylation of cullin-type E3 ligases is necessary for their activation; therefore, drug resistance in the hyponeddylated cells could identify compounds relying on cullin-dependent protein degradation for their activity. Three compounds with a distinct scaffold, dCeMM2, dCeMM3, and dCeMM4, were identified and further investigated. Multi-omics analyses revealed that all the three compounds selectively degraded cyclin K, CDK12, and CDK13 by inducing binding to the DDB1-CUL4B E3 complex. The weak baseline affinity between DDB1 and CDK12 was strongly increased by dCeMM2/3/4, as for CR8.

A third group described a similar compound, HQ461, acting as molecular glue between CDK12 and DDB1 and inducing efficient degradation of cyclin K [73] Also in this case, the compound was initially identified in a phenotypic high-throughput screening. The molecular targets and mechanism of action were then elucidated through a genome-wide clustered regularly interspaced short palindromic repeats-knock-out (CRISPR-KO) screening and a gain-of-function mutagenesis screening in mismatch repair-defective HCT116 cells. HQ461 was shown to bind the ATP-binding pocket of CDK12, thus inducing DDB1 recruitment, while no binding to DDB1 alone was detected.

These compounds are quite interesting as they demonstrate that an undruggable target such as cyclin K can be recruited to an E3 ligase via a ligandable protein partner as CDK12. Although CDK12 is also depleted, data suggest that this is mostly due to the reduction in its partner cyclin K rather than through direct ubiquitylation, which indicates that the geometry of the complex dictates which members are productively ubiquitylated.

11.4.3.2 Target-Based Discovery: Degraders of S37 Mutant β-Catenin

Kyle Simonetta and colleagues at Nurix Therapeutics recently reported the discovery of potent small molecules that stabilize the interaction of a mutant form of β-catenin with its natural E3 ligase β-TrCP [74]. The β-catenin transcription factor can act as an oncogenic driver when the complex process controlling its protein turnover is deregulated in cancer cells [75]. Phosphorylation of a specific set of residues including S33 and S37 is required for binding to the E3 ligase adaptor β-TrCP, leading to ubiquitylation by the $SCF^{\beta\text{-TrCP}}$ cullin-RING ligase and degradation [76]. Not surprisingly, mutations at these residues are often observed in tumors, especially liver hepatocellular carcinomas, and result in the stabilization of β-catenin, which accumulates and translocates to the nucleus to activate the Wnt transcriptional program [77]. After developing a fluorescence polarization-based assay to measure the binding of a mutant β-catenin phospho-degron peptide lacking the S37 phosphorylation and recombinant β-TrCP, Simonetta and colleagues were able to screen a library of 350 000 compounds and identify four structurally related molecules that stabilized the protein–protein interaction. Although the degradation in cells appeared to be highly dependent on the phosphorylation levels of S33, this report is an excellent example of a strategy to prospectively discover molecular glue degraders for a given target. This is particularly interesting in the field of oncology as mutations impairing ubiquitylation and proteasome-dependent degradation are common events in tumors [78].

11.4.4 To Glue or Not to Glue for Targeted Protein Degradation

Although the first oral PROTACs have reached the clinic and are showing encouraging results [14, 79], the development of PROTACs with acceptable bioavailability for therapeutic application remains a challenge for the many reasons explained above. In contrast, molecular glue degraders that are well within Lipinski's "rule of five" space are much more likely to achieve good cellular uptake and bioavailability, making them a safer choice for drug discovery, at least on paper. Why then PROTACs are still occupying the majority of the targeted protein degradation space?

A simple answer is that all the currently known molecular glue degraders have been discovered serendipitously. Even the prospective screening efforts leading to the discovery of cyclin K/CDK12 degraders did not start from a specific target but were based on phenotypic readouts. The S37 mutant β-catenin degraders from Nurix Therapeutics are the only example so far of rational, target-based discovery of molecular glue degraders [65].

Drug discovery efforts for target-specific molecular glue degraders will have to be based on highly robust degradation assays that are able to rule out confounding effects due to nonspecific toxicity. As these are necessarily cellular assays, the suboptimal permeability of early compounds might be a relevant hurdle to finding good starting points for optimization. Kastl et al. at Astra Zeneca have recently suggested a screening approach for molecular glues that they have used to identify degraders of an undisclosed target among more than 100 000 molecules [80]. Furthermore, even if a good starting molecule is discovered through a rational approach, optimization criteria for molecular glues are still relatively unclear, making the whole drug discovery process highly complex. For this reason, many companies still focus mostly if not exclusively on PROTACs.

11.5 Targeted Protein Degradation: Here to Stay

It is not possible to predict if any of the many early preclinical and clinical programs will lead to a successful new treatment option for patients. Failure is routine in drug development. Therefore, could it be that PROTACs and glues will be of transient fashion in drug discovery, as many that we have seen come and go in the past decades? We think that this is unlikely. The big question was whether these unconventional molecules can be optimized for application in humans, and that has already been shown with Arvinas' successful phase I trials. There is little reason to believe that the risk of failure of the current early degrader projects is much different than those of any other new small-molecule drug candidates. There is also ample space for addressing unmet medical needs that only now becomes accessible with the advent of PROTACs. We expect that this will foster the development of many new protein degrading drug candidates, many of which are likely to fail, while some of them can be expected to succeed.

References

1 Hoffman, G.R., Rahal, R., Buxton, F. et al. (2014). Functional epigenetics approach identifies BRM/SMARCA2 as a critical synthetic lethal target in BRG1-deficient cancers. *Proc. Natl. Acad. Sci. U. S. A.* 111: 3128–3133.

2 Oike, T., Ogiwara, H., Tominaga, Y. et al. (2013). A synthetic lethality-based strategy to treat cancers harboring a genetic deficiency in the chromatin remodeling factor BRG1. *Cancer Res.* 73 (17): 5508–5518.

3 Wilson, B.G., Helming, K.C., Wang, X. et al. (2014). Residual complexes containing SMARCA2 (BRM) underlie the oncogenic drive of SMARCA4 (BRG1) mutation. *Mol. Cell. Biol.* 34 (6): 1136–1144.

4 Vangamudi, B., Paul, T.A., Shah, P.K. et al. (2015). The SMARCA2/4 ATPase domain surpasses the bromodomain as a drug target in SWI/SNF-mutant cancers: insights from cDNA rescue and PFI-3 inhibitor studies. *Cancer Res.* 75 (18): 3865–3878.

5 Farnaby, W., Koegl, M., Roy, M.J. et al. (2019). BAF complex vulnerabilities in cancer demonstrated via structure-based PROTAC design. *Nat. Chem. Biol.* 15 (7): 672–680.

6 Mashtalir, N., D'Avino, A.R., Michel, B.C. et al. (2018). Modular organization and assembly of SWI/SNF family chromatin Remodeling complexes. *Cell* 175 (5): 1272–1288.e20.

7 Gatchalian, J., Malik, S., Ho, J. et al. (2018). A non-canonical BRD9-containing BAF chromatin remodeling complex regulates naive pluripotency in mouse embryonic stem cells. *Nat. Commun.* 9 (1): 5139.

8 Zoppi, V., Hughes, S.J., Maniaci, C. et al. (2019). Iterative design and optimization of initially inactive proteolysis targeting chimeras (PROTACs) identify VZ185 as a potent, fast, and selective von Hippel–Lindau (VHL) based dual degrader probe of BRD9 and BRD7. *J. Med. Chem.* 62 (2): 699–726.

9 Brien, G.L., Remillard, D., Shi, J. et al. (2018). Targeted degradation of BRD9 reverses oncogenic gene expression in synovial sarcoma. *eLife* 7: e41305.

10 Remillard, D., Buckley, D.L., Paulk, J. et al. (2017). Degradation of the BAF complex factor BRD9 by heterobifunctional ligands. *Angew. Chem. Int. Ed.* 56 (21): 5738–5743.

11 Komm, B.S. and Mirkin, S. (2014). An overview of current and emerging SERMs. *J. Steroid Biochem. Mol. Biol.* 143: 207–222.

12 D'Souza, A., Spicer, D., and Lu, J. (2018). Overcoming endocrine resistance in metastatic hormone receptor-positive breast cancer. *J. Hematol. Oncol.* 11 (1): 80.

13 Lin, X., Xiang, H., and Luo, G. (2020). Targeting estrogen receptor alpha for degradation with PROTACs: a promising approach to overcome endocrine resistance. *Eur. J. Med. Chem.* 206: 112689.

14 Snyder, L.B., Flanagan, J.J., Qian, Y. et al. (2021). Abstract 44: the discovery of ARV-471, an orally bioavailable estrogen receptor degrading PROTAC for the treatment of patients with breast cancer. *Exp. Mol. Ther.* 44–44.

15 Ehsani, M., David, F.O., and Baniahmad, A. (2021). Androgen receptor-dependent mechanisms mediating drug resistance in prostate cancer. *Cancers* 13 (7): 1534.

16 Petrylak, D.P., Gao, X., Vogelzang, N.J. et al. (2020). First-in-human phase I study of ARV-110, an androgen receptor (AR) PROTAC degrader in patients (pts) with metastatic castrate-resistant prostate cancer (mCRPC) following enzalutamide (ENZ) and/or abiraterone (ABI). *J. Clin. Oncol.* 38 (15_suppl): 3500–3500.

17 Motshwene, P.G., Moncrieffe, M.C., Grossmann, J.G. et al. (2009). An oligomeric signaling platform formed by the toll-like receptor signal transducers MyD88 and IRAK-4*. *J. Biol. Chem.* 284 (37): 25404–25411.

18 Ngo, V.N., Young, R.M., Schmitz, R. et al. (2011). Oncogenically active MYD88 mutations in human lymphoma. *Nature* 470 (7332): 115–119.

19 Zarrin, A.A., Bao, K., Lupardus, P., and Vucic, D. (2021). Kinase inhibition in autoimmunity and inflammation. *Nat. Rev. Drug Discov.* 20 (1): 39–63.

20 Mullard, A. (2021). Targeted protein degraders crowd into the clinic. *Nat. Rev. Drug Discov.* 20 (4): 247–250.

21 Schneider, M., Radoux, C.J., Hercules, A. et al. (2021). The PROTACtable genome. *Nat. Rev. Drug Discov.* 20 (10): 789–797.

22 Bondeson, D.P., Smith, B.E., Burslem, G.M. et al. (2018). Lessons in PROTAC design from selective degradation with a promiscuous warhead. *Cell Chem. Biol.* 25 (1): 78–87.e5.

23 Burslem, G.M., Smith, B.E., Lai, A.C. et al. (2017). The advantages of targeted protein degradation over inhibition: an RTK case study. *Cell Chem. Biol.* 25 (1): 67–77.e3.

24 Huang, H.T., Dobrovolsky, D., Paulk, J. et al. (2017). A chemoproteomic approach to query the degradable kinome using a multi-kinase degrader. *Cell Chem. Biol.* 25 (1): 88–99.e6.

25 Gadd, M.S., Testa, A., Lucas, X. et al. (2017). Structural basis of PROTAC cooperative recognition for selective protein degradation. *Nat. Chem. Biol.* 13 (5): 514–521.

26 Smith, B.E., Wang, S.L., Jaime-Figueroa, S. et al. (2019). Differential PROTAC substrate specificity dictated by orientation of recruited E3 ligase. *Nat. Commun.* 10 (1): 131.

27 Donovan, K.A., Ferguson, F.M., Bushman, J.W. et al. (2020). Mapping the degradable kinome provides a resource for expedited degrader development. *Cell* 183 (6): 1714–1731 e10.

28 Pillow, T.H., Adhikari, P., Blake, R.A. et al. (2020). Antibody conjugation of a chimeric BET degrader enables in vivo activity. *ChemMedChem* 15 (1): 17–25.

29 Han, X., Wang, C., Qin, C. et al. (2019). Discovery of ARD-69 as a highly potent proteolysis targeting chimera (PROTAC) degrader of androgen receptor (AR) for the treatment of prostate cancer. *J. Med. Chem.* 62 (2): 941–964.

30 Mares, A., Miah, A.H., Smith, I.E.D. et al. (2020). Extended pharmacodynamic responses observed upon PROTAC-mediated degradation of RIPK2. *Commun. Biol.* 3 (1): 140.

31 Miah, A.H., Smith, I.E.D., Rackham, M. et al. (2021). Optimization of a series of RIPK2 PROTACs. *J. Med. Chem.* 64 (17): 12978–13003.

32 Pike, A., Williamson, B., Harlfinger, S. et al. (2020). Optimising proteolysis-targeting chimeras (PROTACs) for oral drug delivery: a drug metabolism and pharmacokinetics perspective. *Drug Discov. Today* 25 (10): 1793–1800.

33 Amidon, G.L., Lennernäs, H., Shah, V.P., and Crison, J.R. (1995). A theoretical basis for a biopharmaceutic drug classification: the correlation of in vitro drug product dissolution and in vivo bioavailability. *Pharm. Res.* 12 (3): 413–420.

34 Collins, D.S., Sánchez-Félix, M., Badkar, A.V., and Mrsny, R. (2020). Accelerating the development of novel technologies and tools for the subcutaneous delivery of biotherapeutics. *J. Control. Release* 321: 475–482.

35 Cantrill, C., Chaturvedi, P., Rynn, C. et al. (2020). Fundamental aspects of DMPK optimization of targeted protein degraders. *Drug Discov. Today* 25 (6): 969–982.

36 Bricelj, A., Steinebach, C., Kuchta, R. et al. (2021). E3 ligase ligands in successful PROTACs: an overview of syntheses and linker attachment points. *Front. Chem.* 9: 707317.

37 Ishida, T. and Ciulli, A. (2020). E3 ligase ligands for PROTACs: how they were found and how to discover new ones. *SLAS Discov.* 26 (4): 484–502.

38 Atilaw, Y., Poongavanam, V., Nilsson, C.S. et al. (2020). Solution conformations shed light on PROTAC cell permeability. *ACS Med. Chem. Lett.* 12 (1): 107–114.

39 Benowitz, A.B., Scott-Stevens, P.T., and Harling, J.D. (2021). Challenges and opportunities for in vivo PROTAC delivery. *Future Med. Chem.* 14 (3): 119–121.

40 Schiemer, J., Horst, R., Meng, Y. et al. (2021). Snapshots and ensembles of BTK and cIAP1 protein degrader ternary complexes. *Nat. Chem. Biol.* 17 (2): 152–160.

41 Nowak, R.P., DeAngelo, S.L., Buckley, D. et al. (2018). Plasticity in binding confers selectivity in ligand-induced protein degradation. *Nat. Chem. Biol.* 14 (7): 706–714.

42 Testa, A., Hughes, S.J., Lucas, X. et al. (2020). Structure-based design of a macrocyclic PROTAC. *Angew. Chem. Int. Ed.* 59 (4): 1727–1734.

43 Stanton, B.Z., Chory, E.J., and Crabtree, G.R. (2018). Chemically induced proximity in biology and medicine. *Science* 359 (6380): eaao5902.

44 Schreiber, S.L. (1992). Immunophilin-sensitive protein phosphatase action in cell signaling pathways. *Cell* 70 (3): 365–368.

45 Liu, J., Farmer, J.D., Lane, W.S. et al. (1991). Calcineurin is a common target of cyclophilin-cyclosporin A and FKBP-FK506 complexes. *Cell* 66 (4): 807–815.

46 Michnick, S., Rosen, M., Wandless, T. et al. (1991). Solution structure of FKBP, a rotamase enzyme and receptor for FK506 and rapamycin. *Science* 252 (5007): 836–839.

47 Kissinger, C.R., Parge, H.E., Knighton, D.R. et al. (1995). Crystal structures of human calcineurin and the human FKBP12–FK506–calcineurin complex. *Nature* 378 (6557): 641–644.

48 Griffith, J.P., Kim, J.L., Kim, E.E. et al. (1995). X-ray structure of calcineurin inhibited by the immunophilin-immunosuppressant FKBP12-FK506 complex. *Cell* 82 (3): 507–522.

49 Bartlett, J.B., Dredge, K., and Dalgleish, A.G. (2004). The evolution of thalidomide and its IMiD derivatives as anticancer agents. *Nat. Rev. Cancer* 4 (4): 314–322.

50 Ito, T., Ando, H., Suzuki, T. et al. (2010). Identification of a primary target of thalidomide teratogenicity. *Science* 327 (5971): 1345–1350.

51 Gandhi, A.K., Kang, J., Havens, C.G. et al. (2014). Immunomodulatory agents lenalidomide and pomalidomide co-stimulate T cells by inducing degradation of T cell repressors Ikaros and Aiolos via modulation of the E3 ubiquitin ligase complex CRL4CRBN. *Brit. J. Haematol.* 164 (6): 811–821.

52 Lu, G., Middleton, R.E., Sun, H. et al. (2014). The myeloma drug lenalidomide promotes the cereblon-dependent destruction of Ikaros proteins. *Science* 343 (6168): 305–309.

53 Chamberlain, P.P., Lopez-Girona, A., Miller, K. et al. (2014). Structure of the human cereblon–DDB1–lenalidomide complex reveals basis for responsiveness to thalidomide analogs. *Nat. Struct. Mol. Biol.* 21 (9): 803–809.

54 Fischer, E.S., Böhm, K., Lydeard, J.R. et al. (2014). Structure of the DDB1–CRBN E3 ubiquitin ligase in complex with thalidomide. *Nature* 512 (7512): 49–53.

55 Krönke, J., Udeshi, N.D., Narla, A. et al. (2014). Lenalidomide causes selective degradation of IKZF1 and IKZF3 in multiple myeloma cells. *Science* 343 (6168): 301–305.

56 Krönke, J., Fink, E.C., Hollenbach, P.W. et al. (2015). Lenalidomide induces ubiquitination and degradation of CK1α in del(5q) MDS. *Nature* 523 (7559): 183–188.

57 Owa, T., Yoshino, H., Okauchi, T. et al. (1999). Discovery of novel antitumor sulfonamides targeting G1 phase of the cell cycle. *J. Med. Chem.* 42 (19): 3789–3799.

58 Raymond, E., ten Bokkel Huinink, W.W., Taieb, J. et al. (2002). Phase I and pharmacokinetic study of E7070, a novel chloroindolyl sulfonamide cell-cycle inhibitor, administered as a one-hour infusion every three weeks in patients with advanced cancer. *J. Clin. Oncol.* 20 (16): 3508–3521.

59 Han, T., Goralski, M., Gaskill, N. et al. (2017). Anticancer sulfonamides target splicing by inducing RBM39 degradation via recruitment to DCAF15. *Science* 356 (6336): eaal3755.

60 Uehara, T., Minoshima, Y., Sagane, K. et al. (2017). Selective degradation of splicing factor CAPERα by anticancer sulfonamides. *Nat. Chem. Biol.* 13 (6): 675–680.

61 Ting, T.C., Goralski, M., Klein, K. et al. (2019). Aryl sulfonamides degrade RBM39 and RBM23 by recruitment to CRL4-DCAF15. *Cell Rep.* 29 (6): 1499–1510.e6.

62 Faust, T.B., Yoon, H., Nowak, R.P. et al. (2020). Structural complementarity facilitates E7820-mediated degradation of RBM39 by DCAF15. *Nat. Chem. Biol.* 16 (1): 7–14.

63 Bussiere, D.E., Xie, L., Srinivas, H. et al. (2020). Structural basis of indisulam-mediated RBM39 recruitment to DCAF15 E3 ligase complex. *Nat. Chem. Biol.* 16 (1): 15–23.

64 Li, L., Mi, D., Pei, H. et al. (2020). in vivo target protein degradation induced by PROTACs based on E3 ligase DCAF15. *Signal Transduct. Target. Ther.* 5 (1): 129.

65 Kerres, N., Steurer, S., Schlager, S. et al. (2017). Chemically induced degradation of the oncogenic transcription factor BCL6. *Cell Rep.* 20 (12): 2860–2875.

66 Słabicki, M., Yoon, H., Koeppel, J. et al. (2020). Small-molecule-induced polymerization triggers degradation of BCL6. *Nature* 588 (7836): 164–168.
67 Wang, C., Zhang, Y., Wu, Y., and Xing, D. (2021). Developments of CRBN-based PROTACs as potential therapeutic agents. *Eur. J. Med. Chem.* 225: 113749.
68 Robbins, D.W., Kelly, A., Tan, M. et al. (2020). Nx-2127, a degrader of BTK and IMiD neosubstrates, for the treatment of B-cell malignancies. *Blood* 136 (Supplement 1): 34–34.
69 Mayo, M., Karnik, R., Klaus, C. et al. (2021). KT-413, a novel IRAKIMID degrader of IRAK4 and IMID substrates, has a differentiated moa that leads to single-agent and combination regressions in MYD88MT lymphoma models. *Hematol. Oncol.* 39 (S2): 37–38.
70 Zhang, J., Fu, L., Shen, B. et al. (2020). Assessing IRAK4 functions in ABC DLBCL by IRAK4 kinase inhibition and protein degradation. *Cell Chem. Biol.* 27 (12): 1500–1509.e13.
71 Słabicki, M., Kozicka, Z., Petzold, G. et al. (2020). The CDK inhibitor CR8 acts as a molecular glue degrader that depletes cyclin K. *Nature* 585 (7824): 293–297.
72 Mayor-Ruiz, C., Bauer, S., Brand, M. et al. (2020). Rational discovery of molecular glue degraders via scalable chemical profiling. *Nat. Chem. Biol.* 16 (11): 1199–1207.
73 Lv, L., Chen, P., Cao, L. et al. (2020). Discovery of a molecular glue promoting CDK12-DDB1 interaction to trigger cyclin K degradation. *eLife* 9: e59994.
74 Simonetta, K.R., Taygerly, J., Boyle, K. et al. (2019). Prospective discovery of small molecule enhancers of an E3 ligase-substrate interaction. *Nat. Commun.* 10 (1): 1402.
75 Clevers, H. and Nusse, R. (2012). Wnt/β-catenin signaling and disease. *Cell* 149 (6): 1192–1205.
76 Liu, C., Li, Y., Semenov, M. et al. (2002). Control of β-catenin phosphorylation/ degradation by a dual-kinase mechanism. *Cell* 108 (6): 837–847.
77 Sanchez-Vega, F., Mina, M., Armenia, J. et al. (2018). Oncogenic signaling pathways in the cancer genome atlas. *Cell* 173 (2): 321–337.e10.
78 Tokheim, C., Wang, X., Timms, R.T. et al. (2021). Systematic characterization of mutations altering protein degradation in human cancers. *Mol. Cell* 81 (6): 1292–1308.
79 Snyder, L.B., Neklesa, T.K., Chen, X. et al. (2021). Abstract 43: discovery of ARV-110, a first in class androgen receptor degrading PROTAC for the treatment of men with metastatic castration resistant prostate cancer. *Exp. Mol. Ther.* 115: 43–43.
80 Kastl, J.M., Davies, G., Godsman, E., and Holdgate, G.A. (2021). Small-molecule degraders beyond PROTACs—challenges and opportunities. *SLAS Discov. Adv. Sci. Drug Discov.* 26 (4): 524–533.

12

Taming the Beast: How to Optimize DMPK–PD Properties of Oral Degraders

Caroline Rynn, Arthur Van De Vyver, Antje Walz, Carina Cantrill and Matthias Wittwer

Roche Pharma Research and Early Development, Pharmaceutical Sciences, Roche Innovation Center Basel, F. Hoffmann-La Roche Ltd, Grenzacherstrasse 124, CH-4070, Basel, Switzerland

Targeted protein degraders (degraders, PROTACs, or degronomids) belong to a nascent class of promising therapeutic modalities that have garnered a lot of attention from the clinical space, thanks to their unique mechanism of action. Degraders are heterobifunctional molecules and have two different binding sites, one on the ligand to bind the target protein and the second on the ligand binding the ubiquitin–protein ligase (E3). Both these functional groups are connected by a linker [1]. Degraders are distinct in their ability to target the so-called "undruggable" target space [2], which puts them at a therapeutic advantage over classical small-molecule inhibitors [3]. Successful development of these compounds relies on good characterization and understanding of the mechanism of action and the drug properties that govern the pharmacology of degraders. This chapter explores the properties related to drug metabolism, pharmacokinetics, and pharmacodynamics (DMPK–PD) of degraders. It is intended to give a broad outline of the fundamental concepts relating to the physicochemical properties and their impact on the absorption, distribution, metabolism, and excretion (ADME) profiles of degraders as well as to provide an overview of the available tools to characterize and quantify these properties. Additionally, the importance of good experimental design and the role of computational models in characterizing and predicting the PK/PD profiles of degraders, both in early development and in the clinics, are discussed. Gathering this information and insights is crucial to allow the selection of a degrader dose that is both safe and efficacious to the patient.

Inducing Targeted Protein Degradation: From Chemical Biology to Drug Discovery and Clinical Applications, First Edition. Edited by Philipp Cromm.

12.1 Physicochemical and ADME Properties of Degraders

12.1.1 Physicochemical Properties

Protein degraders are a unique class of small molecules in their own right, not in the least because of their unique mechanism of action and relatively large size. These compounds usually do not adhere to Lipinski's rule of 5 (Ro5). This Ro5 has long been the industry standard for rational drug design of small molecules in order to achieve favorable oral drug disposition characteristics [4]. Lately, an increasing number of small-molecule compounds that do not strictly adhere to this have been developed. They possess physicochemical and DMPK properties that extend or go beyond the rule of 5 (respectively called bRo5 compounds) but still exhibit adequate oral bioavailability [5–7]. Increasingly, the special role of degraders within the bRo5 space has been recognized and discussed, and several research groups have focused on gaining a better understanding of the degrader chemical space [8]. As the degrader field is rapidly advancing and more data becomes publicly available, the boundaries of the degrader chemical space and the definition of optimal compound properties are still subject to considerable change. A database of published degraders has been compiled and classified according to different criteria (including chemical structures, degradation effectiveness, and physicochemical properties) with the aim to provide an overview from the chemical perspective with a special focus on modulation of properties during the development of degraders [9]. In order to assess degradation effectiveness, these authors introduced the degrader score (Deg_S), which is a single overall measure of degrader efficacy. Interestingly, physicochemical properties did not correlate with Deg_S with the exception of lipophilicity (clogP), which shows a positive correlation with degradation efficiency. The authors also suggest that the number of hydrogen bond donors (HBDs) is kept at or below 5 and that the total polar surface area (TPSA) does not exceed 250 $Å^2$ as these limitations are respected by degraders with the highest Deg_S. However, Deg_S does not directly consider the bioavailability, a composite parameter that is key for orally dosed degraders (see Section 12.1.8). Nevertheless, several authors also found HBD count to be an important descriptor regarding oral availability [10, 11]. Finally, Garcia Jimenez used the PROTAC database and focused on seven rationally selected 2D molecular descriptors [11]. By comparing the overall chemical space with the space occupied by orally available degraders, the authors conclude that the number of carbon atoms (nC), TPSA, and Kier's index of flexibility help to identify property spaces with the potential for oral absorption [12]. The subregion with the best drug-like properties showed smaller size, lower polarity, and flexibility. Other authors also suggested composite analyses with different parameters, and one prominent example is AbbVie's multiparametric score (AB-MPS), which worked well for early assessment of bRo5 compounds. However, the applicability still needs to be shown for degraders [9, 10].

Overall, the number of H-bond donors emerges in several analyses as an important parameter regarding oral availability with a general recommendation to keep this number below 5 or at least generally low [9, 10, 13]. Interestingly, the number of H-bond acceptors seems to be less critical as long as it is not excessively high [10]. Additionally, the degrader's TPSA is generally lower than that for other bRo5 compounds, suggesting that this parameter is optimized during drug discovery and development [9].

Lipophilicity is considered as a key parameter that influences many compound properties including permeability, transporters, solubility, plasma protein binding, drug–drug interaction (DDI) potential, clearance, and oral absorption (see Sections 12.1.2–12.1.8). Generally, lipophilicity needs to be kept in check even for larger molecules to improve the permeability and solubility interplay [10, 13, 14]. An elegant solution to combine both good solubility and permeability already in the design stage would be to design chameleonic behavior [15], or dynamic solubility as highlighted by Tinworth and Young [10], where the general principle around a so-called physicochemical "sweet spot," to make a drug as hydrophilic as possible without losing potency, should also be applicable to degraders.

However, lipophilicity of degraders is not straightforward to assess because of solubility limitation. The general recommendation by several research groups to derive reliable early estimations is to use chromatographic methods such as chromLogD [10, 16–18] or delta log Kow using immobilized artificial membranes [19].

12.1.2 Permeability

Based on Lipinski's rules established for small molecules, molecules such as degraders would not be expected to have significant membrane permeability and, consequently, good oral bioavailability. However, given the entry into clinical trials for Arvinas' orally dosed degraders, ARV-110 and ARV-471 [20], optimization of permeability is, in fact, feasible and efforts are widespread. Permeability methods for early screening need to be carefully considered and validated in support of successful degraders. To assess this in early development, a number of *in vitro* experimental models with high-throughput capacity have been utilized. Two of the most commonly used assays are the parallel artificial membrane permeability assay (PAMPA) [21–23] and the transcellular permeability screens such as Caco-2, MDCKII, or LLC-PK1 [13, 24, 25]. PAMPA is a cell-free, simple phospholipid bilayer model. Because of its simplistic nature, PAMPA allows for the assessment of passive membrane permeability without the presence of convoluting factors such as active transport mechanisms present in cell-based models.

In the context of degrader development, a number of publications have described challenges associated with the early permeability screening of degraders [14, 24, 26, 27], particularly with a focus on degrader molecular properties. For example, a study by Kihlberg and colleagues [28] provided the first mechanistic insights into how degraders adapt to their solution environment, confirming that degraders can behave as molecular chameleons and permeate membranes because of the formation of intramolecular hydrogen bonds and a folded structure in a chloroform solution, mimicking the plasma membrane. This highlights the need for robust *in vitro* assays at the design stage in order to identify the most promising candidates in terms of permeability properties. Recent literature has described a number of different approaches where PAMPA in combination with new techniques proposed as a feasible strategy to support the optimal design of oral degraders.

Although it is widely recognized that there is a higher rate of invalid data for bRo5 molecules (14%) compared to the compliant Ro5 molecules (8%) when assessed in PAMPA, this is likely attributed to the poor physicochemical properties. A recent study by Klein et al. [13] using a combination of PAMPA and an assay termed lipophilic permeability efficiency (LPE) provided mechanistic insights into the permeability of 11 structurally similar Von Hippel–Lindau (VHL) degraders to support the design and improvement in structural conformations to improve the permeability. However, PAMPA ranks inherent permeability, and LPE provides an insight into how structural changes affect permeability measurements in these systems. Among the degraders tested, there was a 300-fold difference in permeability estimates, which reflected the differences in physical properties, outside of those that are typically considered. However, compounds with a lower molecular weight (MW) and fewer hydrogen bond acceptors or HBDs were significantly more permeable. As observed in other studies [24], it is important to highlight that degraders with an atomic partition coefficient (ALogP) up to four possessed a good correlation with permeability, whereas for degraders with ALogP values beyond this threshold, confounding factors such as solubility and membrane retention would diminish the parameter estimate reliability.

Because of the potential limitations of PAMPA in early screening, a number of studies do not recommend PAMPA as a tool to support accurate ranking of degraders during preclinical development [16, 25, 29] without careful consideration of the experimental setup. It has been proposed that because of the challenging physicochemistry of degraders, cellular models may be better suited for the characterization of these molecules for the assessment of permeability and subsequent prediction of oral bioavailability [24, 26]. It is however also recognized that these models require adaptations of the assay conditions to overcome some of the limitations such as nonspecific binding and low aqueous solubility. Most studies conducted have utilized "standard" screening conditions with reports of degraders showing very low permeability or outside of detectable limits [16, 24, 25]. Nonetheless, a potential approach adoptable during early development was described by Cui et al. [30] for bRo5 compounds, whereby adaptation of transcellular permeability assays to include a 1 μM preincubation with compound for 24 hours followed by washing and subsequent standard incubation resulted in significant improvements in permeability estimates. Using this approach, the authors demonstrated that the peptides were in fact moderate to highly permeable under those assay conditions. While this has not yet been demonstrated for degraders specifically, it is not unreasonable to expect improvements in detectability using this approach. However, this requires further investigation to ensure that adequate viability of cells is retained, and sufficient translation can be established to understand the barriers to oral absorption for degraders between solubility and permeability.

12.1.3 Transporters

For a detailed summary of transporter impact in the "beyond rule of five" chemical space, the authors refer readers to a review by Matsson et al. [7]. In general, the bRo5 space is largely unexplored in terms of drug–transporter interactions. An analysis undertaken by Mak et al. [31], however, demonstrated that molecules within the Ro5 space could be substrates of ATP-binding cassette (ABC) and solute carrier (SLC) transporters. To date, the most widely reported interactions are with *P*-glycoprotein (*P*-gp), a 170 kDa member of the ABC transporter superfamily (ABCB1). This transporter is widely recognized as a major determinant for the low or variable oral absorption of several drugs via efflux at the intestine. Compounds possessing high passive permeability have the least potential to be influenced by *P*-gp, likely because of the high local concentration in the gut following oral dose. However, transport of molecules with high MW and poor passive cell permeability are more likely to be subject to transporter-mediated efflux, whose influence increases in a size-dependent manner [32]. In particular, for degraders, publications have highlighted the potential contribution of *P*-gp in limiting the efficacy of degraders, whereby inclusion of *P*-gp inhibitors, cyclosporine A, or tariquidar elicited an increase in observed potency in cell lines, leading to the assumption that this is therefore limited by *P*-gp [33, 34]. However, this only applies to inherent target cell permeability as opposed to potential limitations of oral bioavailability.

New reports are emerging, whereby *P*-gp has been assessed as a means to guide the orally available degrader design. The results are, however, somewhat varied with those of Chessum et al. [34], stating that because of poor solubility and permeability, measurement of the thalidomide protein degradation probes (PDPs) was not possible. On the other hand, Rathod et al. [35] demonstrated the preclinical assessment of a degrader in Caco-2 cells, where permeability was assessed and derived to be in a very low range, i.e. <10 nm/s [35]. The dynamic range in cellular assays of apparent permeability (P_{app}) was significantly higher than that of PAMPA and allowed for the identification of many low-permeability compounds (<10 nm/s) as well as permeable compounds within the series (up to 100 nm/s) [16]. Moreover, as the permeability estimate is in general low to medium (<50 nm/s), the certainty in the accuracy of passive transcellular permeability estimations is reduced, and in this range, the correlation between permeability and fraction absorbed (F_{abs}) is very steep [36]. Compounds with MW > 700 Da tended to show a higher efflux and in some cases an incomplete inhibition of the observed flux. For this, it should be considered that the efflux ratio (ER) is a composite of bidirectional permeability. Assuming that there is a high uncertainty in the P_{app} estimation if experimental conditions are not optimized, this can result in a likely overestimation of the *P*-gp or transporter effect and should be interpreted with caution when ranking series.

With some consideration for SLC transporters and in the context of the extended clearance classification system (ECCS) [37], many degrader molecules would likely be classed as Class 1B or 3B whereby hepatic clearance (CL) could be driven by the interplay of active uptake and metabolism. The full extent of organic-anion transporting polypeptide (OATP) transporters, a transporter class in the SLC superfamily, in particular, and their impact in bRo5 space is, at present, not possible to assess because of the limited data available. Nonetheless, using an internal example molecule whereby biliary CL was the main route of clearance *in vivo*, we conducted hepatic uptake studies in the presence and absence of inhibitors, where active uptake was estimated to be approximately 65% of total uptake (data not shown). Furthermore, recent clinical data from ARV-110 showed a clinically significant drug–drug interaction (see Section 12.1.6) in two patients co-dosed with rosuvastatin (RSV, a known OATP substrate). Although the patients suffered from grade 3/4 increases in liver enzyme levels, upon withdrawal of RSV, no further clinical findings were noted, and as a consequence, RSV is prohibited [38] for co-dosing with ARV-110. At present, there are no reported *in vitro* data indicating substrate or perpetrator interactions for ARV-110. However, it is evident that the influence of SLCs on the disposition and potential interaction of degraders with SLCs, particularly OATPs, requires further investigation.

12.1.4 Solubility

As previously mentioned, only sparse literature has emerged treating the solubility issues of degraders. However, some authors consider the rules derived for bRo5 molecules to be also applicable for degraders. Generally, the solubility of degraders is considered low and challenging to assess with standard methodology [9, 16]. In addition, changes in solubility will be frequently observed during development because of the changes in the availability of amorphous and crystalline forms of the material and because of the increasing sophistication of solubility methodologies used during the development process [10]. For oral degraders, low solubility (even when combined with low permeability) should be considered in context of oral bioavailability and if it is sufficient to elicit efficacious exposure in the tumor. Additionally, modern formulation optimization, for example, nanoformulations, may be employed to boost solubility [39].

12.1.5 Plasma Protein Binding

Plasma protein binding (PPB) of drug molecules influences the free drug concentration that is available to reach the therapeutic target and determines the *in vivo* efficacy and pharmacokinetics [40]. Owing principally to high lipophilicity, degraders in general display very high binding to plasma proteins, yielding a low unbound fraction in the plasma (fu_p). In practice, low fu_p values can be problematic to measure with good accuracy as issues to reach binding equilibrium or poor recovery may confound accurate fu_p measurement for large lipophilic molecules like degraders. Therefore, the PPB method applied for degraders needs to be carefully considered, and adaptations may be required to make them fit for purpose [16, 17].

12.1.6 Drug–Drug Interactions

Pharmacokinetic DDIs caused by the co-administration of multiple drugs are common and may result in reduction in the treatment efficacy or even serious or fatal adverse events. Pharmacokinetic DDIs, which can affect all aspects of absorption, distribution, metabolism, and excretion, are typically mediated by cytochrome P450's (CYP450s), and strategies have been developed to assess DDI risks early in drug discovery [41, 42]. A more systematic assessment of CYP450- and transporter-mediated DDIs of degraders has yet to be shared in the public domain. As degraders can access the catalytic sites of phase 1 and phase 2 enzymes, including those of CYP450s [16, 43, 44], and interact with transporters [34], it is the authors' opinion that there is a similar potential for DDI as for traditional small molecules. This highlights the need for a systematic assessment of DDI potential and must be considered in the benefit–risk evaluation for degraders. Comprehensive guidance [45, 46] should be followed to mitigate drug–drug interaction with concomitant medications and costly developmental failures.

12.1.7 Clearance

The clearance rate of a drug describes the irreversible elimination of drug molecules from the systemic circulation, i.e. the volume of blood cleared of drug per unit time. The total body clearance of a drug refers to the sum of all the different clearance processes occurring, with the main organs of elimination being the liver and kidney, and metabolism and/or drug transporters as principal drivers of clearance [47]. As clearance is a determinant of other pharmacokinetic parameters such as half-life, oral bioavailability, and efficacious dose, it is a key pharmacokinetic optimization parameter for which structural modification strategies to improve clearance and elimination profiles of traditional small molecules are well defined in the literature [48, 49].

The pharmacokinetic profile of degrader molecules needs to provide adequate unbound exposure at the target site, which facilitates target protein–degrader–E3 ternary complex formation and target protein knockdown, leading to the desired biological effect, for example, tumor shrinkage in the oncology setting (see Section 12.2.2). Once inside the body, degrader molecules must remain intact and reach the target site in order to elicit degradation of the target protein. The extent to which the physicochemical properties of degraders affect drug clearance pathways is now becoming clearer owing to a number of publications on this topic [9, 11, 19, 50, 51].

Degraders that are metabolically labile could break into fragments resulting in ineffective binding of the target protein or E3 ligase, which will preclude effective ternary complex formation and proteasomal dependent degradation, and the fragments may be eliminated from the body without eliciting the pharmacodynamic effect. Despite their large size, degraders can be substrates of both Phase 1 and Phase 2 metabolizing enzymes and thus share similar metabolic liabilities with more traditional bRo5 molecules. The chemical nature of the linker connecting the protein of interest (POI) and E3 ligands has been extensively modified with time to adapt the degrader to its biological function. However, the linker is also commonly playing an important role in determining the overall metabolic stability of degraders [50], as demonstrated in metabolic studies with microsomes and cryopreserved hepatocytes and in rodent pharmacokinetic studies [16, 17, 43, 44]. It has previously been proposed that a shorter aliphatic linker may provide steric hindrance to the catalytic site of metabolizing enzymes, leading to increased metabolic stability, while the site of attachment of the linker to the ligands may also impact the metabolic liability [51]. Even though secondary amide bonds are abundantly present in degraders because of the easy chemical coupling reaction, from a stability perspective, these are not found to be beneficial [9]. Further attempts to better understand the metabolism of degraders were made using cryopreserved human hepatocytes, and it was concluded that the overall metabolism of a degrader cannot be predicted by just considering the metabolism of the individual ligands because the overall structure influences the metabolism significantly [51]. In addition, it has been shown that, in addition to CYP450 and UDP-glucuronosyltransferase (UGT) enzymes, human aldehyde oxidase (hAOX) can also metabolize degraders *in vitro*, thus expanding the known enzyme repertoires involved in metabolic degradation of degraders. As discussed in the transporter section of this chapter (see Section 12.1.3), evidence has emerged, which indicates that SLC drug transporters influence the disposition of the clinical candidate ARV-110, but this is currently the only case of transporter-mediated drug disposition of degraders that has been well documented in the literature [38].

12.1.8 Oral Absorption

The oral administration route remains one of the most common systemic drug delivery routes for patients undergoing chronic therapy owing to its noninvasiveness, ease of use convenience, and the feasibility to achieve stable, solid formulations. Despite the clear advantages offered by this route, the human gastrointestinal (GI) tract is complex, and many barriers exist, which can limit drug delivery from the stomach across the GI tract into portal blood. Drug absorption is largely controlled by solubility and dissolution rate, which determine how fast the drug reaches the peak concentration in the stomach, and inherent permeability, which determines the rate at which dissolved drug molecules diffuse across the GI wall [50, 52]. As indicated in Figure 12.1, drug absorption can be influenced by metabolism and drug efflux at the site of the gut wall, which are principally mediated by CYP3A4 catalysis and *P*-gp, respectively. However, the liver, which is considered the main organ of drug clearance, can also influence drug elimination via metabolism and/or drug transport to limit the amount of absorbed drug that reaches the systemic circulation. The CYP450 expression and function at the intestine and liver have been well documented as has drug transporter expression [54–56]. Further barriers to oral

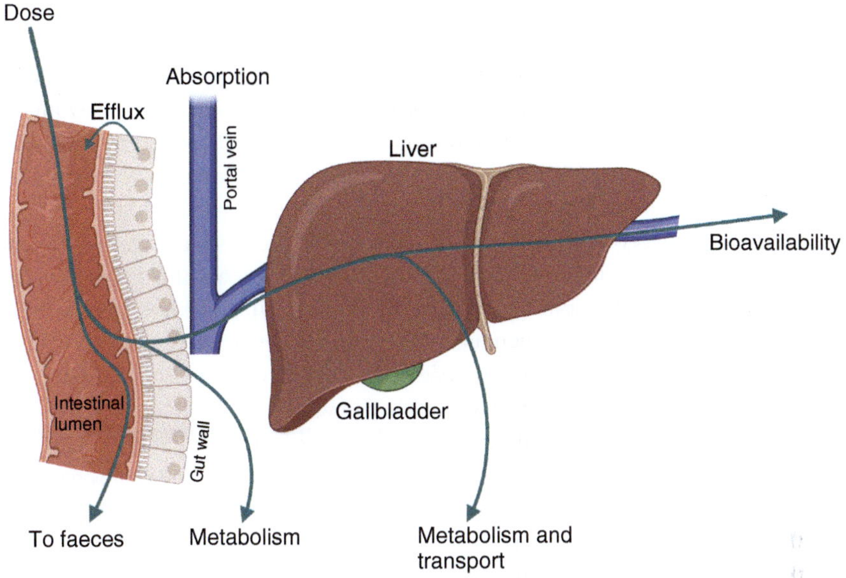

Figure 12.1 Major sites of drug metabolism and drug transport in the gut wall and liver that influence oral bioavailability. *Source:* Figure adapted from Han van de Waterbeemd et al. [53] and created with Biorender.com.

absorption include potential for drug precipitation and pH differences across the GI tract, which can influence the solubility of drug molecules. Improved understanding of the physiology of the GI tract and optimization strategies for more traditional Ro5 molecules have been well documented in the literature in the past [57–59].

Heterobifunctional degraders are a very hot topic in drug discovery, and they are expected to strongly impact the future of drug discovery as they offer an attractive approach for highly potent and selective degradation of proteins of interest, with continued response even at substoichiometric concentrations [1, 3, 60, 61]. However, limited tissue penetration and issues with oral bioavailability are common, owing to their large and flexible structures that lie in the bRO5 chemical space [50]. Despite this extra complexity, much of the earlier peer-reviewed degrader literature appears to focus on degradation kinetics with little regard for the optimization of physicochemical properties to drive the design of improved oral degraders. Unsurprisingly, many of the early *in vivo* efficacy studies detailed in these publications were conducted using parenteral routes of administration, with only few examples of orally efficacious degraders [62], suggesting that the latter may have been a serendipitous finding achieved through empirical efforts. Irrespective of whether these earlier degraders were regarded as *in vivo* tool compounds, knowledge has been gleaned along the way and the degrader toolbox is growing rapidly with several physicochemical guidelines emerging to guide property-based drug discovery strategies producing permeable oral degraders [19], such as establishment of the predictive degrader score Deg_S (see Section 12.1.1) [50]. More recently, databases have been constructed that integrate structural information and experimental data, which facilitates mapping of the degrader chemical space [9, 11, 63]. These have been populated with the recent disclosure of structures of two orally bioavailable degraders that are progressing in the clinic ARV-110 and ARV-471 [64]. ARV-110, the first degrader to enter the clinic in 2019, targets the androgen receptor (AR) for the treatment of metastatic castration-resistant prostate cancer, which was closely followed by ARV-471, a degrader that targets the estrogen receptor (ER) for the treatment of breast cancer. The subregion they occupy has been identified and may be exploited as property-based guidance for permeable, oral degraders [11] Additionally, Arvinas recently shared the medicinal chemistry evolution that led to the identification of these AR and ER degraders [65, 66]. Figure 12.2a highlights an early AR degrader with an aliphatic linker; all the three parts of the molecule were then optimized, E3 recruiting ligands, linker, and AR binders, leading to their front-running degrader ARV-110 (semirigid linker). In Figure 12.2b, the structures of their early ER degrader and the final clinical lead, ARV-471, can be seen. The preclinical *in vivo* data demonstrated that both ARV-110 and ARV-471 are orally efficacious, robustly degrading AR and ER, respectively, which supported their transition into the clinic for further development [67, 68].

Furthermore, at least a further 12 degraders have either entered or are expected to enter the clinic by 2021, indicating a better understanding of the properties required for the developability of degraders (Table 12.1). Likewise, for metabolic stability, existing *in vitro* ADME tools and high-throughput *in vitro* ADME screening can be used to guide efficient test-refine cycles for the optimization of degrader physicochemical properties, such as cellular transport and solubility (see Sections 12.1.3 and 12.1.4), which impact oral absorption. However, the conduct of *in vivo* pharmacokinetic studies with degraders tends to need further adaptation in comparison to Ro5 molecules, specifically in terms of formulation support owing to the limited solubility. Mechanistic investigations may also be warranted to generate the most meaningful and highest quality data to understand the key optimization properties to improve oral absorption [16].

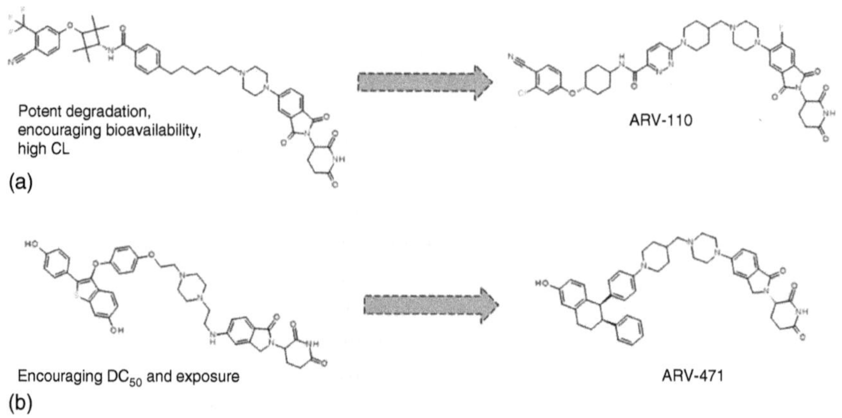

Figure 12.2 Genesis molecules that lead to discovery of Arvinas's clinical candidates (a) ARV-110 and (b) ARV-471.

Table 12.1 Selected heterobifunctional degraders in and approaching the clinic.

Drug	Sponsor	Target POI	Lead indication	Status
ARV-100	Arvinas	Androgen receptor	Prostate cancer	Phase II
ARV-471	Arvinas	Estrogen receptor	Breast cancer	Phase II
ARV-766	Arvinas	Androgen receptor	Prostate cancer	Phase 1
AR-LDD	Bristol Myers Squibb	Androgen receptor	Prostate cancer	Phase 1
DT2216	Dialectic	BCL-XL degrader	Liquid and solid cancers	Phase 1
KT-474	Kymera/Sanofi	IRAK4 degrader	Autoimmune including AD, HS, and RA	Phase 1
KT-413	Kymera	IRAK4 degrader with IMiD activity	MYD88-mutant DLBCL	Phase 1
KT-333	Kymera	STAT3 degrader	Liquid and solid cancers	Phase 1
NX-2127	Nurix	BTK degrader with IMiD activity	B-cell malignancies	Phase 1
NX-5948	Nurix	BTK degrader	B-cell malignancies and autoimmune disorders	Phase 1
CG001419	Cullgen	TRK degrader	Cancer and other diseases	IND
CFT8634	C4 Therapeutics	BRD9 degrader	Synovial sarcoma	IND
FHD-609	Foghorn	BRD9 degrader	Synovial sarcoma	IND

POI, protein of interest; AD, atopic dermatitis; DLBCL, diffuse large B-cell lymphoma; HS, hidradenitis suppurativa; IMiD, immunomodulatory drug; RA, rheumatoid arthritis; IND, investigational new drug. *Source:* Adapted from Mullard [69].

12.2 Degraders: PK/PD challenges and the Role of Modeling and Simulation

12.2.1 Pharmacological Processes of Degraders and PK/PD Aspects

As the original discovery of degraders as a therapeutic modality, it has been demonstrated that these compounds largely fall beyond the rule of 5 (see Section 12.1.1). This means that degraders may display challenging ADME and pharmacokinetic (PK) properties compared to traditional small molecules. When it comes to pharmacodynamics, the distinct event-driven pharmacology of degraders may offer a greater therapeutic benefit in comparison to the classical antagonistic inhibitors [3]. This includes the possibility to exhibit prolonged pharmacodynamic effects and may possibly be less susceptible to drug-induced resistance mechanisms. A good understanding of the pharmacological processes and their quantification are prerequisites for the successful development of degraders as well as to achieve those therapeutic benefits [62]. Degraders facilitate the active removal of target proteins of interest, which is in contrast to the mode of action of small-molecule antagonistic inhibitors that mainly act by blocking the enzyme or receptor activity through binding, otherwise known as occupancy-driven pharmacology [70]. Target protein removal is achieved by binding to the target protein (i.e. POI) followed by the formation of transient ternary complexes with the ubiquitin–proteasome systems. Through linking of the protein to an E3 ligase, the degrader utilizes the cell's own degradation pathway to eliminate the protein. This linking facilitates the ubiquitination of the protein by E3 ligase. This, and other elements of the proteasome machinery, will tag the protein for degradation. Protein degradation will prompt the degrader to dissociate, making it available again to form new ternary complexes with the protein of interest. This mechanism of serial protein tagging and degrading makes degraders an interesting modality [71]. This process has been described as a "catalytic knockdown" of the target protein and is a key feature of its PK/PD properties. With these pharmacological processes in mind, we will discuss how PK/PD aspects can be captured in mathematical models to guide compound optimization strategies as well as to predict efficacious dosing regimens in cancer patients for those modalities.

12.2.2 PK/PD Considerations During Drug Discovery and Development

PK/PD models are widely used tools to guide the development of therapeutic interventions. They enable quantifying the effective drug concentration at the site of action, the subsequent level of target engagement measured as a biomarker, and the pharmacodynamic effects related to efficacy and safety [72, 73]. Those models recapitulate the relevant pharmacological processes and allow prediction of the optimal dosing regimen achieving maximal therapeutic benefit while minimizing the adverse effects. This includes characterization of pharmacologically active (i.e. free or unbound) drug concentration, the corresponding level of target engagement, and the subsequent target modulation, leading to the therapeutic effects. For classical antagonistic small molecules blocking the activity of enzymes or receptors, the drug potency is closely related to its receptor occupancy. The guiding principles in drug development of those drugs have been studied to achieve exposures that are well tolerated and enable high equilibrium target occupancy at the site of action [74]. If much higher doses are administered for those types of drugs, then the beneficial drug effect will not increase, and there is a higher chance that severe adverse effects occur. Those fundamental PK/PD aspects apply to classical antagonistic inhibitors as well as targeted protein degraders. However, there are key differences with regard to the pharmacological processes between these two classes of drugs that need to be considered in PK/PD modeling in order to ensure successful development of degraders. As degraders engage with both the target protein of interest and the E3 ligase simultaneously, the classical concept of receptor occupancy does not apply. Instead, degraders form ternary complexes with their binding partners. Simulation of ternary complex formation as a function of the degraders' concentration shows a bell-shaped curve (Figure 12.3a) [75]. The concentration of complexes increases with increasing degrader concentration up to the optimal concentration at which maximal ternary complex formation occurs. At higher concentrations, the formation of ternary complexes is reduced, while more binary

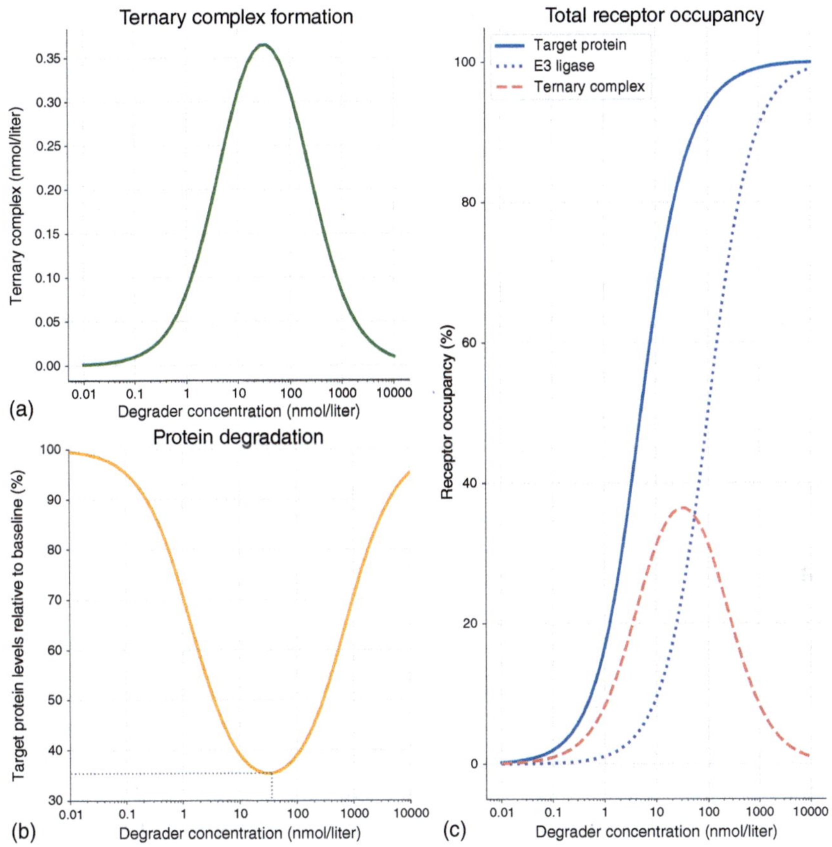

Figure 12.3 Degrader exposure–response relationship on ternary complex formation, protein degradation, and receptor occupancy, as well as ternary complex formation assuming steady-state conditions. (a) Ternary complex formation follows a bell-shaped curve in accordance with the "Hook effect" described for degraders. (b) The level of target protein degradation is proportional to the formation of ternary complexes. A dosing regimen can thus be optimized to yield degrader concentrations at the site of action that lead to maximal ternary complex formation and, as such, maximal protein degradation (D_{max}). (c) Receptor occupancy can be expressed as the total receptor occupancy of the target protein (blue, solid line) and the E3 ligase (blue, dotted line), which reflects the proportion of both ternary and binary complexes from the total protein pool. Alternatively, receptor occupancy can be expressed as the proportion of target protein bound in ternary complexes (red, dashed line).

complexes are formed because of steric hindrances. This bell-shaped curve of ternary complex formation as a function of drug concentration has implications on the anticipated pharmacological activity (Figure 12.3b).

As illustrated, a concentration-dependent decrease of target protein is observed, reaching a maximal effect at concentrations corresponding to the drug concentration (D_{max}, Figure 12.3b) at which maximal trimeric formation occurs. At concentrations above this level, the effectiveness of protein degradation is reduced because of a decrease of ternary complexes and increase in binary complexes. This peculiar concentration–effect relationship is also known as the "hook effect" [76] and suggests that higher dose levels may result in reduced target engagement and hence reduced efficacy [77].

In terms of drug target binding, a distinction can be made between receptor occupancy (i.e. the proportion of E3 Ligase or target protein bound to the drug) and the formation of ternary complexes (i.e. the proportion of target protein bound in ternary complexes) (Figure 12.3c). Receptor occupancy of either the target protein or E3 ligase refers to the proportion bound in either ternary or binary complexes. Higher drug concentrations lead to higher total receptor occupancy, and the binding affinities correspond to the concentration at which half of the target protein or ligase is bound. In order to trigger protein degradation, however, ternary complexes need to be formed. Ternary complex formation only reflects the proteins bound in ternary complexes and follows a bell-shaped curve. In the simulation in Figure 12.3, considerable protein degradation can already be observed at a low percentage of target protein bound in ternary complexes.

In the early phase of lead identification and compound optimization, besides consideration of PK properties (see Sections 12.1.2–12.1.8), cellular assays are typically established to measure target protein degradation as the PD effect. Those data can subsequently be analyzed with PK/PD models. Bartlett and Gilbert [78] have proposed a mechanism-based PK/PD model that describes the kinetics of this multistep process and balances the ternary complex stability against ubiquitin–proteasome system degradation rates. This model is based on the concept of kinetic proofreading that has been proposed to explain the accuracy and specificity of biological processes including protein translation and T-cell receptor signal transduction [79, 80]. It suggests that for efficient protein degradation, the formation of a productive ternary complex is required that is stable for a sufficient amount of time as a sequence of ubiquitination events needs to occur before the proteasome-mediated degradation can be triggered. This process is rapidly reversed if the degrader dissociates to break up the ternary complex and, as a consequence, the process of protein degradation will not be initiated. In line with the experimental data, the degradation potency of a given substrate protein does not correlate with its binding affinity but rather the ability to form a stable ternary complex with the degrader and the recruited E3 ubiquitin ligase [81, 82]. The model also explains how positive cooperativity mitigates the high-dose hook effect [83] and is suited to guide the optimization of binding and degradation efficiency. For illustration of the impact of the kinetics of these multistep processes, Figure 12.4a shows the dose–response curves of two drug candidates with the same affinity (KD = 10 nmol/l) to the target and different dissociation (k_{off}) constants (compound 1 with slow dissociation, $k_{off} = 10$ 1/h, and compound 2 with rapid dissociation, $k_{off} = 1000$ 1/h). In line with the kinetic proofreading theory [79], slow dissociation rates result in the formation of stable complexes with longer half-lives compared to those formed by a compound exhibiting rapid dissociation rates. A longer half-life of the ternary complex increases the chances that there is sufficient time for the ubiquitination process of the target protein and its subsequent degradation (Figure 12.4a, yellow line) and results in higher protein degradation as

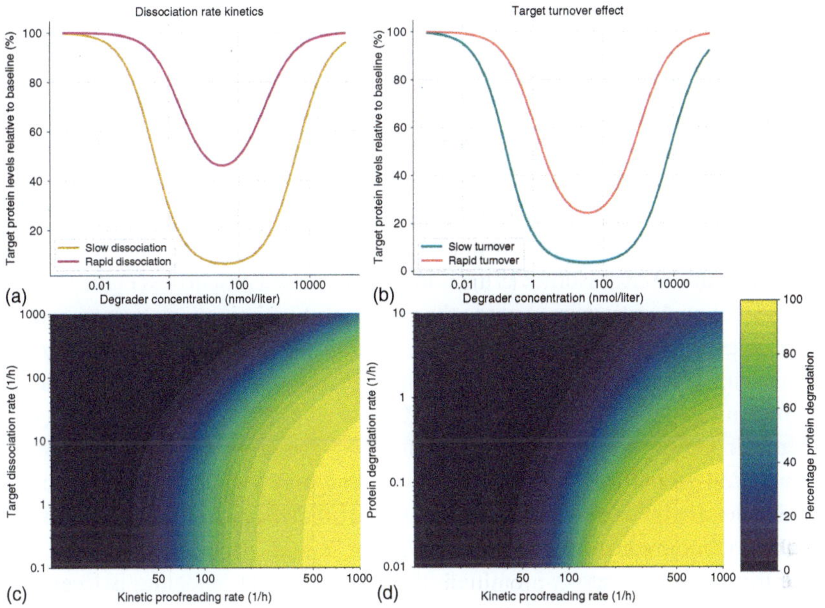

Figure 12.4 Simulated protein degradation as a function of dissociation rate kinetics (a) or target turnover (b), a mechanism-based model as proposed by Bartlett and Gilbert. (a) Impact of target binding dissociation rate on protein degradation. Two hypothetical compounds that have the same affinity are simulated, but with either a slow dissociation rate (compound 1, yellow) or a rapid dissociation rate (compound 2, magenta). Under the assumption of kinetic proofreading activity in the ubiquitination steps, compound 1 will induce a higher level of target degradation. (b) Impact of protein turnover on protein degradation. Two hypothetical target proteins that have either a slow turnover (protein 1, cyan) or a rapid turnover (protein 2, red) are simulated. Protein 1 will be suppressed to a higher extent because of its slower turnover. (c, d) Contour plots are useful to explore the parameter space and may give guidance in either compound design or target candidate selection. Based on the assumptions or information on the expected range of kinetic proofreading, a range of target dissociation rates that will induce sufficient target degradation (c), or a range of turnover rates that highlight a protein as a likely target for degrader treatment (d), can be explored.

compared to drugs with a rapid dissociation (Figure 12.4a, magenta line). Figure 12.4b highlights how system-related properties such as target protein turnover may impact the degradation efficiency and thus the dose–response. A slow turnover protein (Figure 12.4b, teal line), because of its intrinsically slow degradation and synthesis rates, is more susceptible to degrader-mediated degradation as compared to a target protein with a rapid turnover (Figure 12.4b, orange line). Together with the relevant experimental data, mechanistic models, such as the Bartlett–Gilbert model presented here, allow to explore the best compound properties and to assess whether the intended target is therapeutically viable. For instance, if data on the ubiquitination and kinetic proofreading rates are available, this enables *in silico* exploration of the optimal compound properties as illustrated in the contour plots in Figure 12.4c,D. These plots allow simultaneous exploration of a combination of compound properties and are suited to assess at which range the combination of these of compound properties will give maximal degradation (yellow area) versus those combinations that are suboptimal and result in negligible degradation (blue area). Figure 12.4c explores the range of target dissociation rates in order to achieve optimal target degradation over a range of kinetic proofreading rates within a given timeframe (Figure 12.4c, blue-yellow gradient) and can guide medicinal chemistry in lead identification and optimization. Likewise, the intrinsic turnover rate of the target protein may inform the investigators about the therapeutic viability of that target protein under the assumed drug- and system-related properties (Figure 12.4d). Those *in silico* explorations may guide the compound optimization strategy and are suited to identify relevant parameters impacting the efficiency of protein degradation. The combination of tailored *in vitro* experiments analyzed with mathematical modeling as suggested by Bartlett and Gilbert is a suitable screening strategy for degraders. It allows researchers to rank compounds based on the interplay between the compound properties and the target and proteasome biology. The most promising molecules are those that shift the degradation efficiency toward the yellow spectrum of the color gradient as presented in Figure 12.4c,d.

Once the lead candidate is identified, the goal of PKPD modeling is to explore the therapeutic window, quantify the exposure response relationship, and define the optimal dose and dosing regimen. Target engagement and downstream events are evidently driven by the presence of the drug at the site of action. Predicting the drug exposure in patients at a given dose relies on a good understanding of the physicochemical and ADME properties of that drug, such as permeability, solubility, PPB, clearance, and oral absorption (see Sections 12.1.2–12.1.8). Deciphering the pharmacokinetics of a degrader and the link to pharmacodynamic effects is key to anticipate the duration of intended target suppression, which has implications on dosing frequency (Figure 12.5). PK/PD models are useful to explore these relationships. The prolonged drug effect that has been described for degraders is highly dependent on the turnover rate of the target protein (Figure 12.5a). If the natural target turnover is slow, this means that the target synthesis rate is slow as well. Consequently, after maximal degradation of the target protein, it will take some time to replenish the target pool. This is in contrast to target proteins with rapid turnover rates, reaching baseline levels much more rapidly. Figure 12.5a shows the kinetics of target degradation. It illustrates durable drug response even after drug removal, which is the result of the natural target turnover [62]. The target turnover can either be retrieved from the literature or estimated from experimental data from *in vitro* studies. A straightforward experimental setup is to expose the drug to the target for a given period of time at different drug concentrations (e.g. 24–36 hours) and then remove the drug by gently washing the cells and monitor the time course of protein levels throughout the experiments [84–86]. It should be noted that the turnover of a given target varies across the cell lines, and therefore, it is recommended to run these assays with a relevant cell system that is representative to the clinical situation [87]. When predicting target turnover *in vivo* from *in vitro* studies, it is suggested to account for the differences in tumor growth kinetics [86]. Figure 12.5b shows the plasma PK profiles at

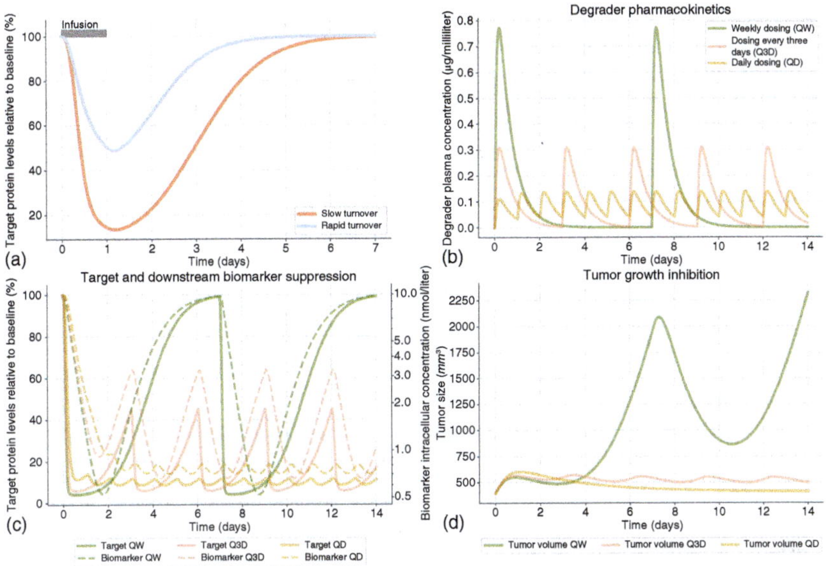

Figure 12.5 Simulated PK/PD profiles for a hypothetical degrader. (a) Percentage of targeted protein degradation for a protein with either a slow (red) or a rapid (blue) turnover after a 24 hour intravenous infusion of degrader. Besides the greater extent of protein degradation (see Figure 12.4b), the suppression of a slow turnover protein is also maintained for a longer period of time after cessation of treatment. (b–d) Influence of dosing regimen on therapeutic effect. (b) Three simulated regimens of daily (QD, yellow), every three days (Q3D, red), or weekly (QW, green) degrader dosing result in different profiles of plasma concentration levels. (c) The kinetics of protein degradation (solid line) and its downstream biomarker response (dashed line) differ based on the chosen dosing regimen. Daily dosing results in a sustained suppression of the response without major fluctuations. (d) Therapeutic effect on tumor growth. Daily dosing results in a sustained tumor growth inhibition, whereas the weekly dosing, besides an initial stronger anti-tumor response, does not prevent tumor growth at later time points. Intermittent dosing such as Q3D will have intermediate results between these extremes.

different dosing regimens reaching the same total exposure. Figure 12.5c represents the corresponding profiles of target protein and its downstream biomarker response, and Figure 12.5d shows the respective tumor growth profiles. While the PK/PD properties may vary from compound to compound, a PK/PD model built on a PK/PD study for a given molecule can be useful to explore the impact of different dosing regimen on target engagement, biomarker response, and therapeutic effect. A thorough understanding of this PK/PD aspect has implications on the experimental design. As it is technically not straightforward to measure the pharmacologically active drug at the site of action [77], the target protein decrease can be regarded as an indirect readout of the pharmacologically active concentration. The collection of total tumor drug concentration in tumor tissue may not provide any meaningful insights as this concentration is a mixture of free and nonspecifically bound drugs and may therefore not be suited for PK/PD characterization [88].

12.2.3 Translational PK/PD and Human Dose Prediction for Targeted Protein Degraders

Robust translation of nonclinical PK (i.e. physicochemical and ADME properties and PK parameters from *in vivo* studies) and PK/PD information to humans is based on two components. It requires two different types of modelings, namely, physiologically based pharmacokinetic (PBPK) for human PK prediction and mechanism-based PK/PD modeling to relate the drug concentration to the dynamics of the target engagement and the downstream PD effects.

For prospective prediction of human PK, PBPK models allow us to account for species differences [89]. The PK of a given drug is predicted based on the physiological and anatomical characteristics of the species of interest and the interplay with its drug-dependent properties (e.g. physicochemical properties, plasma protein binding, and enzymatic activity). For PBPK modeling, there are commercially available software packages such as GastroPlus, SimCyp, and the open-source platform PKSim. Harling et al. demonstrated how this was applied to the degrader PROTAC7 using *in vivo* PK profiles from nonclinical animal species as well as *in vitro* data [90]. In summary, the authors selected the liver as the main clearance organ and used a perfusion-limited PBPK model. A systemic clearance of about 10% of the hepatic blood flow appeared to be consistent among different animal species and was assumed similar for humans. Tissue distribution was described with a permeability-limited tissue model, and the permeability surface area of the tissues was estimated from rat PK data. This parameter was also shown to be consistent across animal species.

The second component of translational PK/PD is to relate the prospective predicted human PK profile to the nonclinical PK/PD model. As outlined in Figure 12.5, the basis of this model can be informed by dynamic *in vitro* PD data allowing the investigator to estimate key parameters such as the drug's potency for target protein degradation in the relevant cell system and the corresponding target turnover. This forms the backbone of the translational PK/PD model to predict target engagement and downstream effects. The PK/PD model can be refined based on dose–response PK/PD studies in relevant pharmacological animal models.

12.3 Gaps and Future Perspectives

As the ADME properties of degraders continue to emerge in the public domain, it is becoming clearer that they share similarities in ADME pathways and fate with more traditional small molecules. As such, degrader discovery projects can address issues such as metabolic instability and drug transporter-mediated elimination using the existing *in vitro* ADME tools and high-throughput *in vitro* ADME screening previously reported [91] to guide efficient test-refine optimization cycles. Despite considerable advances in degrader design and an increasing number of molecules moving into development and clinical trials, some knowledge gaps remain at this point of time. For example, certain aspects of rational drug design, such as how to achieve orally available degraders by chemical structural modifications, remain elusive, and despite promising initial publications in this direction, more work needs to be done to further our understanding. Owing in part to their unique mechanism of action, there is still relatively little known about safety considerations and the suitability of early toxicity screening assays. Along the same lines, only little information is available on DDIs and the translatability of preclinical *in vitro* findings to clinical DDI studies. Finally, more work is required on tissue distribution and tissue selectivity of degraders, particularly regarding exposures in areas that are difficult to reach with larger molecules, such as the central nervous system. Future research and emerging insights should shed light on these important aspects to determine the similarities of degraders with other bRo5 compounds and to what extent, if any, they go into unchartered ADME territory.

As discussed throughout this chapter, solid experimental design and assay selection play a crucial part in achieving success in the development of these compounds. The use of state-of-the-art modeling approaches enables investigators to optimally leverage the experimental data, allowing them to explore optimal compound properties during lead selection or dosing regimens when going into clinics. A model-based framework can assist in establishing the required level of target engagement and subsequent target modulation, linking it to the anticipated therapeutic effect, which allows bridging from *in vitro* and animal studies to the patients. This stepwise process serves to improve the chances of success at any stage in development. Ultimately, the selection of a good dosing regimen is crucial to ensure the safety and efficacy of degraders.

References

1 Scudellari, M. (2019). The protein slayers. *Nature* 567 (7748): 298–300.

2 Dale, B. et al. (2021). Advancing targeted protein degradation for cancer therapy. *Nat. Rev. Cancer* 21 (10): 638–654.

3 Neklesa, T.K., Winkler, J.D., and Crews, C.M. (2017). Targeted protein degradation by PROTACs. *Pharmacol. Ther.* 174: 138–144.

4 Benet, L.Z. et al. (2016). BDDCS, the rule of 5 and drugability. *Adv. Drug Delivery Rev.* 101: 89–98.

5 Doak, B.C. et al. (2014). Oral druggable space beyond the rule of 5: insights from drugs and clinical candidates. *Chem. Biol.* 21 (9): 1115–1142.

6 Shultz, M.D. (2019). Two decades under the influence of the rule of five and the changing properties of approved oral drugs. *J. Med. Chem.* 62 (4): 1701–1714.

7 Matsson, P., Doak, B.C., Over, B., and Kihlberg, J. (2016). Cell permeability beyond the rule of 5. *Adv. Drug Delivery Rev.* 101: 42–61.

8 Ermondi, G., Vallaro, M., and Caron, G. (2020). Degraders early developability assessment: face-to-face with molecular properties. *Drug Discovery Today* 25 (9): 1585–1591.

9 Maple, H.J. et al. (2019). Developing degraders: principles and perspectives on design and chemical space. *MedChemComm* 10 (10): 1755–1764.

10 Tinworth, C. and Young, R. (2020). Facts, patterns, and principles in drug discovery: appraising the rule of 5 with measured physicochemical data. *J. Med. Chem.* 63 (18): 10091–10108.

11 Jimenez, D.G. (2021). Are we ready to design oral PROTACs®?

12 Caron, G. et al. (2020). Flexibility in early drug discovery: focus on the beyond-rule-of-5 chemical space. *Drug Discovery Today* 25 (4): 621–627.

13 Klein, V.G. et al. (2020). Understanding and improving the membrane permeability of VH032-based PROTACs. *ACS Med. Chem. Lett.* 11 (9): 1732–1738.

14 Lokey, R.S., Liras, J., Liras, S., and Jacobson, M.P. (2013). Designing molecules to cross biological membranes. *Curr. Top. Med. Chem.* 13 (7): 775.

15 Rossi Sebastiano, M. et al. (2018). Impact of dynamically exposed polarity on permeability and solubility of chameleonic drugs beyond the rule of 5. *J. Med. Chem.* 61 (9): 4189–4202.

16 Cantrill, C. et al. (2020). Fundamental aspects of DMPK optimization of targeted protein degraders. *Drug Discovery Today* 25 (6): 969–982.

17 Pike, A. et al. (2020). Optimising proteolysis-targeting chimeras (PROTACs) for oral drug delivery: a drug metabolism and pharmacokinetics perspective. *Drug Discovery Today* 25 (10): 1793–1800.

18 Young, R.J., Green, D.V., Luscombe, C.N., and Hill, A.P. (2011). Getting physical in drug discovery II: the impact of chromatographic hydrophobicity measurements and aromaticity. *Drug Discovery Today* 16 (17): 822–830.

19 Ermondi, G., Jimenez, D.G., Sebastiano, M.R., and Caron, G. (2021). Rational control of molecular properties is mandatory to exploit the potential of PROTACs as oral drugs. *ACS Med. Chem. Lett.* 12 (7): 1056–1060.

20 Neklesa, T. et al. (2018). An oral androgen receptor PROTAC degrader for prostate cancer. *J. Clin. Oncol.* 36 (6_Suppl): 381–381.

21 Kansy, M., Avdeef, A., and Fischer, H. (2004). Advances in screening for membrane permeability: high-resolution PAMPA for medicinal chemists. *Drug Discov. Today Technol.* 1 (4): 349–355.

22 Volpe, D.A. (2011). Drug-permeability and transporter assays in Caco-2 and MDCK cell lines. *Fut. Med. Chem.* 3 (16): 2063–2077.

23 Hubatsch, I., Ragnarsson, E.G., and Artursson, P. (2007). Determination of drug permeability and prediction of drug absorption in Caco-2 monolayers. *Nat. Protoc.* 2 (9): 2111–2119.

24 Foley, C.A. et al. (2020). Assessing the cell permeability of bivalent chemical degraders using the chloroalkane penetration assay. *ACS Chem. Biol.* 15 (1): 290–295.

25 Scott, D.E. et al. (2020). Systematic investigation of the permeability of androgen receptor PROTACs. *ACS Med. Chem. Lett.* 11 (8): 1539–1547.

26 Ahlbach, C.L. et al. (2015). Beyond cyclosporine A: conformation-dependent passive membrane permeabilities of cyclic peptide natural products. *Fut. Med. Chem.* 7 (16): 2121–2130.

27 DeGoey, D., Chen, H.J., Cox, P.B., and Wendt, M.D. (2018). Beyond the rule of 5: lessons learned from AbbVie's drugs and compound collection. *J. Med. Chem.* 61 (7): 2636–2651.

28 Atilaw, Y. et al. (2021). Solution conformations shed light on PROTAC cell permeability. *ACS Med. Chem. Lett.* 12 (1): 107–114.

29 Guo, W.H. et al. (2020). Enhancing intracellular accumulation and target engagement of PROTACs with reversible covalent chemistry. *Nat. Commun.* 11 (1): 4268.

30 Cui, Y. et al. (2021). A bidirectional permeability assay for beyond rule of 5 compounds. *Pharmaceutics* 13 (8): 1146.

31 Mak, L. et al. (2015). Metrabase: a cheminformatics and bioinformatics database for small molecule transporter data analysis and (Q)SAR modeling. *J. Cheminf.* 7: 31.

32 Desai, P.V., Sawada, G.A., Wastson, I.A., and Raub, T.J. (2013). Integration of in silico and in vitro tools for scaffold optimization during drug discovery: predicting *P*-glycoprotein efflux. *Mol. Pharmaceutics* 10 (4): 1249–1261.

33 Powell, C.E. et al. (2018). Chemically induced degradation of anaplastic lymphoma kinase (ALK). *J. Med. Chem.* 61 (9): 4249–4255.

34 Chessum, N.E.A. et al. (2018). Demonstrating in-cell target engagement using a pirin protein degradation probe (CCT367766). *J. Med. Chem.* 61 (3): 918–933.

35 Rathod, D., Fu, Y., and Patel, K. (2019). BRD4 PROTAC as a novel therapeutic approach for the treatment of vemurafenib resistant melanoma: Preformulation studies, formulation development and *in vitro* evaluation. *Eur. J. Pharm. Sci.* 138: 105039.

36 Artursson, P. and Karlsson, J. (1991). Correlation between oral drug absorption in humans and apparent drug permeability coefficients in human intestinal epithelial (Caco-2) cells. *Biochem. Biophys. Res. Commun.* 175 (3): 880–885.

37 Umehara, K. et al. (2020). Application of the extended clearance classification system (ECCS) in drug discovery and development: selection of appropriate *in vitro* tools and clearance prediction. *Drug Metab. Dispos.* 48 (10): 849–860.

38 Petrylak, D. et al. (2020). First-in-human phase I study of ARV-110, an androgen receptor (AR) PROTAC degrader in patients (pts) with metastatic castrate-resistant prostate cancer (mCRPC) following enzalutamide (ENZ) and/or abiraterone (ABI). *J. Clin. Oncol.* 38 (15): 3500.

39 Minko, T. (2020). Nanoformulation of BRD4-degrading PROTAC: improving druggability to target the 'Undruggable' MYC in pancreatic cancer. *Trends Pharmacol. Sci.* 41 (10): 684–686.

40 Smith, D., Di, L., and Kerns, E. (2010). The effect of plasma protein binding on in vivo efficacy: misconceptions in drug discovery. *Nat. Rev. Drug Discovery* 9 (12): 929–939.

41 Lu, C. and Di, L. (2020). *in vitro* and *in vivo* methods to assess pharmacokinetic drug–drug interactions in drug discovery and development. *Biopharm. Drug Dispos.* 41 (1–2): 3–31.

42 Zakharov, A. et al. (2016). QSAR modeling and prediction of drug–drug interactions. *Mol. Pharmaceutics* 13 (2): 545–556.

43 Luo, G. et al. (2021). Discovery of an orally active VHL-recruiting PROTAC that achieves robust HMGCR degradation and potent hypolipidemic activity. *Acta Pharm. Sin. B* 11 (5): 1300–1314.

44 Disch, J. et al. (2021). Bispecific estrogen receptor a degraders incorporating novel binders identified using DNA-encoded chemical library screening. *J. Med. Chem.* 64 (8): 5049–5066.

45 EMA (2012). *Guideline on the Investigation of Drug Interactions.* Committee for Human Medicinal Products (CHMP).

46 FDA (2020). *Clinical Drug Interaction Studies – Cytochrome P450 Enzyme- and Transporter-Mediated Drug Interactions.* Guidance for Industry.

47 Smith, D.A., Beaumont, K., Maurer, T.S., and Di, L. (2019). Clearance in drug design. *J. Med. Chem.* 62 (5): 2245–2255.

48 Gleeson, M.P. (2008). Generation of a set of simple, interpretable ADMET rules of thumb. *J. Med. Chem.* 51 (4): 817–834.

49 Lombardo, F. et al. (2017). *In silico* absorption, distribution, metabolism, excretion, and pharmacokinetics (ADME-PK): utility and best practices. An industry perspective from the international consortium for innovation through quality in pharmaceutical development. *J. Med. Chem.* 60 (22): 9097–9113.

50 Edmondson, S.D., Yang, B., and Fallan, C. (2019). Proteolysis targeting chimeras (PROTACs) in 'beyond rule-of-five' chemical space: recent progress and future challenges. *Bioorg. Med. Chem. Lett.* 29 (13): 1555–1564.

51 Goracci, L. et al. (2020). Understanding the metabolism of proteolysis targeting chimeras (PROTACs): the next step toward pharmaceutical applications. *J. Med. Chem.* 63 (20): 11615–11638.

52 Gomez-Orellana, I. (2005). Strategies to improve oral drug bioavailability. *Expert Opin. Drug Deliv.* 2 (3): 419–433.

53 van De Waterbeemd, H., Smith, D.A., Beaumont, K., and Walker, D.K. (2001). Property-based design: optimization of drug absorption and pharmacokinetics. *J. Med. Chem.* 44 (9): 1313–1333.

54 Xie, F., Ding, X., and Zhang, Q. (2016). An update on the role of intestinal cytochrome P450 enzymes in drug disposition. *Acta Pharm. Sin. B* 6 (5): 374–383.

55 Hammer, H. et al. (2021). Cross-species analysis of hepatic cytochrome P450 and transport protein expression. *Arch. Toxicol.* 95 (1): 117–133.

56 Giacomini, K. et al. (2010). Membrane transporters in drug development. *Nat. Rev. Drug Discovery* 9 (3): 215–236.

57 Lipinski, C.A. (2000). Drug-like properties and the causes of poor solubility and poor permeability. *J. Pharmacol. Toxicol. Methods* 44 (1): 235–249.

58 Thomas, V.H. et al. (2006). The road map to oral bioavailability: an industrial perspective. *Expert Opin. Drug Metab. Toxicol.* 2 (4): 591–608.

59 Aungst, B.J. (2017). Optimizing oral bioavailability in drug discovery: an overview of design and testing strategies and formulation options. *J. Pharm. Sci.* 106 (4): 921–929.

60 Crews, C., Georg, G., and Wang, S. (2016). Inducing protein degradation as a therapeutic strategy. *J. Med. Chem.* 59 (11): 5129–5130.

61 Fisher, S.L. and Phillips, A.J. (2018). Targeted protein degradation and the enzymology of degraders. *Curr. Opin. Chem. Biol.* 44: 47–55.

62 Watt, G.F., Scott-Stevens, P., and Gaohua, L. (2019). Targeted protein degradation *in vivo* with proteolysis targeting chimeras: current status and future considerations. *Drug Discov. Today Technol.* 31: 69–80.

63 Weng, G. et al. (2021). PROTAC-DB: an online database of PROTACs. *Nucleic Acids Res.* 49 (D1): D1381–D1387.

64 Halford, B. (2021) Arvinas unveils PROTAC structures, https://cen.acs.org/pharmaceuticals/drug-discovery/Arvinas-unveils-PROTAC-structures/99/i14.

65 Snyder, L. (2021). The discovery of ARV-471, an orally bioavailable estrogen receptor degrading PROTAC®for the treatment of patients with breast cancer. *AACR.*

66 Snyder, L. (2021). Discovery of ARV-110, a first in class androgen receptor degrading PROTAC® for the treatment of men with metastatic castration resistant prostate cancer, AACR Annual Meeting 2021.

67 Snyder, L. (2021). Abstract 43: Discovery of ARV-110, a first in class androgen receptor degrading PROTAC for the treatment of men with metastatic castration resistant prostate cancer. *AACR.*

68 Snyder, L. (2021). Abstract 44: The discovery of ARV-471, an orally bioavailable estrogen receptor degrading PROTAC for the treatment of patients with breast cancer. *AACR.*

69 Mullard, A. (2019). First targeted protein degrader hits the clinic. *Nat. Rev. Drug Discovery* 18: 237–239.

70 Salahudeen, M.S. and Nishtala, P.S. (2017). An overview of pharmacodynamic modelling, ligand-binding approach and its application in clinical practice. *Saudi Pharm. J.* 25 (2): 165–175.

71 Bondeson, D. et al. (2015). Catalytic *in vivo* protein knockdown by small-molecule PROTACs. *Nat. Chem. Biol.* 11 (8): 611–U120.

72 Morgan, P. et al. (2012). Can the flow of medicines be improved? Fundamental pharmacokinetic and pharmacological principles toward improving phase II survival. *Drug Discovery Today* 17 (9-10): 419–424.

73 Lavé, T. et al. (2016). Translational PK/PD modeling to increase probability of success in drug discovery and early development. *Drug Discov. Today Technol.* 21–22: 27–34.

74 Churcher, I. (2018). Protac-induced protein degradation in drug discovery: breaking the rules or just making new ones? *J. Med. Chem.* 61 (2): 444–452.

75 Schropp, J. et al. (2019). Target-mediated drug disposition model for bispecific antibodies: properties, approximation, and optimal dosing strategy. *CPT: Pharm. Syst. Pharmacol.* 8 (3): 177–187.

76 Pettersson, M. and Crews, C.M. (2019). PROteolysis TArgeting Chimeras (PROTACs) – past, present and future. *Drug Discov. Today Technol.* 31: 15–27.

77 Nowak, R.P. and Jones, L.H. (2021). Target validation using PROTACs: applying the four pillars framework. *SLAS Discov* 26 (4): 474–483.

78 Bartlett, D.W. and Gilbert, A.M. (2020). A kinetic proofreading model for bispecific protein degraders. *J. Pharm. Pharmacodyn.* 48 (1): 149–163.

79 McKeithan, T.W. (1995). Kinetic proofreading in T-cell receptor signal transduction. *Proc. Natl. Acad. Sci. U.S.A.* 92 (11): 5042.

80 Hopfield, J.J., Yamane, T., Yue, V., and Coutts, S.M. (1976). Direct experimental evidence for kinetic proofreading in amino acylation of tRNAIle. *Proc. Natl. Acad. Sci. U.S.A.* 73 (4): 1164–1168.

81 Bondeson, D.P. et al. (2018). Lessons in PROTAC design from selective degradation with a promiscuous warhead. *Cell Chem. Biol.* 25 (1): 78–87.e5.
82 Roy, M.J. et al. (2019). SPR-measured dissociation kinetics of PROTAC ternary complexes influence target degradation rate. *ACS Chem. Biol.* 14 (3): 361–368.
83 Zorba, A. et al. (2018). Delineating the role of cooperativity in the design of potent PROTACs for BTK. *Proc. Natl. Acad. Sci. U.S.A.* 115 (31): E7285.
84 Higgins, B. et al. (2014). Preclinical optimization of MDM2 antagonist scheduling for cancer treatment by using a model-based approach. *Clin. Cancer Res.* 20 (14): 3742–3752.
85 Smith, B.E. et al. (2019). Differential PROTAC substrate specificity dictated by orientation of recruited E3 ligase. *Nat. Commun.* 10 (1): 131.
86 Bouhaddou, M. et al. (2020). Predicting in vivo efficacy from in vitro data: quantitative systems pharmacology modeling for an epigenetic modifier drug in cancer. *Clin. Transl. Sci.* 13 (2): 419–429.
87 Ross, A.B., Langer, J.D., and Jovanovic, M. (2020). Proteome turnover in the spotlight: approaches, applications, and perspectives. *Mol. Cell. Proteomics* 20: 100016.
88 Eigenmann, M.J. et al. (2016). Combining nonclinical experiments with translational PKPD modeling to differentiate erlotinib and gefitinib. *Mol. Cancer Ther.* 15 (12): 3110–3119.
89 Jones, H.M. et al. (2015). Physiologically based pharmacokinetic modeling in drug discovery and development: a pharmaceutical industry perspective. *Clin. Pharmacol. Ther.* 97 (3): 247–262.
90 Harling, J.D., Scott-Stevens, P., and Gaohua, L. (2020). Developing pharmacokinetic/pharmacodynamic relationships with PROTACs. In: *Protein Degradation with New Chemical Modalities: Successful Strategies in Drug Discovery and Chemical Biology*, Chapter 4 (ed. H. Weinmann and C. Crews), 75–93. The Royal Society of Chemistry.
91 Shou, W.Z. (2020). Current status and future directions of high-throughput ADME screening in drug discovery. *J. Pharm Anal.* 10 (3): 201–208.

13

PROTAC® Protein Degraders: Bridging the Divide from Chemical Biology Tools to Clinical Candidates

Erika M.V. Araujo and Keith R. Hornberger

Arvinas, Inc., Department of Chemistry, 5 Science Park, 395 Winchester Ave, New Haven, CT, 06511, USA

13.1 Introduction

The past two decades since the seminal report on proteolysis targeting chimeras (PROTAC® molecules) [1] have seen an explosion of research aimed at transforming the technology from proof-of-concept to a novel clinical therapeutic modality. The advancement of several heterobifunctional degraders to the clinic highlights the rapid pace of discoveries in the field. As advances in targeted protein degradation have been extensively reviewed elsewhere [2, 3], we have herein chosen to focus our attention on the pragmatic drug discovery components required for efficient translation of tool molecules to drug candidates.

PROTAC molecules are designed to induce proteasomal degradation of a protein of interest (POI) by co-opting the ubiquitin proteasome system. The heterobifunctional molecules, composed of ligands that simultaneously target an E3 ubiquitin ligase and a POI connected by a linker, serve as a catalyst to bring the two proteins together (Figure 13.1). Once complexed, the E3 ligase ubiquitinates the POI, causing a cascade that leads to the degradation of the POI via the proteasome. The ability to modify the intracellular levels of disease-causing proteins with a PROTAC can potentially couple the advantages of gene-based medicines with the ease of administration and manufacturing typified by small-molecule inhibitors. Furthermore, the catalytic nature of the ubiquitination event suggests that substoichiometric concentrations can be sufficient to profoundly affect the pharmacodynamics. Herein, we will review some of the unique challenges associated with the optimization and development of heterobifunctional degraders, in particular those designed for oral delivery, that arise from their mechanism of action and physicochemical properties.

Inducing Targeted Protein Degradation: From Chemical Biology to Drug Discovery and Clinical Applications, First Edition. Edited by Philipp Cromm.

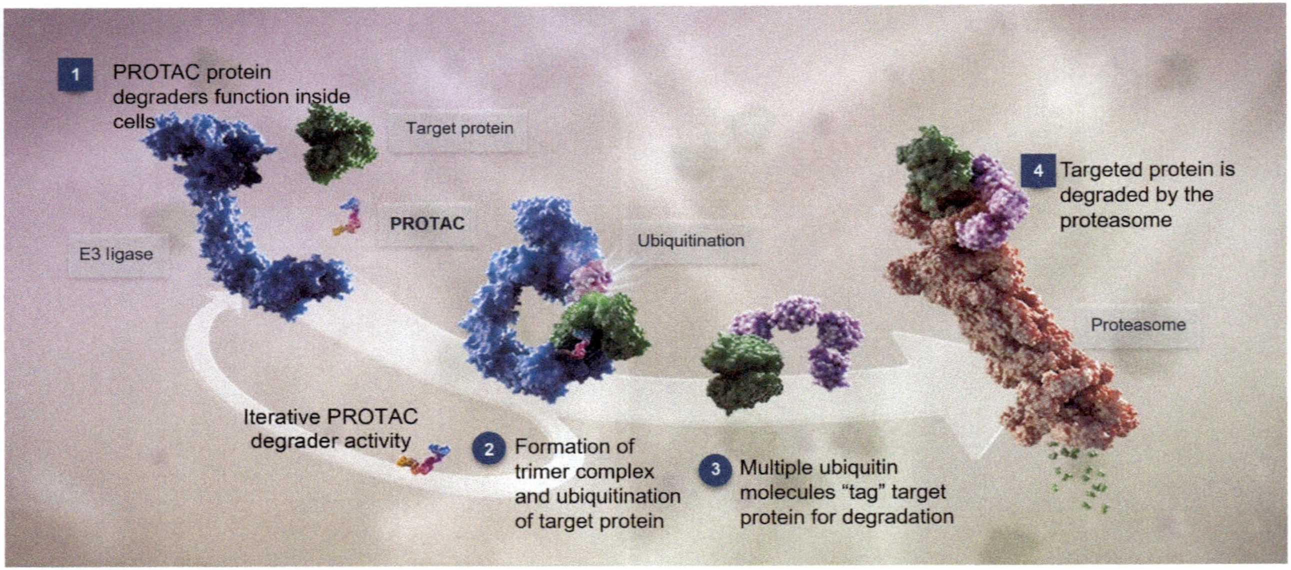

Figure 13.1 Mechanism by which PROTACs induce protein degradation via the proteasome. *Source:* Arvinas, Inc. [38] / with permission of Arvinas, Inc.

13.2 Physicochemical Properties

The "Rule-of-5" (bRo5) mnemonic has been influential in the design of oral drugs since 1997 as it provided simple guidelines to avoid poorly absorbed or permeable compounds: molecular weight (MW)≤500 Da, cLogP ≤5, hydrogen bond donors (HBD)≤5, and hydrogen bond acceptors (HBA)≤10 [4]. As roughly 90% of the orally administered drugs at the time obeyed these cutoffs, it was understood that oral absorption was far more likely in the chemical space defined by these calculated parameters. PROTACs occupy a physiochemical property space classified as beyond Ro5 [5] because of the nature of their tripartite structural architecture. Namely, the larger size (molecular weight typically >650 Da) and higher degree of flexibility (number of rotatable bonds >10) of heterobifunctional degraders negatively impact the features associated with good oral absorption: permeability and solubility. Based on the retrospective analyses of the physicochemical properties of drugs and clinical candidates, Kihlberg and coworkers described instead the upper limits of molecular weight (≤1000 Da), cLogP (≥−2 or≤10), PSA (≤250 Å^2), and numbers of H-bond donors (≤6), acceptors (≤15), and rotatable bonds (≤20), where attaining oral availability is still possible [5–7]. A similar *in silico* analysis of the preclinical drug metabolism and pharmacokinetics (DMPK) database at AbbVie was performed to derive the physicochemical properties most highly correlated with oral bioavailability, leading to the development of the AbbVie multiparametric score: AB-MPS = Abs(cLogD-3) + NAR + NRB (NAR = number of aromatic rings and NRB = number of rotatable bonds) [8]. A greater likelihood for oral absorption is observed from molecules scoring 14 or below.

Figure 13.2 shows that the average calculated chemical descriptors for PROTACs in the literature are overlayed on a map colored by the constraints required for bioavailability as defined by the aforementioned studies on bRo5 compounds [9]. The PROTACs were further characterized by the targeted E3 ligase limited to the handful with known ligands, mouse double minute-2 (MDM2), inhibitor-of-apoptosis (IAP), Von Hippel–Lindau (VHL), or cereblon (CRBN), with the latter two representing the most widely employed. The analysis from Edmondson et al. argues that the recruiting ligands for MDM2 and IAP are too lipophilic and large on their own to have any prospect of eliciting oral absorption once incorporated into a PROTAC (Table 13.1). It is further concluded that CRBN-based degraders have physicochemical properties most closely aligned with the chemical space known to produce orally absorbed drugs. The designer of degraders should therefore seek to minimize the size and polarity during the selection of POI and E3 ligase binders, especially if an oral agent is desired.

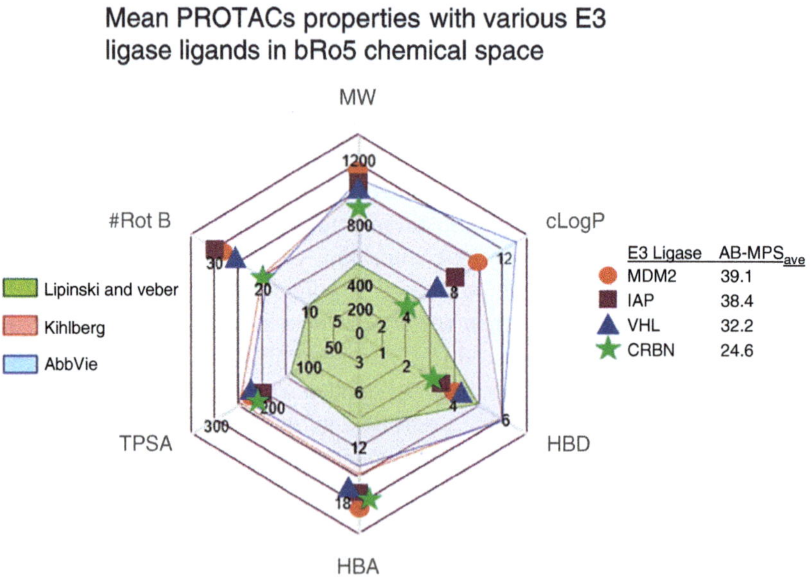

Figure 13.2 The mean physical chemical property descriptors for published PROTACs with various E3 warheads compared with the upper boundary limits for oral bioavailability suggested by Kihlberg and AbbVie. *Source:* Reproduced from Edmondson et al. [9], with permission from Elsevier.

Table 13.1 Representative E3 ligases and their ligands.

	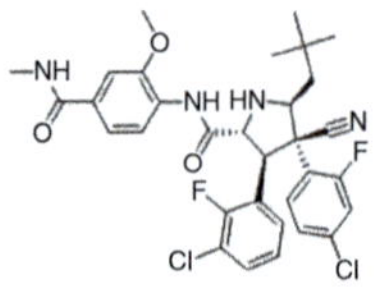	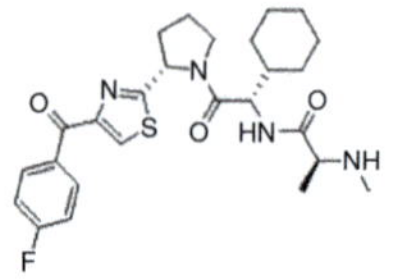	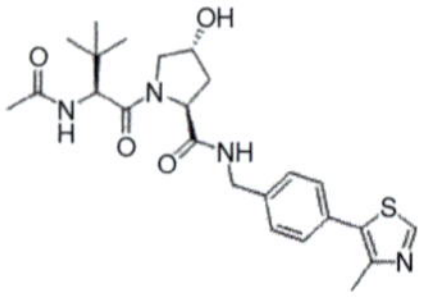	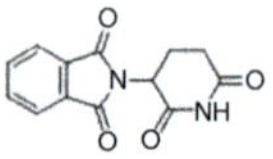
Parameter	**Idasanutlin amide**	**LCL-161**	**HIF1α binder**	**Thalidomide**
	MDM2 ligand	**IAP ligand**	**VHL ligand**	**CRBN ligand**
MW	630	500	472	258
HBD	3	2	3	1
HBA	7	7	8	6
nRotB (number of rotatable bonds)	11	10	10	1
PSA	108	95	118	89
cLogP	6.2	3.6	2.0	0.53
Ar rings	3	2	2	1

Source: Edmonson et al. [9], with permission from Elsevier.

13.3 Pharmacokinetics

Recently, an analysis of the data from pharmacokinetic (PK) studies of orally dosed mice with CRBN- and VHL-recruiting degraders at AstraZeneca has confirmed the prediction that heterobifunctional degraders derived from thalidomide belong to the chemical space with a higher probability for oral absorption. From the molecules studied over a range of five projects (Figure 13.3), only those designed to bind CRBN resulted in robust (≥30 %F) oral absorption [10]. All the tested PROTACs targeting VHL failed to exceed 5 %F in mice in line with the comparably higher molecular weight and numbers of H-bond donors and acceptors limiting permeability. Pike and coworkers further detail that molecules with higher lipophilicity (likely derived from the nature of the POI-targeting moieties) with cLogP and ChromLogD values ranging from 5 to 7 provided the greatest bioavailability. The authors conclude that despite residing in beyond the Ro5 space, PROTACs had better ADME and PK properties than were anticipated based on their physicochemical attributes.

Understanding the factors that govern the ability of PROTACs to traverse cell membranes can assist chemists in the design of compounds with greater opportunity for oral absorption. To this end, NMR spectroscopy has been used to interrogate the conformational flexibility and preferences for an ERK5–VHL PROTAC in polar and apolar solvents [11]. In chloroform, selected to mimic the membrane lipid bilayer, the PROTAC reduced its polar surface area through folding by way of intramolecular H-bonds. On the other hand, conformations found in polar solutions, to simulate the intra- and extracellular environments, were elongated to maximize the solvent-exposed polar surface area. The degree to which PROTACs behave as molecular chameleons [12] in biological systems remains to be evaluated but may provide an insight as to why traditional descriptors associated with permeability may not be suitable for the prediction of PROTAC behavior.

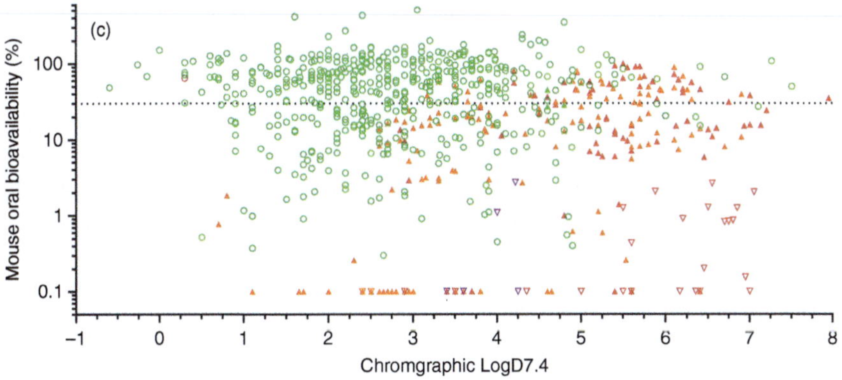

Figure 13.3 Mouse oral bioavailability as a function of ChromlogD for small molecules and PROTACs; shaped by small molecules (open circle ○), cereblon PROTACs (solid triangle ▲), and VHL PROTACs (inverted open triangle ▽); colored by number of Rule-of-5 violations: 0 = dark green, 1 = light green, 2 = orange, 3 = red, and 4 = purple. The dotted line shows a target of 30% for robust oral bioavailability. *Source:* Reproduced from Pike et al. [10], with permission from Elsevier.

Although the calculation of chemical properties of designed PROTACs can point to the space where success is possible, many of the advances in determining which PROTACs are orally absorbed have been derived empirically owing primarily to a lack of a meaningful *in vitro-in vivo* correlation (IVIVC). The next challenge faced in advancing degraders involves the ability to assess the ADME properties *in vitro* to accurately predict for compounds with suitable pharmacokinetic profiles *in vivo*.

13.4 *in vitro* ADME Assays

It has been well documented that the high lipophilicity and poor aqueous solubility of PROTACs impart a significant hurdle to employing the suite of ADME assays developed for screening cascades of small molecules as the interpretation can often be muddled from a high degree of nonspecific binding [10, 13–15]. Routine assays to assess passive permeability such as the cell-free parallel artificial membrane permeability assay (PAMPA) or those using monolayer systems such as Caco-2 have been noted to be uninformative and inconsistent with *in vivo* data [10, 12]. Evaluation of cell penetration using the HaloTag system and chloroalkane-tagged PROTACs and warheads demonstrated that PROTACs can have drastically lower passive permeability than the components from which they are derived [14]. Moreover, the rank order of permeability determined using the chloroalkane penetration assay (CAPA) could not be reproduced using a bidirectional Caco-2 assay.

Determination of plasma protein binding (PPB), a key parameter to interpreting PK/PD relationships in preclinical models of efficacy, has also been reported to have various challenges because of the nature of PROTAC molecules. Researchers from AstraZeneca [10] and Roche [13] have suggested methods to reduce the effects of nonspecific binding and the need to modify assay protocols to ensure data quality. Poor compound recovery from rapid equilibrium dialysis could be attenuated using a presaturation protocol with an 18-h incubation [10]. Use of prolonged incubation times, however, should consider the varied plasma stability of PROTAC molecules. Ultracentrifugation is an alternative suggested approach [13] but may need to be tailored to the issues common with PROTACs, namely, plasma stability and nonspecific binding to plastics. Both groups reported that PROTACs are typically highly protein bound with $f_u < 0.01$, in line with the high lipophilicity, and thus recommend that analytical methods have high sensitivity to ensure accuracy [13].

13.5 Pharmacodynamics

An important aspect in the clinical translation of heterobifunctional degraders is a detailed understanding of their pharmacokinetic–pharmacodynamic-efficacy (PK–PD-efficacy) relationships. Clear knowledge of the drug PK exposure required for PD and efficacy, whether driven by C_{max}, area under the curve (AUC), time over a minimum threshold concentration, or other scenario, is crucial to estimation of an eventual human dose [16, 17]. Although such understanding is not strictly required for basic research studies, it is indispensable in pharmaceutical discovery.

Although there are currently many published examples of *in vivo* proof-of-principle PD experiments for PROTAC molecules, the great majority of these studies measures degradation in a tumor or other tissues at a single compound dose at a single time point. This information is rarely presented together with the PK and PPB data needed to put the observed degradation into context in the framework of the free drug hypothesis [18, 19], nor do these preliminary evaluations typically generate longitudinal data assessing degradation at many time points at several different doses. A greater level of rigor is needed in translational research.

PROTAC molecules are expected, based on their event-driven pharmacology [20], to demonstrate nonlinear PK–PD relationships. This nonlinearity arises for several reasons, all of which are tied to kinetic rather than thermodynamic events. First, in contrast to traditional occupancy-based inhibitors, there is expected to be little correlation between the free drug concentration of a degrader and the pharmacodynamic effect it exerts at a given time point. Low (or zero) target depletion may be observed at a time when drug concentration is high because insufficient time has elapsed for a critical mass of degradation events to occur. Conversely, high target depletion may be observed at a time when drug concentration is low (or zero) because the depletion was driven by higher drug concentrations at an earlier time. Second, once a degradation event occurs and the degrader is cleared from systemic circulation, there can be a profoundly extended duration of action as protein levels recover based on the intrinsic resynthesis rate of the protein (*vide infra*). In essence, there is a push–pull between the kinetics of degradation and the kinetics of protein resynthesis. If the former is faster than the latter at a given point of time, protein concentration, and drug concentration, then protein levels will decline.

A key limitation in developing practical, usable models of degradation pharmacodynamics is a requirement to understand the concentration of the ternary complex among PROTAC, target protein, and E3 ligase. Ternary complexes have been well remarked to exhibit what at first appear to be counterintuitive properties [21]. First, ternary complex concentration follows a bell-shaped dose response. This behavior is a direct consequence of high ligand concentrations outcompeting the ternary complex, giving rise to saturated binary complexes instead. A reduction in ternary complex concentration may be manifested in a degradation assay as a "hook effect" where the extent of protein degradation increases as expected with concentration and then begins to decrease above a certain concentration. Second, because ternary complexes may induce protein–protein interactions between the target protein and the E3 ligase, this interaction may introduce either favorable or unfavorable interactions that add or subtract from the total binding energy of the complex – positive or negative cooperativity (usually represented as α), respectively. It is common for there to be a little direct relationship between a binary K_d for the binding of a PROTAC to either protein of interest or E3 ligase and the K_d for the ternary complex. This behavior also has profound consequences for degradation selectivity versus other proteins. Indeed, in many cases, the selectivity of a PROTAC as a degrader far exceeds the selectivity of the warhead for the protein of interest as an inhibitor (*vide infra*). Thus, any mathematical modeling treatment of degraders must also in some way account for cooperativity.

In a key advance, the Spiegel lab reported in a seminal 2013 publication on a set of equations that govern ternary complex equilibria under a set of different limiting assumptions [22]. This model divides ternary complex behavior into four quadrants depending on where the concentrations of the two proteins in the ternary complex sit relative to the binary equilibrium binding constants with the PROTAC. This work also established that there is no exact analytical solution for ternary complex concentration "as a function of measurable parameters" once cooperativity has been factored in.

In 2020, Han described an analytical solution for ternary complex concentration with the free ligand concentration rather than the more customary total ligand concentration [23]. Although free ligand concentration is not a readily measured parameter, it can be estimated numerically. The underlying assumptions, and novelty, of this analysis have recently been challenged [24].

Moving beyond the understanding of ternary complex formation to a more comprehensive model has been the focus of a recent investigation by scientists at Pfizer [25]. They have reported on modeling the time course of degradation pharmacodynamics using a kinetic proofreading model. The model shown in Figure 13.4 treats the successive transfer of ubiquitin as the proofreading event as multiple ubiquitin units must be transferred to result in successful protein degradation [26]. This biological requirement imposes a thermodynamic demand that a ternary complex among PROTAC, target protein, and E3 ligase be sufficiently long-lived for these transfer events to occur. Cooperativity is explicitly included via adjustment of the rates for the formation of ternary complex. As initial tests, the model was used to predict, for a fixed set of inputs, degradation as a function of PROTAC concentration (including recapitulation of a hook effect) and degradation as a function of time for several PROTAC concentrations.

Ultimately, using the kinetic proofreading model in conjunction with an input pharmacokinetic profile to reflect the change in PROTAC concentration as a function of time can simulate the expected pharmacodynamic response as a function of dose, time, and other variations of the input parameters (Figure 13.5). The model can recapitulate several known, occasionally counterintuitive, properties of heterobifunctional degraders, including profound degradation despite low target occupancy, the lack of correlation between degradation selectivity and various binary binding affinities, and prolonged duration of degradation dependent on the intrinsic half-life of a protein. On the point of selectivity, the authors note that selectivity in degradation can be driven not only by binary binding affinities but also by ternary binding affinities (further influenced by cooperativity) and differences in the intrinsic rates of ubiquitin transfer and proteasomal degradation.

Although there are few detailed experimental reports of PK–PD time course studies for heterobifunctional degraders, a team at GlaxoSmithKline in conjunction with the Crews lab has reported such data extensively for a series of RIPK2 degraders [27–28]. Taking advantage of the long half-life (~50 hours) of RIPK2, a single subcutaneous (SC) dose of a tool IAP-based RIPK2 PROTAC led to profound

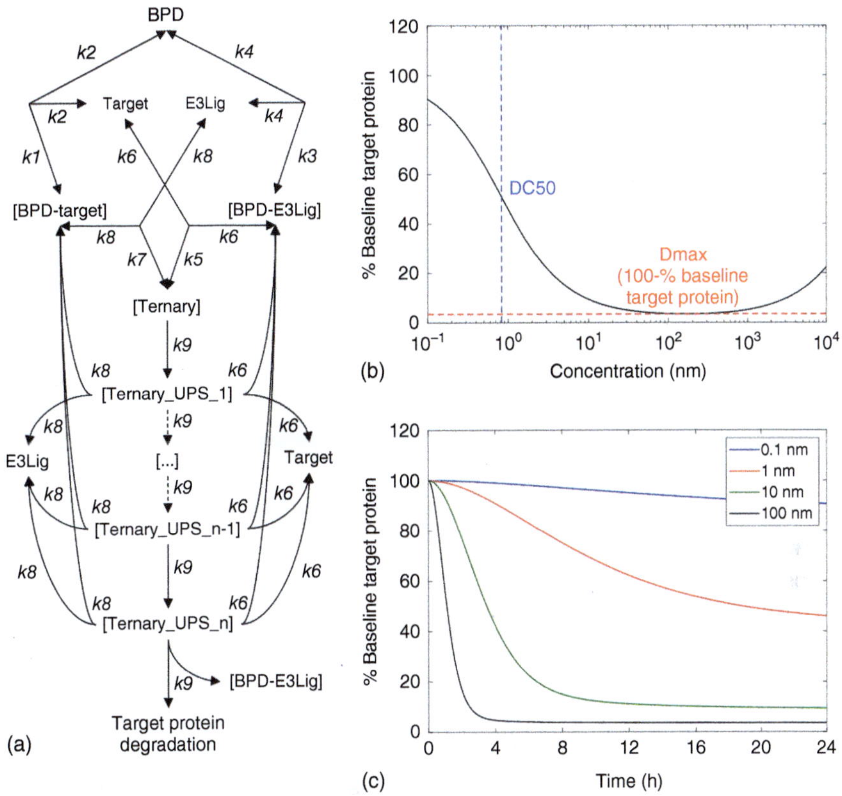

Figure 13.4 A kinetic proofreading model for bifunctional degraders demonstrating (a) the kinetic and thermodynamic events captured in the model, (b) an example of degradation as a function of concentration at 24 hours, and (c) degradation as a function of time at several concentrations. *Source:* Reproduced from Bartlett and Gilbert [25], with permission from Springer Nature.

degradation of RIPK2 in rat whole blood. The degradation of RIPK2 and suppression of the associated cytokine TNFα was sustained for >168 hours despite that the PROTAC blood concentration is below the rat whole blood IC_{90} after 72 hours. With further optimization and the development of a slow-release SC formulation, the duration of action of IAP-based RIPK2 PROTACs was extended to >1 month following a single drug administration [29] (Figure 13.6).

This series of studies with RIPK2 highlight a crucial aspect for translational research with PROTACs: traditional notions of PK–PD-efficacy relationships derived with assumptions from occupancy-based inhibitors may not be valid, or at least require experimental validation, for degraders with event-based pharmacology. Such translational studies would ideally assess the duration of PD response from single and multiple administrations of PROTAC with different doses and schedules. Furthermore, additional studies are required beyond pharmacodynamics to establish a link to efficacy. For inhibitors, there is often a clear 1 : 1 relationship between the degree of target occupancy and the degree of efficacy in a disease model. For degraders, because the protein (and thus any associated scaffolding/noncatalytic

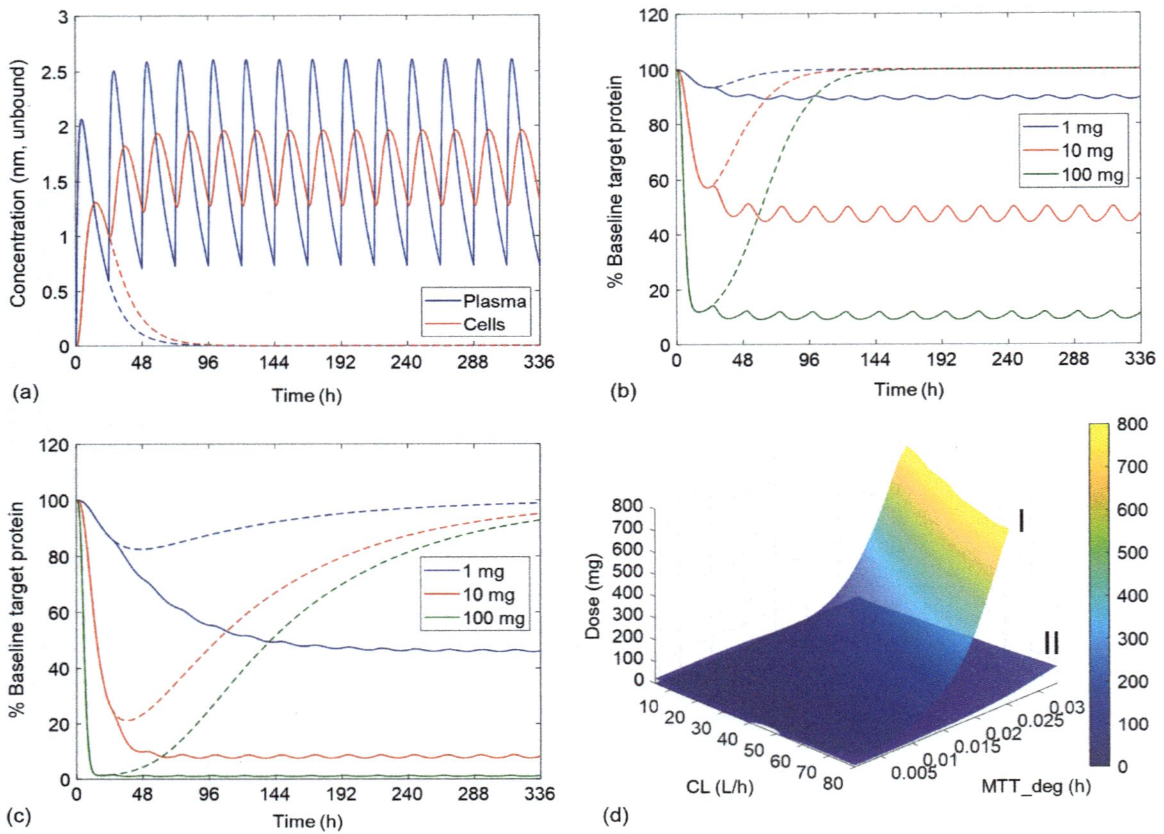

Figure 13.5 Using an (a) input pharmacokinetic profile, the kinetic proofreading model can simulate the extent of protein degradation achieved from single- or multi-day administration for proteins with (b) short or (c) long half-lives. The model can also be used (d) for estimation of the dose required to achieve a predetermined level of degradation as a function of other input parameters. *Source:* Reproduced from Bartlett and Gilbert [25], with permission from Springer Nature.

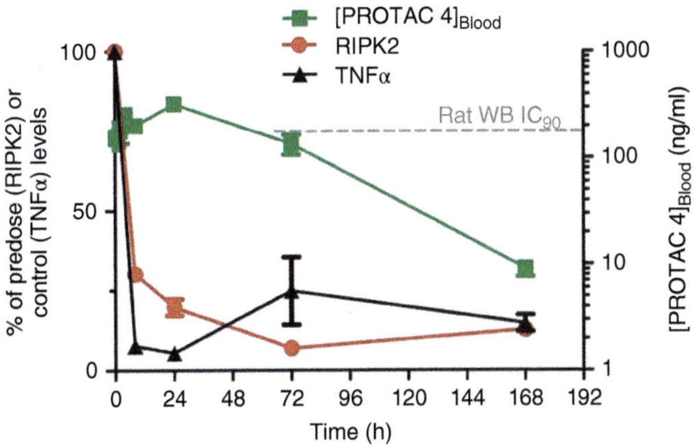

Figure 13.6 Extended duration of action for a VHL-based RIPK2 PROTAC. *Source:* Mares et al. [28] / Springer Nature/ CC BY 4.0.

function) is eliminated, efficacy requires closer interrogation. The extent of protein degradation needed to normalize a disease state may not be the same as the extent of protein inhibitor occupancy for the same disease state. Indeed, there may be cases where degradation of a protein for a few days out of a week may be functionally equivalent to (or even better than) "round the clock" occupancy-based inhibition. These duration of action and efficacy studies are also essential because they may open the door to intermittent clinical administration by a parenteral route (IV, SC, etc.) and challenge the assumption that daily PO administration is the only option.

13.6 Toxicology

In order for the degradation of a targeted protein to occur, a ternary complex must be formed between POI:PROTAC:E3, and the induced proximity allows for the E3 to ubiquitinate a non-native substrate. Stable ternary complex formation and the attendant cooperativity are thought to confer degradation selectivity and suggest that PROTACs may reduce toxicological liabilities. This concept was demonstrated with the transformation of promiscuous kinase inhibitors into PROTACs by the Crews [30] and Gray [31] laboratories. One of the conclusions from these studies was that engagement of PROTACs with various intracellular targets did not guarantee degradation. It is postulated that a steric clash at the protein–protein interface induced by the PROTAC prevents degradation, implying the stability of the ternary complex with a given protein to be more correlative with its degradation than binding affinity. The corollary, however, is that a PROTAC can lead to depletion of a protein even with very weak affinity interactions. Foretinib-based VHL PROTAC **1** degrades p38α with a DC_{50} of 210 nM despite only having a K_d for p38α of 11 μM [30]. Unexpected changes in cellular protein levels such as this one can be identified by profiling the global proteome using mass spectrometry-based proteomics. In fact, proteomics has quickly become a crucial component in the screening funnel to assess degradation selectivity and off-target liabilities [32, 33].

There may also be specific toxicological concerns regarding the engagement of CRBN as the E3 element by PROTACs. The discovery that CRBN was the target for thalidomide was made in 2010 by Handa and coworkers, half a century after the discovery of its teratogenic activity led to its discontinuation [34]. CRBN is the substrate recognition component of a Cul4 E3 ligase and thalidomide, or its analogs pomalidomide and lenalidomide bind a shallow pocket composed of three tryptophan residues on its surface [35]. This interaction functions as a molecular glue imparting neomorphic binding of a whole set of non-native substrates that are ubiquitinated upon complexation and undergo proteasomal degradation. Remarkably, the crystal structure of the ternary complex of CRBN:lenalidomide:CK1α, one of the many neosubstrates, revealed that only 96.8 $Å^2$ of the compound:CRBN surface interface was sufficient to induce novel protein–protein complexes [36]. The molecular mechanism has been fully elucidated, but the list of potentially affected proteins (for example, Ikaros, Aiolos, CK1α, SALL4, and GSPT1) continues to grow and has been shown to be highly dependent on the structure of the thalidomide analog. This elucidation of both mechanism and pharmacology was enabled by employing a suite of proteomics-based experiments [33].

The implications of the discoveries around thalidomide and its mechanism of action on the PROTAC field have been transformational. As discussed in Section 13.2, only a handful of chemical binders to E3 ligases are known and as such thalidomide was opportunistically assimilated into the PROTAC toolbox. The explosion of research on heterobifunctional degraders has demonstrated many benefits of exploiting CRBN as the targeted ligase, including (1) the ability to degrade many classes of proteins, (2) the potential oral bioavailability of the derived PROTACs, and (3) the relatively ubiquitous expression across many cell types and across species. However, there are also several issues that arise specifically when discussing PROTACs incorporating thalidomide (or its analogs): (1) the glutarimide ring present in the E3 binder can be hydrolytically unstable, leading to metabolites or plasma instability, (2) the phthalimide stereocenter can racemize *in vivo*, and (3) the neosubstrate degradation activity can remain even after incorporation into a PROTAC. The latter represents a safety concern as some neomorphic substrates have toxic and teratogenic effects, and thus, programs seeking to deliver a CRBN-recruiting PROTAC should prescribe to global proteomics as a screen for off targets arising from both PROTACs and molecular glue activity.

With the realization that the assays currently available for evaluating secondary pharmacology are designed to evaluate off-target binding of small molecules and do not address alteration of protein levels, researchers at Amgen have proposed the utilization of a mass-spectrometry-based proteomic platform for the evaluation of the safety of PROTACs [37]. As a heterobifunctional degrader can inadvertently affect protein abundance, a comprehensive method to rule out the changes to the "selected off-target proteome," SOTP, was developed to supplement traditional preclinical assessments of toxicology. The platform employs four living human cell lines that endogenously express ~80% of the 2813 proteins identified as important to comprehensively evaluate for human safety. Because of its ability to capture changes in protein levels, whole cell proteomics will undoubtedly continue to serve as an important tool in the development of molecules that induce degradation to address concerns around selectivity.

13.7 Clinical Case Studies

Although the preceding discussion is partially theoretical in nature and primarily focused on preclinical optimization, there are now real-world use cases that begin to shed light on the use of heterobifunctional degraders in the clinic. Table 13.2 illustrates the examples of bifunctional degraders known to be in clinical development. Note that the closely related molecular glues, which are on a continuum of mechanism of action with bifunctional degraders, are not shown here.

The most advanced bifunctional degraders are ARV-110, a CRBN-based androgen receptor (AR) degrader, and ARV-471, a CRBN-based estrogen receptor (ER) degrader from Arvinas. Both agents are now in Phase 2 clinical trials. DT2216 from Dialectic, a VHL-based Bcl-xL degrader, has also recently entered Phase I clinical trials for a variety of liquid and solid tumors. Additional bifunctional degraders of undisclosed structure from Bristol Myers Squibb (targeting AR), Kymera (targeting IRAK4), Nurix (targeting BTK and immunomodulatory imide drugs [IMiD] targets), Foghorn (targeting BRD9), and Accutar (targeting ER) are also reported to be in clinical development.

Arvinas has recently disclosed details regarding the discovery and development of ARV-110 as shown in Figure 13.7 [38]. Several issues were noted for resolution through optimization en route to the eventual candidate compound, including clearance, *in vivo* potency, autoinduction, AR agonism in the AR ligand, and dose escalation exposure.

ARV-110 has also shown preclinical efficacy in an enzalutamide-resistant patient-derived xenograft (PDX) model of disease, which correlated with a significant reduction in prostate-specific antigen (PSA) levels versus enzalutamide treatment (Figure 13.8) [39]. Clinically, it has been reported from dose escalation studies in humans that at a 420 mg dose level, drug exposure has exceeded the exposure threshold associated with efficacy in this enzalutamide-resistant model.

Arvinas has also disclosed details regarding the discovery and development of ARV-471 as shown in Figure 13.9 [39]. Optimization issues highlighted for resolution for this chemical series include cereblon neosubstrate degradation and a suboptimal metabolic clearance profile.

ARV-471 has shown single-agent preclinical efficacy in a patient-derived xenograft model bearing a Y537S mutation and also in the ER+ MCF-7 tumor xenograft model in combination with the CDK4/6 inhibitor palbociclib (Figure 13.10) [39]. Superiority to the estrogen receptor degrader fulvestrant was also established in this model. Clinically, it has been reported from dose escalation studies in humans that at a 60 mg dose level, drug exposure has exceeded the exposure threshold associated with efficacy in the MCF-7 model. Preliminary pharmacodynamic data has also demonstrated potential tumor ER reductions of >90% [40].

Table 13.2 List of bifunctional degraders known to be in clinical development as of October 2021.

Compound (Company)	Structure	Stage of development	Target	Lead indication
ARV-110 (Arvinas)	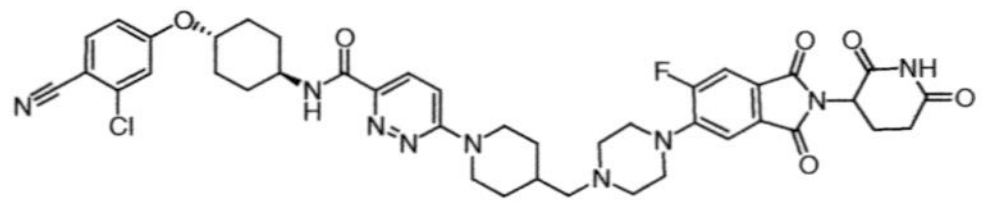	Phase II	AR	Metastatic, castration-resistant prostate cancer
ARV-471 (Arvinas)	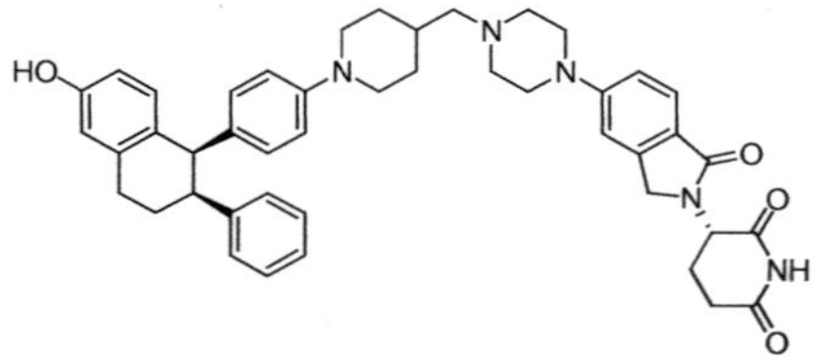	Phase II	ER	ER+/HER2 breast cancer
ARV-766 (Arvinas)	Undisclosed	Phase I	AR	Metastatic, castration-resistant prostate cancer
AR-LDD (Bristol Myers Squibb)	Undisclosed	Phase I	AR	Prostate cancer
DT2216 (Dialectic)	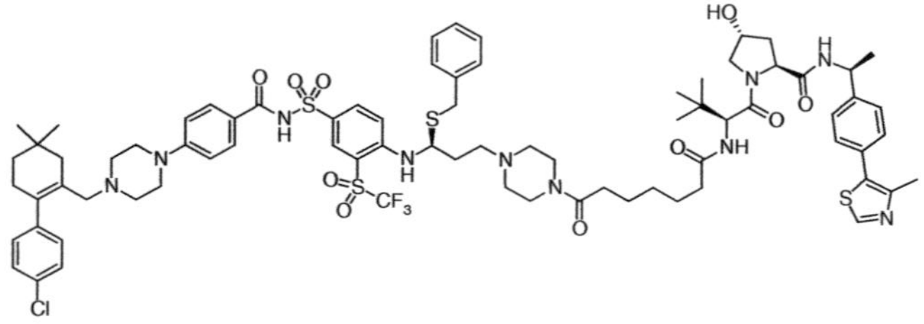	Phase I	Bcl-xL	Liquid and solid tumors
KT-474 (Kymera)	Undisclosed	Phase I	IRAK4	Dermatology, immunology
NX-2127 (Nurix)	Undisclosed	Phase I	BTK + IMiD targets	B-cell malignancies
FHD-609 (Foghorn)	Undisclosed	Phase I	BRD9	Synovial sarcoma
AC0682 (Accutar)	Undisclosed	Phase I	ER	ER+breast cancer

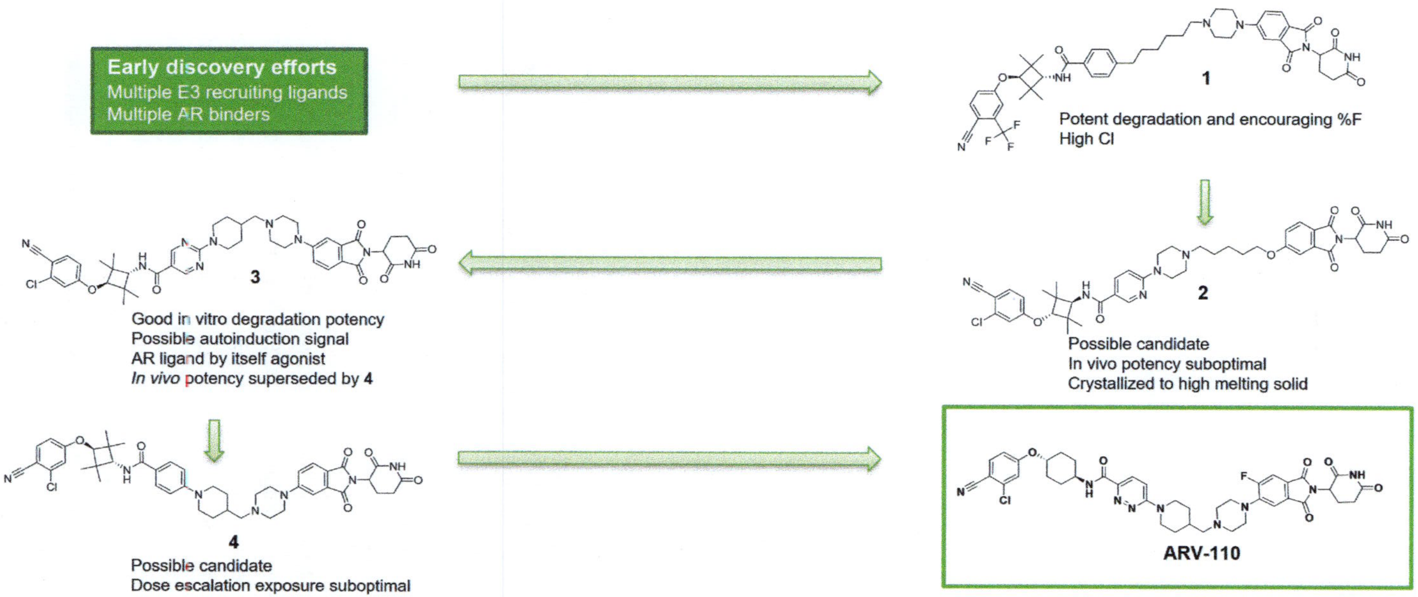

Figure 13.7 Evolution of AR degrading PROTACs leading to ARV-110. *Source:* Arvinas, Inc. [38]/with permission of Arvinas, Inc.

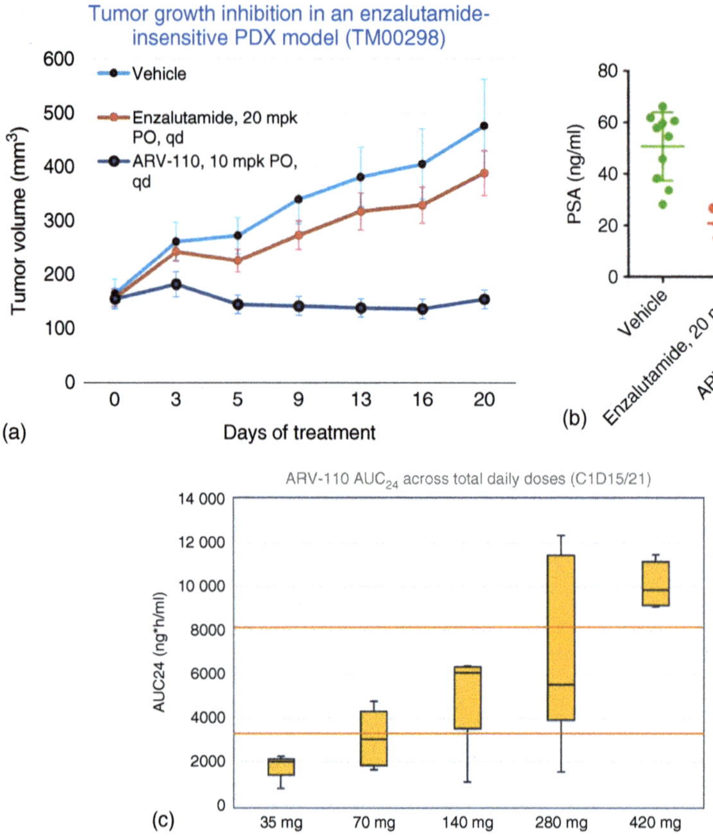

Figure 13.8 (a) Tumor volume versus days of treatment for an enzalutamide-insensitive PDX model following treatment with either enzalutamide (20 mg/kg, po qd) or ARV-110 (10 mg/kg po qd). (b) Reduction in PSA following treatment of tumor-bearing mice in (a). (c) Initial human dose escalation PK data. The 420 mg group includes both qd and bid dosing for a 420 mg total daily dose. The lower horizontal line depicts the minimum preclinical efficacious threshold represented by the AUC associated with tumor growth inhibition in standard VCaP models. The upper horizontal line depicts the AUC associated with tumor growth inhibition in a preclinical enzalutamide-resistant VCaP model. *Source:* Arvinas, Inc. [38]/with permission of Arvinas, Inc.

Kymera Therapeutics has also now reported initial clinical data for the IRAK4 degrader KT-474 in a single ascending dose study in healthy volunteers [41]. In this study, dose-dependent increases in AUC were reported from the 25 mg dose level up to the 1000 mg dose level, after which plateauing was observed at the 1600 mg dose level. KT-474 was reported to have a long human half-life of 25–40 hours. A concomitant dose-dependent pharmacodynamic response 48 hours post-single dose was also reported, reaching >90% degradation in PBMCs at the 600 mg dose level and higher. No serious adverse events were noted in the single ascending dose portion of the trial.

Several common threads emerge from these early clinical stories. First, despite preclinical concerns regarding the pharmacokinetic properties of PROTACs

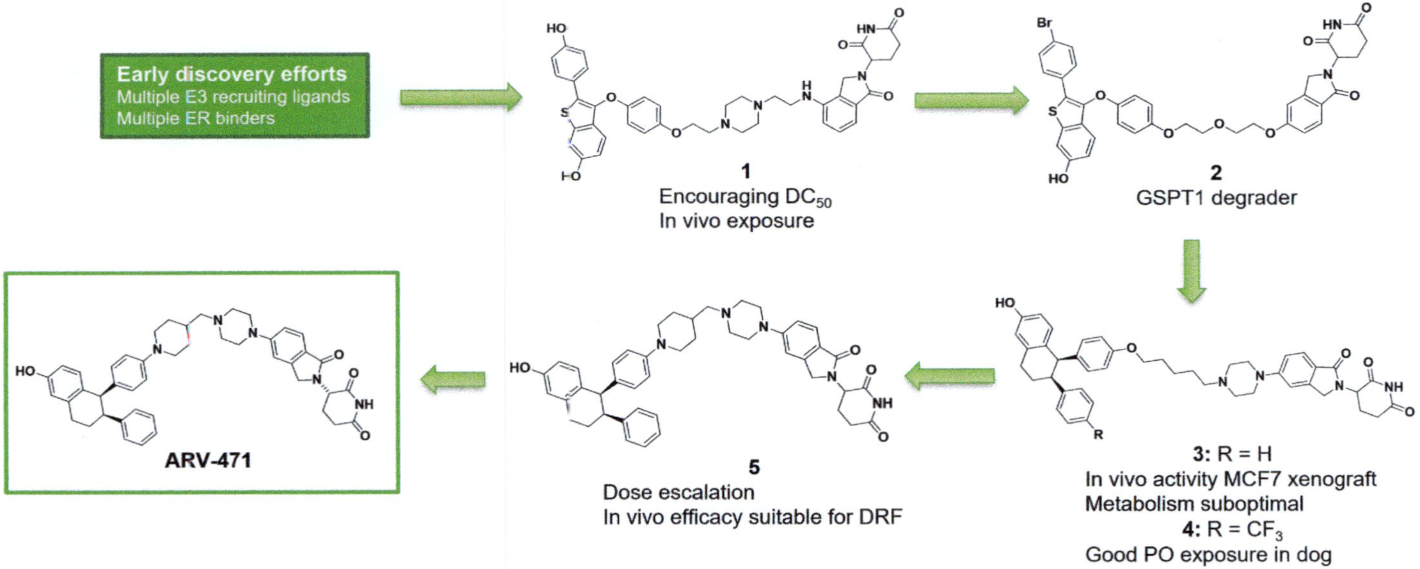

Figure 13.9 Evolution of AR degrading PROTACs leading to ARV-471. *Source:* Arvinas, Inc. [39]/with permission of Arvinas, Inc.

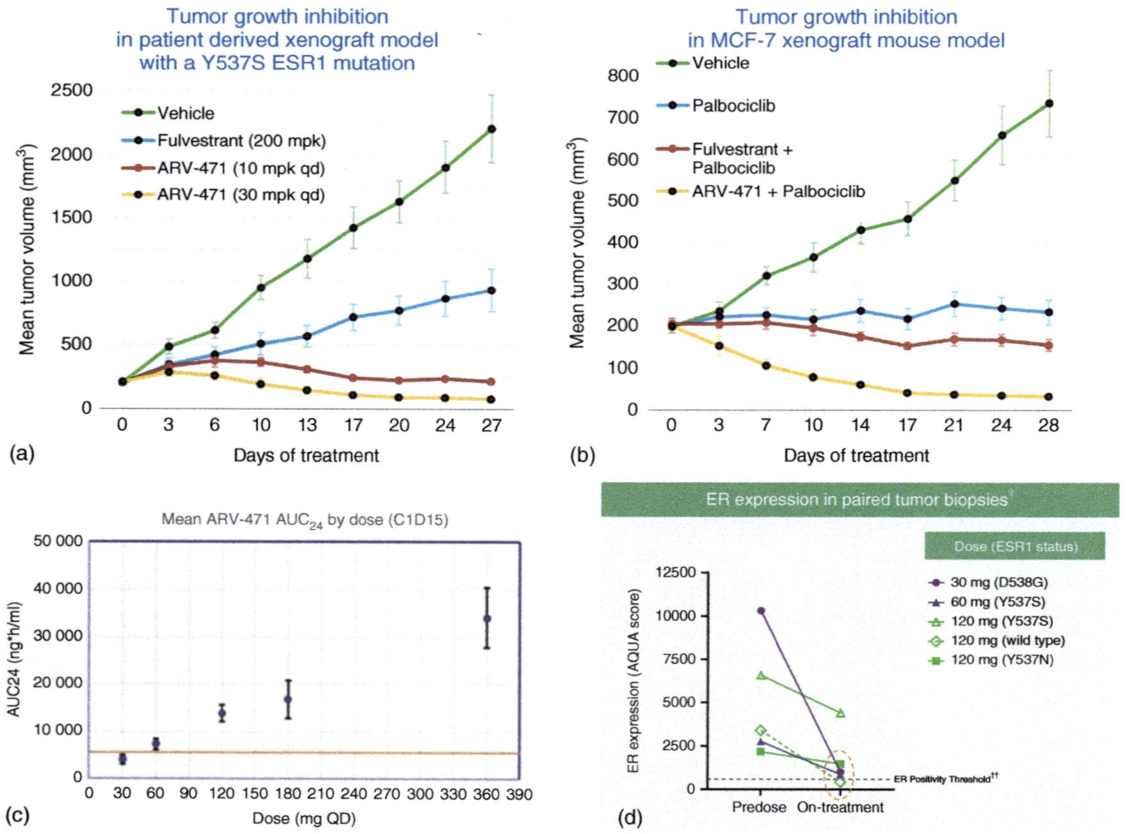

Figure 13.10 (a) Tumor volume versus days of treatment for a patient-derived xenograft model with a Y537S ESR1 mutation following treatment with either fulvestrant or ARV-471. (b) Tumor volume versus days of treatment for an MCF-7 xenograft model following treatment with either palbociclib alone, fulvestrant + palbociclib, or ARV-471 + palbociclib. (c) Initial human dose escalation PK data. The orange line represents the efficacious exposure in a preclinical model. (d) Clinical reduction of ER expression. *Source:* Adapted from [39, 40]/with permission of Arvinas, Inc.

occupying the bRo5 space, the early entrants have been able to establish dose-dependent exposure increases in the clinic. These early successes point to an accessible bRo5 property space that retains compatibility with oral drug exposure. Second, the front-runners have also been able to establish pharmacodynamic responses in either their respective patient populations or healthy volunteers. These findings increase confidence that preclinical *in vivo* animal models assessing target degradation may be translationally useful for understanding human pharmacodynamics. Lastly, concerns regarding severe toxicity from prolonged systemic degradation have not appeared in great abundance with what is admittedly still a small number of patients and targets. The early findings suggest that a well-executed preclinical toxicology program can support safe clinical translation to human. Nonetheless, future efforts to address potential systemic toxicity by exploring tissue- or disease-specific E3 ligase targeting, or even simply expanding the stability of targetable E3 ligases beyond those currently known, remains an attractive strategy [42]. Indeed, Dialectic's VHL-based degrader DT2216 can degrade Bcl-xL in a platelet-sparing manner because of the low expression of VHL in platelets, which may offer a better therapeutic window than Bcl-xL inhibitors in the clinic [43]. Alternative delivery strategies such as tumor targeting with antibody–PROTAC conjugates are also explored [44].

13.8 Conclusion

We have assessed targeted protein degradation with heterobifunctional degraders through the lens of pharmaceutical drug discovery and clinical translation. Heterobifunctional degraders have traveled a tremendous distance in the past 20 years, progressing from unwieldy peptide-based entities to fully small-molecule entities to small molecules with properties suitable for clinical development to early clinical proof of concept.

The path to clinical translation for PROTACs has required surmounting many obstacles in medicinal chemistry, including attaining oral bioavailability in the beyond Rule of 5 physicochemical property space. We have reviewed the rapidly expanding literature on this topic. There are, however, other important aspects of clinical translation that have received relatively little attention in the literature. Foremost among these gaps, there is a dearth of published material on building detailed PK–PD-efficacy relationships, which are fundamental to understanding and predicting the eventual human dose of any compound. A few publications have now surfaced that begin to light the way. Toxicology assessment of PROTACs will also continue to come to the fore. The rapid progress in whole-cell proteomics technology over the past decade has been instrumental for decoding potential off-target effects of PROTACs and highlighting potential risks.

The first clinical stories around PROTACs have begun to emerge, and it is expected that several additional PROTAC programs will report clinical data against a growing list of targets and diseases in the coming years. These early data cast a hopeful picture that the many preclinical challenges and concerns can be rationally met.

References

1 Sakamoto, K.M., Kim, K.B., Kumagai, A. et al. (2001). Protacs: chimeric molecules that target proteins to the Skp1-Cullin-F box complex for ubiquitination and degradation. *Proc. Natl Acad. Sci. USA* 98: 8554–8559. https://doi.org/10.1073/pnas.141230798.

2 Nalawansha, D.A. and Crews, C.M. (2020). PROTACs: an emerging therapeutic modality in precision medicine. *Cell Chem. Biol.* 27: 998–1014. and references cited therein. https://doi.org/10.1016/j.chembiol.2020.07.020.

3 Hughes, S.J., Testa, A., Thompson, N., and Churcher, I. (2021). The rise and rise of protein degradation: opportunities and challenges ahead. *Drug Des. Discov.* 26: 2889–2897. https://doi.org/10.1016/j.drudis.2021.08.006.

4 Lipinski, C.A., Lombardo, F., Dominy, B.W., and Feeney, P.J. (2001). Experimental and computational approaches to estimate solubility and permeability in drug discovery and development settings. *Adv. Drug Deliv. Rev.* 46: 3–26. https://doi.org/10.1016/s0169-409x(00)00129-0.

5 Doak, B.C., Over, B., GIordanetto, F., and Kihlberg, J. (2014). Oral druggable space beyond the rule of 5: insights from drugs and clinical candidates. *Chem. Biol.* 21: 1115–1142. https://doi.org/10.1016/j.chembiol.2014.08.013.

6 Doak, B.C., Zheng, J., Dobritzsch, D., and Kihlberg, J. (2016). How beyond rule of 5 drugs and clinical candidates bind to their targets. *J. Med. Chem.* 59: 2312–2327. https://doi.org/10.1021/acs.jmedchem.5b01286.

7 Poongavanam, V., Doak, B.C., and Kihlberg, J. (2018). Opportunities and guidelines for discovery of orally absorbed drugs in beyond rule of 5 space. *Curr. Opin. Chem. Biol.* 44: 23–29. https://doi.org/10.1016/j.cbpa.2018.05.010.

8 DeGoey, D.A., Chen, H.-J., Cox, P.B., and Wendt, M.D. (2018). Beyond the rule of 5: lessons learned from AbbVie's drugs and compound collection. *J. Med. Chem.* 61: 2636–2651. https://doi.org/10.1021/acs.jmedchem.7b00717.

9 Edmondson, S.D., Yang, B., and Fallan, C. (2019). Proteolysis targeting chimeras (PROTACs) in 'beyond rule-of-five' chemical space: recent progress and future challenges. *Bior. Med. Chem. Lett.* 29: 1555–1564. https://doi.org/10.1016/j.bmcl.2019.04.030.

10 Pike, A., Williamson, B., Harlfinger, S. et al. (2020). Optimising proteolysis-targeting chimeras (PROTACs) for oral drug delivery: a drug metabolism and pharmacokinetics perspective. *Drug Discov. Today* 25: 1793–1800. https://doi.org/10.1016/j.drudis.2020.07.013.

11 Atilaw, Y., Poongavanam, V., Nilsson, C.S. et al. (2021). Solution conformations shed light on PROTAC cell permeability. *ACS Med. Chem. Lett.* 12: 107–114. https://doi.org/10.1021/acsmedchemlett.0c00556.

12 Sebastiano, M.R., Doak, B.C., Backlund, M. et al. (2018). Impact of dynamically exposed polarity on permeability and solubility of chameleonic drugs beyond the rule of 5. *J. Med. Chem.* 61: 4189–4202. https://doi.org/10.1021/acs.jmedchem.8b00347.

13 Cantrill, C., Charurvedi, P., Rynn, C. et al. (2020). Fundamental aspects of DMPK optimization of targeted protein degraders. *Drug Des. Discov.* 25: 969–982. https://doi.org/10.1016/j.drudis.2020.03.012.

14 Foley, C.A., Potjewyd, F., Lamb, K.N. et al. (2020). Assessing the cell permeability of bivalent chemical degraders using the chloroalkane penetration assay. *ACS Chem. Biol.* 15: 290–295. https://doi.org/10.1021/acschembio.9b00972.

15 Cecchini, C., Pannilunghi, A., Tardy, S., and Scapozza, L. (2021). From conception to development: investigating PROTACs features for improved cell permeability and successful protein degradation. *Front. Chem.* 9: 1–23. https://doi.org/10.3389/fchem.2021.672267.

16 Grime, K.H., Barton, P., and McGinnity, D.F. (2013). Application of in silico, in vitro and preclinical pharmacokinetic data for the effective and efficient prediction of human pharmacokinetics. *Mol. Pharm.* 10 (4): 1191–1206. https://doi.org/10.1021/mp300476z.

17 Page, K.M. (2016). Validation of early human dose prediction: a key metric for compound progression in drug discovery. *Mol. Pharm.* 13 (2): 609–620. https://doi.org/10.1021/acs.molpharmaceut.5b00840.

18 Smith, D.A., Di, L., and Kerns, E.H. (2010). The effect of plasma protein binding on in vivo efficacy: misconceptions in drug discovery. *Nat. Rev. Drug Discov.* 9: 929–939. https://doi.org/10.1038/nrd3287.

19 Liu, X., Wright, M., and Hop, C.E.C.A. (2014). Rational use of plasma protein and tissue binding data in drug design. *J. Med. Chem.* 57 (20): 8238–8248. https://doi.org/10.1021/jm5007935.

20 Pettersson, M. and Crews, C.M. (2019). PROteolysis TArgetic chimeras (PROTACs) – past, present and future. *Drug Discov. Today Technol.* 31: 15–27. https://doi.org/10.1016/j.ddtec.2019.01.002.

21 Fisher, S.L. and Phillips, A.J. (2018). Targeted protein degradation and the enzymology of degraders. *Curr. Opin. Chem. Biol.* 44: 47–55. https://doi.org/10.1016/j.cbpa.2018.05.004.

22 Douglass, E.F. Jr., Miller, C.J., Sparer, G. et al. (2013). A comprehensive mathematical model for three-body binding equilibria. *J. Am. Chem. Soc.* 135: 6092–6099. https://doi.org/10.1021/ja311795d.

23 Han, B. (2020). A suite of mathematical solutions to describe ternary complex formation and their application to targeted protein degradation by hetero-bifunctional ligands. *J. Biol. Chem.* 295 (45): 15280–15291. https://doi.org/10.1074/jbc.ra120.014715.

24 Douglass, E.F. Jr. and Spiegel, D.A. (2021). Comment on a suite of mathematical solutions to describe ternary complex formation and their application to targeted protein degradation by heterobifunctional ligands. *J. Biol. Chem.* 296: 100331. https://doi.org/10.1016/j.jbc.2021.100331.

25 Bartlett, D.W. and Gilbert, A.M. (2021). A kinetic proofreading model for bispecific protein degraders. *J. Pharmacokinet. Pharmacodyn.* 48: 149–163. https://doi.org/10.1007/s10928-020-09722-z.

26 Kleiger, G. and Mayor, T. (2014). Perilous journey: a tour of the ubiquitin-proteasome system. *Trends Cell Biol.* 24 (6): 352–359. https://doi.org/10.1016/j.tcb.2013.12.003.

27 Bondeson, D.P., Mares, A., Smith, I.E.D. et al. (2015). Catalytic in vivo protein knockdown by small-molecule PROTACs. *Nat. Chem. Biol.* 11: 611–617. https://doi.org/10.1038/nchembio.1858.

28 Mares, A., Miah, A.H., Smith, I.E.D. et al. (2020). Extended pharmacodynamic responses observed upon PROTAC-mediated degradation of RIPK2. *Commun. Biol.* 3 (1): 140. https://doi.org/10.1038/s42003-020-0868-6.

29 Miah, A.H., Smith, I.E.D., Rackham, M. et al. (2021). Optimization of a series of RIPK2 PROTACs. *J. Med. Chem.* 64 (17): 12978–13003. https://doi.org/10.1021/acs.jmedchem.1c01118.

30 Bondeson, D.P., Smith, B.E., Burslem, G.M. et al. (2018). Lessons in PROTAC design from selective degradation with a promiscuous warhead. *Cell Chem. Biol.* 25: 78–87. https://doi.org/10.1016/j.chembiol.2017.09.01.

31 Huang, H.-T., Dobrovolsky, D., Paulk, J. et al. (2018). A chemoproteomic approach to query the degradable kinome using a multi-kinase degrader. *Cell Chem. Biol.* 25: 88–99. https://doi.org/10.1016/j.chembiol.2017.10.005.

32 Zhang, A.X., Cassidy, K., Dahl, G. et al. (2021). The vital role of proteomics in characterizing novel protein degraders. *SLAS Discov.* https://doi.org/10.1177/2472555220985776.

33 Scholes, N.S., Mayor-Ruiz, C., and Winter, G.E. (2021). Identification and selectivity profiling of small-molecule degraders via multi-omics approaches. *Cell Chem. Biol.* 28: 1048–1060. https://doi.org/10.1016/j.chembiol.2021.03.007.

34 Ito, T., Ando, H., Suzuki, T. et al. (2010). Identification of a primary target of thalidomide teratogenicity. *Science* 237: 1345–1350. https://doi.org/10.1126/science.1177319.

35 Chamberlain, P.P. and Cathers, B.E. (2019). Cereblon modulators: low molecular weight inducers of protein degradation. *Drug Discov. Today Technol.* 31: 29–34. https://doi.org/10.1016/j.ddtec.2019.02.004.

36 Petzold, G., Fishcer, E.S., and Thomä, N.H. (2016). Structural basis of lenalidomide-induced CK1a degradation by the $CRL4^{CRBN}$ ubiquitin ligase. *Nature* 532: 127–130. https://doi.org/10.1038/nature16979.

37 Liu, X., Zhang, Y., Ward, L.D. et al. (2021). A proteomic platform to identify off-target proteins associated with therapeutic modalities that induce protein degradation or gene silencing. *Sci. Rep.* 11: 15856. https://doi.org/10.1038/s41598-021-95354-3.

38 Arvinas, Inc. (2021a). Discovery of ARV-110, a first in class androgen receptor degrading PROTAC for the treatment of men with metastatic castration resistant prostate cancer. https://ir.arvinas.com/static-files/99279395-e91e-44d1-8ad9-88db2024c1fa (accessed 30 October 2021).

39 Arvinas, Inc. (2021b). The discovery of ARV-471, an orally bioavailable estrogen receptor degrading PROTAC for the treatment of patients with breast cancer. https://ir.arvinas.com/static-files/7a4db470-3d7f-4d4b-98a4-481b8c573169 (accessed 30 October 2021).

40 Arvinas, Inc. (2021c). Pioneering the future of targeted protein degradation therapeutics. https://ir.arvinas.com/static-files/ae957f0c-ac1a-42c7-883a-4aca15c06762 (accessed 30 October 2021).

41 Kymera Therapeutics (2021). Safety, PK and PD from single ascending dose portion of KT-474 Phase 1 trial in healthy volunteers. https://investors.kymeratx.com/static-files/951b6272-8bdf-4ce6-95dc-23c422587705 (accessed 30 October 2021).

42 Ishida, T. and Ciulli, A. (2021). E3 ligase ligands for PROTACs: how they were found and how to discover new ones. *SLAS Discov.* 26 (4): 484–502. https://doi.org/10.1177/2472555220965528.

43 Khan, S., Zhang, X., Lv, D. et al. (2019). A selective BCL-xL PROTAC degrader achieves safe and potent antitumor activity. *Nat. Med.* 25: 1938–1947. https://doi.org/10.1038/s41591-019-0668-z.

44 Maneiro, M.A., Forte, N., Shchepinova, M.M. et al. (2020). Antibody-PROTAC conjugates enable HER2-dependent targeted protein degradation of BRD4. *ACS Chem. Biol.* 15: 1306–1312. https://doi.org/10.1021/acschembio.0c00285.

Index

Inducing Targeted Protein Degradation: From Chemical Biology to Drug Discovery and Clinical Applications, First Edition. Edited by Philipp Cromm.